D1034180

Breast Pathology
Diagnosis by Needle Core Biopsy

Breast Pathology
Diagnosis by Needle Core Biopsy

Paul Peter Rosen, M.D.
Senior Consultant Pathologist
Dickstein Cancer Treatment Center
White Plains Hospital Center
White Plains, New York;
Adjunct Professor of Pathology
New York Medical College
Valhalla, New York

Former Attending Pathologist
Memorial Sloan-Kettering Cancer Center
New York, New York

with contributions by

D. David Dershaw, M.D.

and

Laura Liberman, M.D.

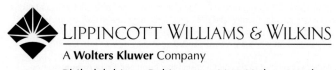

LIPPINCOTT WILLIAMS & WILKINS
A **Wolters Kluwer** Company
Philadelphia • Baltimore • New York • London
Buenos Aires • Hong Kong • Sydney • Tokyo

Acquisitions Editor: Anne S. Patterson
Developmental Editor: Rebecca Diehl
Manufacturing Manager: Dennis Teston
Production Manager: Liane Carita
Production Editor: Kimberly Monroe
Cover Designer: Wanda Kossack
Indexer: Cynthia Bertelsman
Compositor: Maryland Composition Inc.

Printed and bound in China

9 8 7 6 5 4 3 2 1

Library of Congress Cataloging-in-Publication Data
Rosen, Paul Peter.
    Breast pathology : diagnosis by needle core biopsy / Peter Paul
Rosen ; with contributions by D. David Dershaw and Laura Liberman.
        p.   cm.
    Includes bibliographical references and index.
    ISBN 0-397-58790-2
    1. Breast—Diseases—Diagnosis.   2. Breast—Tumors—Diagnosis.
3. Breast—Needle biopsy.   4. Histology, Pathological.   I. Dershaw,
D. David.   II. Liberman, Laura.   III. Title.
[DNLM: 1. Breast Neoplasms—diagnosis.   2. Biopsy, Needle.
3. Fibrocystic Disease of Breast—diagnosis.   4. Breast—pathology.
WP 870R813b 1999]
RG493.5.B56R67   1999
618.1′90758—dc21
DNLM/DLC
for Library of Congress
                                                                98-31090
                                                                CIP

Care has been taken to confirm the accuracy of the information presented and to describe generally accepted practices. However, the authors, editors, and publisher are not responsible for errors or omissions or for any consequences from application of the information in this book and make no warranty, expressed or implied, with respect to the contents of the publication.
  The authors, editors, and publisher have exerted every effort to ensure that drug selection and dosage and procedures set forth in this text are in accordance with current recommendations and practice at the time of publication. However, in view of ongoing research, changes in government regulations, and the constant flow of information relating to drug therapy and drug reactions, the reader is urged to check the package insert for each drug for any change in indications and dosage and for added warnings and precautions. This is particularly important when the recommended agent is a new or infrequently employed drug.
  Some drugs and medical devices presented in this publication have Food and Drug Administration (FDA) clearance for limited use in restricted research settings. It is the responsibility of the health care provider to ascertain the FDA status of each drug or device planned for use in their clinical practice.

In memory of

Flora Caspari and Paul Caspari, M.D.
Rose Rosen and Morris Rosen

and for
Mary Sue Rosen
Deborah, Graham, Madelyn
Jon, Karen, Jordan
Stacy, Paige

Legends to the illustrations on the front cover.

Upper left: A mammographically detected nonpalpable spiculated lesion with calcifications.

Upper right: Core biopsy samples obtained with a 14-gauge needle from a lesion similar to the one shown in the previous illustration.

Lower left: Needle core biopsy samples in histologic section.

Lower right: Infiltrating duct carcinoma in a needle core biopsy.

Contents

Contributing Authors

D. David Dershaw, M.D.   *Professor, Department of Radiology, Cornell University Medical College, 525 East 68th Street, New York, New York, 10021; Director, Breast Imaging Section, Department of Radiology, Memorial Sloan-Kettering Cancer Center, 1275 York Avenue, New York, New York 10021*

Laura Liberman, M.D.   *Associate Professor, Department of Radiology, Cornell University Medical College, 525 East 68th Street, New York, New York, 10021; Associate Attending Radiologist, Breast Imaging Section, Department of Radiology, Memorial Sloan-Kettering Cancer Center, 1275 York Avenue, New York, New York 10021*

The development of modern medical specialism during the latter part of the nineteenth century and the early part of the present century...would hardly have taken place had not physicians accustomed themselves to the idea of distinct disease entities consisting of localized organic lesions connected with certain clinical pictures....The development and application of a concept of localized pathology laid the groundwork for modern specialism by providing a number of foci of interest in the field of medicine. Each such focus of interest, that is, a disease or the diseases of an organ or region of the body, provided a nucleus around which could gather the results of clinical and pathological investigation.

On the technological side the influences represented in specialization manifest themselves in the multiplicity of technical skills, devices, and theories applied to the achievement of human aims in the field of medicine.

From *The Specialization of Medicine* by George Rosen, M.D., 1944

Preface

Prior to the widespread implementation of breast conservation therapy, the role of the pathologist in breast cancer care was limited to making the diagnosis and documenting the extent of the disease after a mastectomy was performed. These two events typically centered around a single operative procedure in which the diagnosis was made by a frozen section biopsy followed by a mastectomy and axillary dissection. Presently, considerably more information is required to recommend breast cancer treatment that may employ more than one of the major existing therapeutic modalities: surgery, radiation, and chemotherapy. An important part of the data used for therapeutic decisions is generated by the pathologist using routine histopathologic procedures and immunohistochemistry.

The complex multifactorial description of breast pathology now considered to be standard practice has expanded the diagnostic report from a brief one- or two-line statement, such as "Infiltrating duct carcinoma, grade II; negative lymph nodes" to a catalogue of data one or more pages in length, often including many statements indicating the absence as well as the presence of features regarded as relevant to therapeutic decisions and to prognosis. A partial list of this information includes classification of the carcinoma, histologic grade, nuclear grade, tumor size, and statements about vascular invasion, proportion of *in situ* component in invasive lesions, subtype of *in situ* carcinoma, multifocality, and proximity of carcinoma to margins of excision. Immunohistochemistry has now replaced biochemistry as the method of choice for characterizing the distribution of estrogen and progesterone receptors as well as other biomarkers and oncogene expression in pathology reports. Proliferative activity may be estimated by the pathologist using immunohistochemistry (Ki-67) and by flow cytometry.

As we approach the end of the 20th century, other advances have added to the complexity of the pathologist's role in breast cancer treatment. Most recent among these is the growing use of needle core biopsy, especially for the diagnosis of nonpalpable mammographically detected lesions. Needle core biopsy has become a routine method to sample nonpalpable breast lesions as a result of the widespread availability of stereotaxic localizing devices coupled with improvements in the technology of biopsy instruments. Progress has occurred so rapidly that this procedure, introduced and currently approved for diagnostic purposes, is also under investigation as a therapeutic tool for the excision of small carcinomas. Stereotactic needle core biopsy is an extremely valuable tool in planning breast conservation therapy because it can establish the diagnosis of nonpalpable lesions before operative surgical intervention.

Many mammographically detected nonpalpable lesions present the pathologist with challenging diagnostic problems when excised intact and viewed in context with surrounding tissues. The appearance of such lesions in the incomplete and sometimes disrupted form of needle core biopsy samples can substantially increase the degree of difficulty. The major differential diagnostic problems encountered in these specimens include:

- reactive changes vs. recurrent carcinoma after lumpectomy
- benign sclerosing lesions (radial scar) vs. infiltrating carcinoma
- papilloma vs. papillary carcinoma
- fibroadenoma vs. cystosarcoma
- atypical duct hyperplasia vs. intraductal carcinoma (DCIS)
- DCIS vs. DCIS with (micro)invasion
- spindle cell tumors (metaplastic carcinoma vs. sarcoma)
- vascular lesions (angioma vs. angiosarcoma)

Although self-evident, it is important to understand that the diagnosis made with a needle core biopsy can only be based on the samples available to the pathologist and that these samples may not be representative of all of the pathologic findings in a given case. Consequently, carcinoma may be found in up to 50% of surgical biopsies after a needle core biopsy diagnosis of atypical hyperplasia, and microinvasion may be present in about 20% of surgical excisions after a needle core diagnosis of intraductal carcinoma. Three principles offer guidance in the use of needle core biopsy for the diagnosis and treatment of breast lesions:

- Anything can turn up.
- What you see is what you have and it may not be all there is.
- What you have may be all there is.

The emergence of needle core biopsy as a major diagnostic tool epitomizes the growing complexity of the interaction of radiologists and pathologists in the diagnosis and management of mammary diseases, especially in the era of breast conservation therapy. Specialization in medicine has created circumstances in which the specialist is increasingly dependent on the assistance of colleagues who have acquired complementary expertise. This evolving situation has contributed to the team approach to disease management reflected in this volume. The intentional limited scope of this presentation, which focuses on diagnosis, does not permit inclusion of contributions from other important members of the team, including surgeons, radiotherapists, and medical oncologists who depend on these diagnoses to implement therapy.

An astute reader of this volume will note infrequent differences in diagnostic terminology from my prior book (*Breast Pathology*, Lipincott-Raven Publishers, 1996). Two of the deviations deserve a comment here because they reflect changes in the appreciation of specific lesions due in large measure to growing experience with needle core biopsy which has focused attention on these abnormalities. In Chapter 9 of *Breast Pathology*, Figure 1 illustrates "ductal hyperplasia in terminal duct lobular unit," a lesion now best classified as "columnar cell ductal hyperplasia in terminal duct lobular unit" (see Chapters 8 and 13 in this volume). Chapter 35 of *Breast Pathology* refers to "lobular carcinoma in situ and intraductal carcinoma" in Figure 30, a lesion cited as "lobular carcinoma *in situ* in ducts" in Chapter 21, Figure 15 of this volume.

Acknowledgments

The potential for the team approach to cancer treatment is perhaps best epitomized in the management of patients with mammographically detected breast lesions, the most likely candidates for needle core biopsy. This effort draws upon the skills of mammographers, pathologists, and surgeons, as well as radiation therapists and medical oncologists. Many of the needle core biopsy procedures that provided samples illustrated in this book were performed by the Breast Imaging Service at Memorial Sloan-Kettering Cancer Center directed by David Dershaw, M.D., including Andrea Abramson, M.D., Laura Liberman, M.D., and Elizabeth Morris, M.D., or by Drs. Michael Cohen and Steven Sferlazza at the Gutman Diagnostic Center in New York. We are also grateful to the hundreds of pathologists, surgeons, and radiologists throughout the United States and abroad who contributed cases for pathology consultation, which may be illustrated in this book.

Some of the histologic sections illustrated herein were prepared in the Pathology Laboratory at Memorial Hospital by the superb technical staff supervised by Debra Harrigan-Jokisch or in the Breast Pathology Laboratory under the supervision of Crispinita Arroyo.

Although this volume deals principally with issues of diagnosis that involve pathologists and radiologists, we are indebted to many colleagues who contributed to the stimulating environment that has made this work possible; particularly Breast Medical Oncology at Memorial Sloan-Kettering Cancer Center headed by Larry Norton, M.D. (Violante Currie, M.D., Teresa Gilewski, M.D., Clifford Hudis, M.D., Mark Moasser, M.D., Mark Robson, M.D., Andrew Seidman, M.D., Nancy Sklarin, M.D., Antonella Surbone, M.D., and Maria Theodoulou, M.D.), Breast Surgery at Memorial Sloan-Kettering Cancer Center headed by Patrick Borgen, M.D. (Hiram S. Cody, III, M.D., Angelo Depalo, M.D., Alexandra Heerdt, M.D., Michael Paglia, M.D., Jeanne Petrek, M.D., and Kimberly Van Zee, M.D.), and Breast Radiation Oncology at Memorial Sloan-Kettering Cancer Center headed by Beryl McCormick, M.D.

We also acknowledge the superb support of the publisher from the earliest discussions of the concept for this book to the final publication. Editors for this project were Vickie Thaw, and subsequently, Anne Patterson with the support of Rebecca Diehl, Kimberly Monroe, and Deirdre Marino-Vasquez.

I am deeply indebted to Ms. Tammy Son for her loyal commitment and assistance in innumerable projects, including two books over the past five years. The timely completion of this volume is in no small measure a tribute to her dedicated, meticulous collaboration in this undertaking.

Introduction

Noninvasive techniques have been used to study breast lesions since the beginning of the 20th century. The usefulness of this approach in the clinical setting has been dependent on technical advances, which permitted the radiologist to detect lesions that are inapparent to the patient and physician, including clinically occult carcinomas. A consequence of this advance has been the need for a close working relationship between the practitioners of several medical specialties. The result is certainly one of the important examples of "team" management that requires the cooperative efforts of medical specialists to provide effective patient care.

Two methods of nonsurgical investigation of the breast were studied in the 1920s and early 1930s, namely, transillumination and radiography. As Cutler reported, the idea for transillumination as a means of diagnosis "...was first developed among the members of the laboratory staff of Memorial Hospital during the routine examination of breast specimens" (1). Cutler also stated that "...at the suggestion of Dr. Ewing,...Adair attempted to transilluminate breasts but encountered technical difficulties, chiefly due to the excessive heat developed by the transilluminating lamp." Although Cutler improved upon the light source, it is clear that transillumination offered little as a method of diagnosis except possibly as a way to distinguish between cystic and solid lesions. With widespread acceptance of needle aspiration of cysts, transillumination was abandoned and it has now been replaced by ultrasound.

The earliest radiologic studies of the breast reported in the United States in the 1930s by Warren and Fray, by Seabold, and by Lockwood were contemporaneous with similar investigations in Europe (2–7). When first employed clinically, it was apparent that roentgenography might prove helpful in the diagnosis of so-called early breast carcinoma. The definition of "early" has changed appreciably since this concept was introduced. This change is exemplified in a 1932 report by Fray and Warren that described a 54-year-old woman who, on clinical examination, was thought to have chronic cystic mastitis (2). Roentgenologic examination revealed "...a small area of dense tissue with irregular margins...in the left breast." The lesion proved on biopsy to be a carcinoma "...the size of a walnut...." It was concluded by the authors that the early status...(of the tumor) was reflected not only by its small size but in the absence of macroscopic involvement of pectoral muscles. Today, the case described by Fray and Warren would be considered operable and potentially curable but not "early." Within a relatively short period of time, the term early has come to be used for lesions of microscopic dimensions, often detectable only by mammography.

The initial mammography studies were met with skepticism. In 1931, Seabold described the mammographic findings in a series of cases to the Philadelphia Academy of Surgery (5). The summary of the discussion that followed his report included the following comment:

> Dr. J. Stewart Rodman said that any attempt to make the diagnosis more exact is certainly praiseworthy. Being a surgeon, however, he is not sure but that sometimes x-ray men have somewhat vivid imaginations.... The clinical diagnosis of carcinoma of the breast and chronic cystic mastitis is not ordinarily difficult, and therefore until we have x-ray evidence of a more positive value we had best go a little slow in accepting evidence which is contrary to clinical findings.

Gunsett and Sichel stated in 1934 that their x-ray images might be useful in some cases, but that radiologic distinctions between benign and malignant lesions were not precise enough to form a basis for surgical treatment (7). Consequently, they concluded that mammography would not replace biopsy as a diagnostic procedure. The warning offered in these comments is applicable today. The clinician faced with a palpable abnormality in the breast should not depend only on mammography to decide whether biopsy is required. On the other hand, advances in clinical mammography and the development of stereotactic biopsy instruments have made it possible to detect and perform biopsies on nonpalpable lesions found by "x-ray men" who "have vivid imaginations" (5).

The need to relate radiologic findings to the histopathologic examination of breast tissue has been appreciated since the earliest x-ray images of the breast were obtained. Albert Salomon, a surgeon at the University of Berlin, described a method for obtaining roentgenograms of serial sections of surgical breast specimens in order to correlate histologic sections with the specimen x-rays (8). The histologic appearance of calcification within a mammary carcinoma was described in his paper. Salomon may be credited with the first reported example of breast specimen radiography and he deserves recognition for investigations that anticipated later developments in mammography and specimen radiography.

Detailed pathologic–radiologic correlations were carried out in the late 1920s by Dominguez in Montevideo, Uruguay (9–11). Dominguez was especially interested in studying the properties of calcifications in breast lesions. In addition to specimen radiography, he undertook biochemical analyses of the calcium content of breast tissue. Conway described the clinical radiologic appearance of calcification in breast cysts and sarcomatous tumors, but failed to appreciate calcification as a potential x-ray marker for carcinoma (12). Lockwood stressed the importance of correlating pathologic and radiologic findings, but did not obtain x-rays of specimens, and there was no mention of mammary calcification as an indicator of carcinoma in his report (3). Warren described two cases thought roentgenologically to be carcinoma but reported to be benign on pathologic examination that "...could not be studied because the specimens were thrown out before films could be made to locate the supposed small area of malignancy seen at the original examination" (6).

The observations of Salomon, and later Dominguez, that calcium deposits in mammary carcinoma could be visualized radiologically remained largely unappreciated for nearly two decades. They were again brought to attention by Leborgne in Montevideo who developed a technique for soft tissue roentgenography that made it possibly to visualize smaller tumors and calcifications in clinical mammograms (13,14). He noted that "the roentgenographic study of the operative specimen also permitted the localization of the tiny calcifications for histopathologic study, and thus aided in finding a small cancer that would otherwise have been overlooked." As had Gershon-Cohen some years earlier (15), Leborgne anticipated the role of mammography for detecting preclinical cancer:

> We firmly believe that the recognition and demonstration of this roentgenographic sign constitutes one of the easily observed aspects in which mammary cancer is presented, especially in its ductal form...and (is) therefore susceptible of detection in prophylactic examinations of women who do not yet present clinical tumor symptomology. With a systematic prophylactic roentgenographic examination of all women with antecedents of cancer in their family, we enter a new stage in the fight against mammary cancer.

The origin of modern needle core biopsy of the breast to obtain a tissue sample for histologic diagnosis is entwined with the history of needle aspiration biopsy and parallels the development of clinical mammography. Needles have been used to obtain samples for diagnosis from various anatomic sites since the middle of the 19th century (16). Needle aspiration biopsies of the lung (17,18) and lymph nodes (19–21) were described by 1914. Many of the early biopsy attempts involved aspirating cells with a needle attached to a syringe. The aspirated blood and cellular material were expressed onto a slide and spread thinly to create a cytologic preparation.

The application of needle aspiration biopsy to the diagnosis of neoplastic conditions attracted attention early in the 20th century. In 1921, Guthrie reported that needle aspiration could be employed to evaluate the causes of lymph node enlargement (22). A method for aspirating cells from lymph nodes and the preparation of stained slides from this material was described in detail by Forkner (23) who also reported his experience using these samples for the diagnosis of cancer, including three women with adenocarcinoma in axillary lymph nodes (24).

The first concerted effort to employ needle aspiration and biopsy for the diagnosis of cancer was undertaken at Memorial Hospital in New York. In 1922, E.B. Ellis, a technician working under Dr. James Ewing, described cancer cells in cell block specimens of pleural fluid (25). Ellis concluded that "the diagnosis of cancer from direct smears is hazardous, but when one has made thin paraffin sections of suspected material and their evidence is fortified by some confirmatory clinical data, positive diagnosis may often be obtained." Four years later, Hayes Martin, a surgeon at Memorial Hospital, Fred Stewart, then the junior associate of Dr. Ewing, and Ellis began to use aspiration biopsy in patients with head and neck cancer (26). In succeeding publications, they documented the applicability of aspiration biopsy to a variety of tumors and defined the role of this procedure in the clinical management of cancer patients (27,28). The Memorial Hospital technique proved to be the forerunner of what are now two largely separate methods of diagnosis: fine-needle aspiration (FNA) and needle core biopsy.

The specimens obtained by Martin and his clinical colleagues included disaggregated cells for cytologic examination, equivalent to FNA today, and fragments of tissue that they described as the clot, a counterpart of the modern needle core biopsy. Ewing, Stewart, and their colleagues were not prepared to rely entirely on cytologic smears as evidenced by the importance they attached to the "clot," described in following commentary by Godwin (29):

After the material is obtained in the syringe, the negative pressure is released to obviate splattering of the aspirate in the syringe. With the rake, the material is placed on several slides and gently smeared by approximating two slides and pulling them apart. The remaining material is placed on a small piece of blotting paper or fibrin foam and put in formalin for later paraffin section. This is designated as the clot.

The clot was ". . . helpful in many instances where the smear is not diagnostic and in making a more definitive diagnosis as to the type of tumor" (29). In retrospect, it is not possible to determine how frequently tissue fragments in the clot proved to be crucial for making a diagnosis.

The system of aspirating tumors for diagnosis implemented at Memorial Hospital in the 1920s and 1930s evolved as a result of experience gained by the participants in this effort. In a later review, Godwin (30) observed that:

> The interpretation of aspirates, as with other pathological material, is certainly not without pitfalls. It requires experience. It is necessary that a sufficient number of cases be available for both clinician and pathologist to maintain their efficiency. The pathologist must know the clinical setting, the normal cells of the region, and the nature of lesions to be anticipated in the area.

The importance of clinical correlation in the diagnosis of aspiration cytology specimens, emphasized by Martin, Stewart, Godwin, and others, appears to have played a role in the further development of needle biopsy as a diagnostic method. The procedures were invariably performed by surgeons, radiation therapists, and other clinicians. Consequently, the pathologist had only second-hand clinical information and rarely participated in the procedure, a situation that probably contributed to resistance by pathologists to accept needle aspiration. On the other hand, the impetus for renewed interest in needle aspiration biopsy grew from the achievements of clinicians with training in hematology and cytopathology who began to perform the procedures and interpreted the specimens they obtained (31).

Technologic developments in imaging have played a major role in advancing the use of needles to biopsy lesions in superficial and visceral locations. The impetus for improving needle biopsy techniques for breast lesions began with the increasing utilization of mammography in the 1960s and 1970s. The mammographic detection of nonpalpable lesions presented a diagnostic challenge to the radiologist, surgeon, and pathologist and led to the development of methods to localize nonpalpable lesions so that they could be found and excised by surgeons and sampled in the pathology laboratory. Various localizing procedures were introduced, employing needles, wires, dyes, and other markers in or near the lesion under mammographic or ultrasound guidance. After localization by the radiologist, the surgeon was guided by the marker. Radiographic examination of the specimen (specimen radiography) has been employed to confirm excision of the nonpalpable abnormality and to help the pathologist pinpoint the lesion for histologic examination (32–34). Specimen radiography has been particularly useful for lesions containing calcifications.

Under optimal conditions where biopsy was recommended for mammographic abnormalities with calcifications considered to be suspicious for carcinoma, 25% to 30% of the excised lesions proved to be carcinoma (33,34). Thus, for each patient with a biopsy that revealed carcinoma, three underwent surgical excision of a benign lesion. The surgical management of nonpalpable breast lesions without calcifications was more difficult because specimen radiography is not very effective for confirming the adequacy of excision. The availability of needle core biopsy to sample these lesions now makes it possible to omit surgical biopsy in a substantial number of women.

The introduction of stereotaxic devices in the 1970s resulted in improved needle localization and made it possible to perform needle biopsies of nonpalpable lesions more efficiently (35). One of the first papers described a "stereotaxic instrument" that facilitated "percutaneous needle biopsy of the breast for microscopic diagnosis" (36). The authors reported that "the sampling site can be located at a precision of ± 1 mm. The instrument can also be used for positioning of metal and dye indicators for guiding surgery and for post-operative identification of excised tumors." Linkage of this computer-guided localization system with the automated biopsy gun introduced in the 1980s (37) led to the development of modern stereotaxic core biopsy instruments (38). Ultrasound-guided core biopsy has proven to be particularly effective for nonpalpable lesions without calcifications. Stereotaxic and ultrasound-guided core biopsy of the breast are now utilized with increasing frequency for the diagnosis of breast diseases. These technologies provide efficient methods for sampling small areas rapidly with less morbidity and expense than surgical excision (39–41). Multifocal lesions are also accessible with this approach (42).

Needle core biopsies give the pathologist specimens that are processed with other tissue biopsy samples to produce histologic sections. While satisfying the pathologist's preference for a tissue sample, core biopsies create new diagnostic problems and challenges. To some extent, these difficulties arise from the partial view of a lesion in the core biopsy. The context of surrounding tissue afforded by sections of surgical biopsies, important in some instances, is largely lacking. The lesions are frequently small abnormalities that can be difficult to interpret, even in a complete excisional biopsy, including nonpalpable lesions for which frozen section is not recommended (43). Unusual tumors previously encountered only in surgical specimens such, as pseudoangiomatous stromal hyperplasia, myofibroblastoma, metaplastic carcinoma, and hemangiomas, are now the targets of stereotaxic biopsy procedures. Today, virtually any lesion that occurs in the breast may appear on the pathologist s microscope as a core biopsy. The purpose of this book is to provide guidance in the interpretation and diagnosis of needle core biopsies and the pathologic changes that occur in the breast as a result of these procedures.

REFERENCES

1. Cutler M. Transillumination as an aid in the diagnosis of breast lesions, with special reference to its value in cases of bleeding nipple. *Surg Gynecol Obstet* 1929;48:721–729.
2. Fray WW, Warren SL. Stereoscopic roentgenography of breasts. An aid in establishing the diagnosis of mastitis and carcinoma. *Ann Surg* 1932;95:425–432.
3. Lockwood IH. Roentgen ray evaluation of breast symptoms. *Am J Roentgenol* 1933;29:145–155.
4. Seabold PS. Roentgenographic diagnosis of diseases of the breast. *Surg Gynecol Obstet* 1931;53:461–468.
5. Seabold PS. Diagnosis of breast disease by x-ray. *Ann Surg* 1931;94:443.
6. Warren SL. Roentgenologic study of the breast. *Am J Roentgenol* 1930;24:113–124.
7. Gunsett A, Sichel G. Sur la valeur praticque de la radiographie du sein. *J de radiol et d électrol* 1934;18:611–614.
8. Salomon A. Beiträge zur Pathologie und Klinik der Mammacarcinome. *Archiv für Klin Chirurgie* 1913;101:573–668.
9. Dominguez CM. Estudio sistematizado del cancer del seno. *Boll Liga Uruguay contra el cancer genit gemen* 1929;1:23.
10. Dominguez CM. Estudio radiologico de los descalcifadores. *Boll Soc Anatomia Patologica* 1930;1:175.
11. Dominiguez CM, Lucas A. Investigacion radiografica y quimica sobre el calcio precipitado en tumores del aparato genital feminio. *Boll Soc Anatomia Patologica* 1930;1:217.
12. Conway JH. Calcified breast tumors. *Am J Surg* 1936;31:72–76.
13. Leborgne R. Diagnostico de los tumores de la mamma por la radiografia simple. *Boll Cir Uruguay* 1949;20:407.
14. Leborgne R. Diagnosis of tumors of the breast by simple roentgenography. Calcifications in carcinomas. *Am J Roentgenol* 1951;65:1–11.
15. Gershon-Cohen J, Colcher AE. An evaluation of the roentgen diagnosis of early carcinoma of the breast. *JAMA* 1937;108:867–871.
16. Webb AJ. Through a glass darkly. (The development of needle aspiration biopsy). *Bristol Med Chir J* 1974;89:59–68.
17. Horder TJ. Lung puncture: a new application of clinical pathology. *Lancet* 1909;2:1345–1346;1539–1540.
18. Leyden OO. Ueber infectiöse Pneumonie. *Dtsch Med Wochenschr* 1883;9:52–54.
19. White WC, Pröscher F. Spirochaetes in acute lymphatic leukemia and in chronic benign lymphomatosis (Hodgkin's disease). *JAMA* 1907;69:1115.
20. Grieg EDW, Gray ACH. Note on the lymphatic glands in sleeping sickness. *Lancet* 1914;1:1570.
21. Chatard JA, Guthrie CG. Human trypanosomiasis: report of a case observed in Baltimore. *Am J Trop Dis Prev Med* 1914;1:493–505.
22. Guthrie CG. Gland puncture as a diagnostic measure. *Bull Johns Hopkins Hosp* 1921;32:266–269.
23. Forkner CE. Material from lymph nodes in man. I. Method to obtain material by puncture of lymph nodes for study with supravital and fixed stains. *Arch Intern Med* 1927;40:532–537.
24. Forkner CE. Material from lymph nodes of man. Studies on living and fixed cells withdrawn from lymph nodes of man. *Arch Intern Med* 1927;40:647–660.
25. Ellis EB. Cancer cells in pleural fluid. *Bull Int Assoc Med Museums J Tech Methods* 1922;8:126–127.
26. Martin HE, Ellis EB. Biopsy by needle puncture and aspiration. *Ann Surg* 1930;92:169–181.
27. Martin HE, Ellis EB. Aspiration biopsy. *Surg Gynecol Obstet* 1934;59:578–589.
28. Stewart FW. The diagnosis of tumors by aspiration. *Am J Pathol* 1933;9:801–812.
29. Godwin JT. Aspiration biopsy: technique and application. *Ann NY Acad Sci* 1956;63:1348–1373.
30. Godwin JT. Cytologic diagnosis of aspiration biopsies of solid and cystic tumors. *Acta Cytol* 1964;8:206–215.
31. Fox CH. Innovation in medical diagnosis: the Scandinavian curiosity. *Lancet* 1979;1:1387–1388.
32. Rosen PP, Snyder PE, Foote Jr., FW, Wallace T. Detection of occult carcinoma in the apparently benign breast biopsy through specimen radiography. *Cancer* 1970;26:944–953.
33. Rosen PP, Snyder RE, Urban J, Robbins G. Correlation of suspicious mammograms and x-rays of breast biopsies during surgery: Results of 60 cases. *Cancer* 1973;31:656–660.
34. Snyder R, Rosen PP. Radiography of breast specimens. *Cancer* 1971;28:1608–1611.
35. Nordenström B. New instruments for biopsy. *Radiology* 1975;117:474–475.
36. Bolmgren J, Jacobson B, Nordenström B. Stereotaxic instrument for needle biopsy of the mamma. *Am J Roentgenol* 1977;129:121–125.
37. Lindgren PG. Percutaneous needle biopsy: a new technique. *Acta Radiol Diagn* 1982;23:653–656.
38. Burbank F. Stereotactic breast biopsy: its history, its present, and its future. *Am Surg* 1996;2:128–150.
39. Nields MW. Cost-effectiveness of image-guided core needle biopsy versus surgery in diagnosing breast cancer. *Acad Radiol* 1996;3:S138–S140.
40. Liberman L, Fahs MC, Dershaw DD, Bonaccio E, Abramson AF, Cohen MA, Hann LE. Impact of stereotactic core biopsy on cost of diagnosis. *Radiology* 1995;195:633–637.
41. Fajardo LL. Cost-effectiveness and outcome studies: example of research. Cost-effectiveness of stereotaxic breast core needle biopsy. *Acad Radiol* 1996;3:S21–S23.
42. Rosenblatt R, Fineberg SA, Sparano JA, Kaleya RN. Stereotactic core needle biopsy of multiple sites in the breast: efficacy and effect on patient care. *Radiology* 1996;201:67–70.
43. Association of Directors of Anatomic and Surgical Pathology. Immediate management of mammographically detected breast lesions. *Am J Surg Pathol* 1993;12:850–851.

Breast Pathology
Diagnosis by Needle Core Biopsy

CHAPTER 1

Anatomy and Physiologic Morphology

EMBRYOLOGY AND INFANTILE BREAST DEVELOPMENT

The mammary glands develop from the mammary ridges, or milk lines. These are thickenings of the epidermis that appear on the ventral surface of the 5-week fetus, extending from the axilla to the upper medial region of the thigh. In the human, most of the ridge does not develop further and disappears during fetal development. Persistence of segments of the milk line is the embryologic anlage for the development of ectopic mammary glandular tissue, which occurs most often at the extreme ends of the mammary ridge in the axilla or vulva.

In most girls, breast development does not begin until puberty. *Premature thelarche* is the unilateral or bilateral appearance of a discoid subareolar thickening before puberty. The incidence in white female infants and children up to 7 years old in the United States in 1980 was 20.8/100,000 (1). The nodular breast tissue formed in premature thelarche, which measures 1.0 to 6.5 cm, tends to regress slowly during the subsequent 6 months to 6 years (1). Excision of this tissue is inappropriate because of the resultant amastia after puberty. Histologically, the breast tissue in premature thelarche resembles that of gynecomastia in that it is characterized by epithelial hyperplasia in the duct system with a solid and micropapillary configuration. Growth and branching of the proliferating ducts result in an increased number of duct cross sections surrounded by moderately cellular stroma.

With the onset of cyclical secretion of estrogen and progesterone at puberty, adolescent female breast development commences (Fig. 1). The growth of ducts and periductal stroma is estrogen-dependent (2). Lobules are derived from solid masses of cells that form at the ends of terminal ducts. Whereas the greatest amount of breast glandular differentiation occurs during puberty, the process may continue into the twenties and is enhanced by pregnancy.

ANATOMY AND HISTOLOGY

The functional glandular and ductal elements are embedded in fibrofatty tissue, which forms the bulk of the mammary gland. The relative proportions of fat and collagenous stroma vary greatly among individuals and with age. The combination of stromal and epithelial components is responsible for the radiographic appearance of breast structure in normal and pathologic states. Magnetic resonance (MR) imaging provides a relatively precise method for discriminating between fatty and fibroglandular tissue in the breast. By comparing images obtained with mammography and MR, Lee et al. (3) found a mean fat content of 42.5% (SD ± 30.3%) in mammograms and 66.5% (SD ± 18%) in MR images. The ranges of fat content obtained by mammography and MR imaging were 7.5% to 90% and 17% to 89%, respectively. The correlation coefficient for estimates of fat content obtained by both methods was 0.63, with the strongest correlation ($r = .81$) in postmenopausal women.

Each of the major lactiferous ducts terminates and exits from the breast at the nipple via a secretory pore forming the lactiferous duct orifice. The squamocolumnar junction, where the squamous epithelium joins the glandular duct epithelium, is normally distal to a dilated segment of the lactiferous duct, the lactiferous sinus, located just beneath the nipple surface. Extension of squamous epithelium into or beyond the lactiferous sinus is a pathologic condition termed squamous metaplasia. This may result in obstruction of the affected duct system.

Lactiferous ducts in the nipple are surrounded by circular and longitudinal arrays of smooth-muscle fibers embedded in fibrocollagenous stroma. The lactiferous ducts extend distally through a series of branches that diminish in caliber from the nipple to the terminal ductal-lobular units, which are embedded in specialized, hormonally responsive stroma. Extralobular ducts are lined by columnar epithelium that is supported by myoepithelial cells, a basement membrane, and surrounding elastic fibers. In a breast that is not lactating, the major ducts cut in cross section have contours marked by numerous folds or indentations, which create a foliate or serrate border. The epithelium in the baylike extensions of the duct lumen can give rise to ductular branches. Fully formed lobules can originate directly from this anatomic arrangement in the nipple and at deeper levels of the mammary duct system (4).

The majority of the cells that form the duct epithelium are columnar cells lining the lumen. Their cytoplasm is endowed with abundant organelles involved in secretion. Myoepithelial cells lie between the epithelial layer and the basal lamina. The cytoplasm of the myoepithelial cells, distributed in

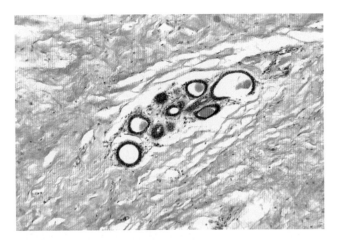

FIGURE 1. Immature breast. Breast tissue at the onset of puberty in an 11-year-old girl showing early lobular differentiation with glandular secretion and intralobular stroma.

a network of slender processes that invest the overlying epithelial cells, is rich in myofibrils. The histologic appearance and immunoreactivity of myoepithelial cells is variable, especially in pathologic conditions, and depends on the degree to which the myoid or epithelial phenotype is accentuated in a particular situation.

The normal periductal stroma contains fibroblasts, elastic fibers, a sparse scattering of lymphocytes, plasma cells, mast cells, and histiocytes. Ochrocytes are periductal histiocytes with a cytoplasmic accumulation of lipofuscin pigment. These pigmented cells become more numerous in the postmenopausal breast and in association with inflammatory or proliferative conditions (5).

Mammary secretion originates in the lobules. These structures are composed of groups of alveolar glands encompassed by specialized vascularized stroma. The alveoli are connected by intralobular ductules; these combine to form a single terminal lobular duct that drains into the extralobular duct system. The resting lobular gland is lined by a single layer of cuboidal epithelial cells supported by loosely connected myoepithelial cells. The normal microscopic anatomy of the lobules is not constant because the structure and histologic appearance of the lobule in the mature breast are subject to changes associated with the menstrual cycle, pregnancy, lactation, exogenous hormone administration, and the menopause. Furthermore, the functional state of individual lobules varies regardless of the physiologic circumstances, which suggests that there are intrinsic differences in individual lobules or regions of the breast in response to hormonal stimuli. This is reflected in the substantial variability in labeling indices indicating different proliferative rates among lobules in a given individual (6).

PHYSIOLOGIC MORPHOLOGY

Histologic cellular and structural alterations occur in the normal breast during the *menstrual cycle*. The proliferative phase, days 3 through 7, is characterized by the highest rate

of epithelial mitoses and apoptosis (7,8). Lobular glands at this time are lined by crowded, poorly oriented epithelial cells with little or no lumen formation and secretion. Myoepithelial cells are inconspicuous. The lobular stroma is relatively dense and hypovascular, with plump fibroblasts ringing lobular glands.

Mitotic activity is decreased in the follicular phase (days 8 through 14). At this stage, the myoepithelial cells have a polygonal shape and clear cytoplasm. Epithelial cells become columnar, with increasingly basophilic cytoplasm and basally oriented, darkly stained nuclei. An acinar lumen without secretion is evident.

During the luteal phase, comprising days 15 through 20, myoepithelial cells become more prominent because of increased glycogen accumulation that results in cytoplasmic clearing. The glandular lumen is clearly defined by epithelial cells with basophilic cytoplasm. A small amount of secretion is present in a few glands.

The secretory phase, corresponding to days 21 through 27, is characterized by heightened secretion with distension of glandular lumina by accumulated secretory material. The epithelium consists of epithelial cells and myoepithelial cells with clear cytoplasm (Fig. 2).

In the menstrual phase, comprising days 28 through 2, the stroma becomes compact, with loss of intralobular edema. Lymphocytes, macrophages, and plasma cells are most conspicuous in the lobular stroma at this stage (7). Some glandular lumina remain, and others appear collapsed. Mitotic activity is absent.

Estrogen and progesterone receptors are expressed in the nuclei of epithelial cells in the normal breast. Immunohistochemical staining reveals a higher proportion of reactive nuclei in lobular than in ductal cells (9). Considerable heterogeneity exists in nuclear hormone receptor activity among lobules, with maximal expression in the follicular phase (10). No consistent menstrual cycle-related pattern has been found in the expression of estrogen and progesterone recep-

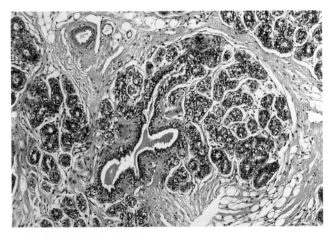

FIGURE 2. Secretory phase lobule. Secretion is present in the intralobular ductules and terminal duct. Myoepithelial cells with clear cytoplasm outline the lobular glands, and stromal edema is present.

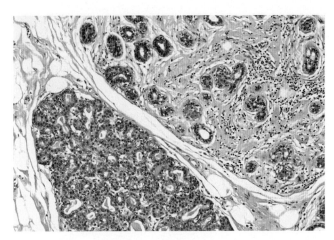

FIGURE 3. Lactational hyperplasia. This needle core biopsy specimen from a 31-year-old woman in her thirty-fourth week of pregnancy shows lactational hyperplasia in one lobule (*lower left*) and another, unaltered lobule with fibroadenomatoid change.

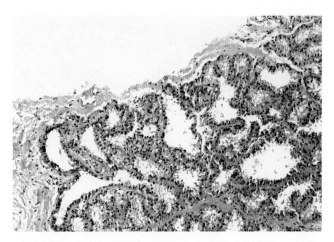

FIGURE 5. Lactating breast. This needle core biopsy specimen obtained from a 36-year-old nursing woman 8 months post partum also contained invasive ductal carcinoma. The lactating glands shown here are larger and more irregular in shape than those seen in lactational hyperplasia. The cytoplasm has prominent apical blebs and a frayed appearance at the luminal border.

tors in breast carcinomas that arise in premenopausal women (11,12).

Secretory changes associated with *pregnancy* occur unevenly throughout the breast (Fig. 3). There is progressive recruitment of lobules with successive pregnancies. Early in pregnancy, terminal ducts and lobules grow rapidly, resulting in lobular enlargement with some coincidental depletion of the fibrofatty stroma (13,14). Stromal vascularity increases, accompanied by infiltration by mononuclear inflammatory cells. During the second and third trimesters, lobular growth progresses through the enlargement of cells as well as by cellular proliferation. The cytoplasm of lobular epithelial cells becomes vacuolated, and secretion accumulates in lobular glands (Fig. 4). Lactation features markedly distended, irregularly shaped lobular glands formed by cells with hyperchromatic nuclei (Fig. 5).

Hormonal alterations that occur during and after the *menopause* are manifested by a decrease in the cellularity and number of lobules, mainly as a result of epithelial atrophy. Coincidental with the loss of glandular epithelium, there is a tendency to thickening of lobular basement membranes and collagenization of intralobular stroma. The process of menopausal atrophy occurs in a heterogeneous fashion, often leaving some lobules relatively unaffected in comparison with neighboring glands. Atrophy tends to spare lobular myoepithelial cells, which frequently persist even in a late stage of the process. Most lobular glands appear to collapse and shrink, but cystic distension may also occur, and calcifications are sometimes formed in atrophic lobular glands. In many women over 65 years of age, lobular integrity is progressively lost, leaving ducts and glands that

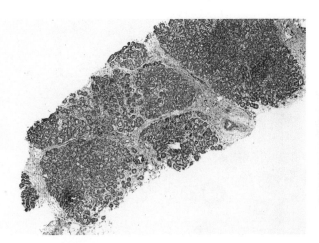
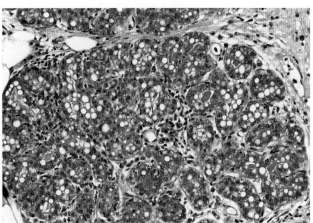

A   B

FIGURE 4. Lactational hyperplasia. A: The patient was 8 months pregnant when the needle core biopsy was performed for a mass that proved to be nodular lactational hyperplasia. **B:** Basophilic, vacuolated cytoplasm, luminal secretion, nuclei with prominent nucleoli, and inconspicuous myoepithelial cells are characteristic features.

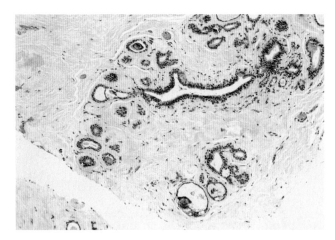

FIGURE 6. Atrophy. An atrophic lobule with a calcification in fibrous breast stroma. The needle core biopsy was performed on a 78-year-old woman with mammographically detected calcifications.

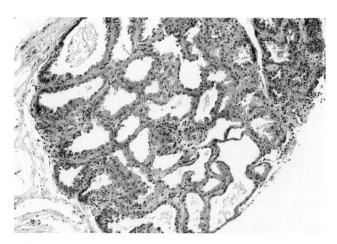

FIGURE 8. Pregnancy-like change. This lobule was present in a needle core biopsy specimen from a 49-year-old woman with invasive carcinoma. The enlarged lobule is composed of irregularly shaped glandular acini that contain small amounts of secretion. Crowding and hyperchromasia are apparent in the epithelium, formed largely by a single layer of cells.

may contain calcifications embedded in fibrocollagenous stroma (Fig. 6). The relative proportions of fat and stroma vary greatly in the atrophic breast. In advanced atrophy, calcifications may be found in the stroma unaccompanied by epithelium, and pronounced elastotic change in the stroma may be a source of calcifications (Fig. 7).

Pregnancy-like change (pseudolactational hyperplasia) is a microscopic alteration characterized by lobules that resemble those of lactational hyperplasia. It occurs in breast tissue from patients who are neither pregnant nor lactating when the specimen is obtained. Many of the patients are parous premenopausal or postmenopausal women, but similar changes have been observed in nulliparous women (15). The reported frequency of pregnancy-like change is 1.7% to about 3% in surgical pathology and autopsy series (15–17). The etiology of pregnancy-like change is unknown, and it remains to be determined whether this is a physiologic alteration or a hyperplastic change.

Glands and terminal ducts with pregnancy-like change usually contain little or no secretion, although they are dilated (Fig. 8). The glandular cells are swollen with abundant, pale-to-clear, finely granular or vacuolated cytoplasm. The nuclei are usually small, uniform, round, and darkly stained. The luminal cytoplasmic borders of glandular cells are frayed, and small cytoplasmic blebs are formed. The nucleus may be contained in a bleb of cytoplasm extruded into the glandular lumen. Diastase-resistant granules that stain positively with periodic acid–Schiff (PAS) are present in the cytoplasm, which is also immunoreactive for alpha-lactalbumin and S-100 (18). Calcifications can be formed in pregnancy-like change (Fig. 9).

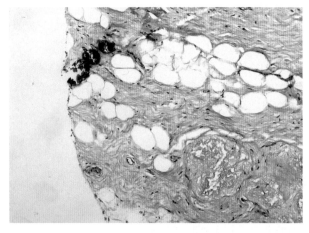

FIGURE 7. Atrophy. Calcification appears in fibrofatty stroma at the edge of a needle core biopsy from a 73-year-old woman. Note the stromal elastotic nodules (*lower right*).

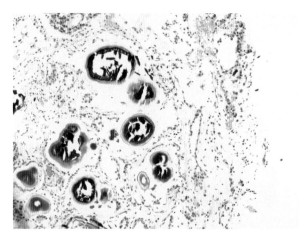

FIGURE 9. Pregnancy-like change with calcification. Large, laminated calcifications are present in pregnancy-like change in this needle core biopsy specimen from a 53-year-old woman with mammographically detected calcifications.

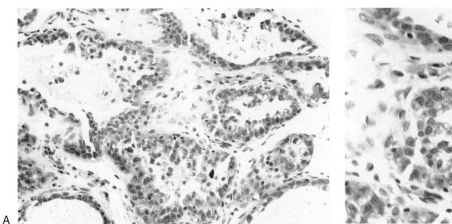
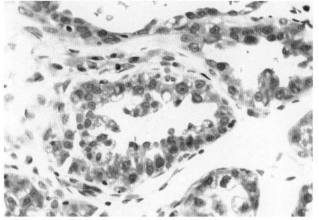

FIGURE 10. Pregnancy-like hyperplasia. A,B: Micropapillary fronds composed of hyperplastic epithelium protrude into some glandular lumina. Note the slightly uneven, crowded distribution of nuclei. Some nuclei have prominent nucleoli. Pale, eosinophilic secretion is present. This appearance resembles that of cystic hypersecretory hyperplasia in a lobule, but the epithelium does not have the appearance of micropapillary carcinoma, and the secretion lacks the intense eosinophilia and linear parallel cracks that characterize a cystic hypersecretory lesion.

In most instances, the epithelium in lobules altered by pregnancy-like change retains a thickness of one or two cell layers, thus simulating the architecture of the lactating breast. *Pregnancy-like hyperplasia* is the occurrence of pregnancy-like change in hyperplastic epithelium, which usually has a papillary configuration (Fig. 10). The epithelium is arranged in irregular fronds composed entirely of glandular cells. Although the cytologic appearance may duplicate the findings in pregnancy-like change, some of these lesions feature nuclear atypia, manifested in most instances by a degree of pleomorphism. Rarely, these atypical cytologic changes may be extreme, in which case they warrant a diagnosis of *atypical pregnancy-like hyperplasia* (Fig. 11).

Clear-cell change, also referred to as lamprocytosis or *hellenzellen* ("clear cells"), is a cytologic alteration in lobular and terminal duct epithelium (19). The affected lobules tend to be larger than adjacent uninvolved lobules. The lobular gland epithelium is composed of swollen cells with abundant clear or pale cytoplasm (Fig. 12). The cells have well-defined borders. Some glands have dilated lumina with PAS-positive, diastase-resistant secretion, but more often the lobular gland lumina are obliterated by the swollen cells (20). Calcifications are very uncommon in clear-cell change. The small, round, and darkly stained nuclei are often displaced toward the center of the gland. The clear cells are immunoreactive for cytokeratin but not for actin.

The etiology of clear-cell change is not known. It is encountered in premenopausal and postmenopausal women.

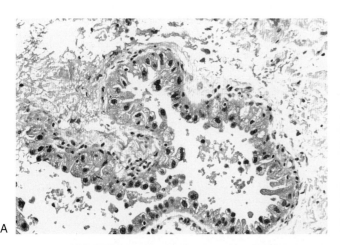
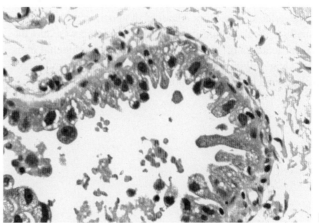

FIGURE 11. Atypical pregnancy-like hyperplasia. A,B: Enlarged, hyperchromatic, and pleomorphic nuclei in pregnancy-like change in a needle core biopsy specimen from a 48-year-old woman. Despite the cytologic atypia, the cells tend to be distributed in a single layer. Extrusion of nuclei is shown at the luminal border.

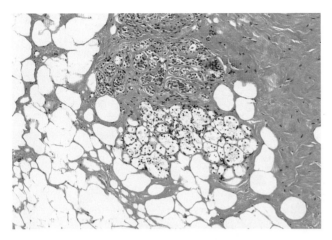

FIGURE 12. Clear-cell change. The lower lobule is composed of cells with clear cytoplasm and small dark nuclei in this needle core biopsy specimen from a 54-year-old woman with mammographically detected calcifications associated with intraductal carcinoma. The upper lobule has isolated, prominent myoepithelial cells.

There is no association with pregnancy or exogenous hormone use (20,21). Foci of clear-cell change have been identified retrospectively in breast tissue obtained before exogenous hormones were available. Viña and Wells (18) reported finding clear-cell change in 15 of 934 (1.6%) biopsy specimens. Specimens that contain clear-cell change may harbor carcinoma or benign changes, there being no association with any other particular breast lesions (18). Rarely, clear-cell change and pregnancy-like change may coexist in the same breast (21).

The differential diagnosis of clear-cell change includes pregnancy-like change, cytoplasmic clearing in apocrine metaplasia, cytoplasmic clearing in myoepithelial cells, and clear-cell forms of carcinoma. Pregnancy-like change is most readily distinguished from clear-cell change by the presence of "decapitation" secretion at the luminal borders of the cells. Cytoplasmic clearing in apocrine metaplasia is usually a focal change in epithelium that otherwise has the typical features of apocrine metaplasia. Myoepithelial cells with clear-cell change retain their position between the epithelium and basement membrane.

REFERENCES

1. van Winter JT, Noller KL, Zimmerman D, Melton JL III. Natural history of premature thelarche in Olmsted County, Minnesota, 1940 to 1984. *J Pediatr* 1990;116:278–280.
2. Topper YJ, Freeman CS. Multiple hormone interactions in the developmental biology of the mammary gland. *Physiol Rev* 1980;60:1049–1106.
3. Lee NA, Rusinek H, Weinreb J, et al. Fatty and fibroglandular tissue volumes in the breasts of women 20–83 years old: comparison of x-ray mammography and computer-assisted MR imaging. *AJR Am J Roentgenol* 1997;168:501–506.
4. Rosen PP, Tench W. Lobules in the nipple. *Pathol Annu* 1985;20(Pt1):317–322.
5. Davies JD. Pigmented periductal cells (ochrocytes) in mammary dysplasias: their nature and significance. *J Pathol* 1974;114:205–216.
6. Christov K, Chew KL, Ljung B-M, et al. Proliferation of normal breast epithelial cells as shown by *in vivo* labeling with bromodeoxyuridine. *Am J Pathol* 1991;138:1371–1377.
7. Longacre TA, Bartow SA. A correlative morphologic study of human breast and endometrium in the menstrual cycle. *Am J Surg Pathol* 1986;10:382–393.
8. Ferguson DJP, Anderson TJ. Morphological evaluation of cell turnover in relation to the menstrual cycle in the "resting" human breast. *Br J Cancer* 1981;4:177–181.
9. Petersen OW, Hoyer PE, van Deurs B. Frequency and distribution of estrogen receptor-positive cells in normal, nonlactating human breast tissue. *Cancer Res* 1987;47:5748–5751.
10. Fabris G, Marchetti E, Marzola A, Bagni A, Querzoli P, Nenci I. Pathophysiology of estrogen receptors in mammary tissue by monoclonal antibodies. *J Steroid Biochem* 1987;27:171–176.
11. Markopoulos C, Berger U, Wilson P, Gazet J-C, Coombes RC. Oestrogen receptor content of normal breast cells and breast carcinoma throughout the menstrual cycle. *Br Med J* 1988;296:1349–1351.
12. Smyth CM, Benn DE, Reeve TS. Influence of the menstrual cycle on the concentrations of estrogen and progesterone receptors in primary breast cancer biopsies. *Breast Cancer Res Treat* 1988;11:45–50.
13. McCarty KS Jr, Tucker JA. Breast. In: Sternberg SS, ed. *Histology for pathologists*. New York: Raven Press, 1992:893–902.
14. Salazar H, Tobon H, Josimovich JB. Developmental gestational and postgestational modifications of the human breast. *Clin Obstet Gynecol* 1975;18:113–137.
15. Kiaer HW, Andersen JA. Focal pregnancy-like changes in the breast. *Acta Pathol Microbiol Scand [A]* 1977;85:931–941.
16. Frantz VK, Pickren JW, Melcher GW, Auchencloss H Jr. Incidence of chronic cystic disease in so-called normal breasts: a study based on 225 postmortem examinations. *Cancer* 1951;4:762–783.
17. Sandison AT. An autopsy study of the adult human breast. *Natl Cancer Inst Monograph* 1962;8:58–59.
18. Viña M, Wells CA. Clear cell metaplasia of the breast: a lesion showing eccrine differentiation. *Histopathology* 1989;15:85–92.
19. Skorpil F. Uber das Vorkommen von sog. hellen Zellen (Lamprocyten) in der Milchdruse. *Beitr Pathol Anat* 1943;108:378–393.
20. Barwick KW, Kashigarian M, Rosen PP. "Clear-cell" change within duct and lobular epithelium of the human breast. *Pathol Annu* 1982;17(Pt 1):319–328.
21. Tavassoli FA, Yeh IT. Lactational and clear cell changes of the breast in nonlactating, nonpregnant women. *Am J Clin Pathol* 1987;87:23–29.

CHAPTER 2

Inflammatory and Reactive Tumors

FAT NECROSIS

Fat necrosis may result from incidental trauma, but presently the most frequent causes are prior surgery and radiation therapy. Patients typically present with a painless mass located superficially in the breast, accompanied by retraction or dimpling of the overlying skin. Any part of the breast may be affected. The tumors average 2 cm. The clinical problem of distinguishing between fat necrosis and recurrent carcinoma is especially difficult in patients who have undergone breast-conserving surgery and radiation therapy (1). Fat necrosis has been reported after external beam therapy and at the site of iridium implantation (2,3). Hemorrhagic necrosis of the skin, subcutaneous tissue, and breast parenchyma associated with warfarin (Coumadin) anticoagulant treatment is an uncommon form of fat necrosis (4). Pain and breast swelling appear within a week of the start of therapy, usually progressing to gangrene of most or all of the breast (5).

Mammography of fat necrosis usually reveals a spiculated mass that may contain punctate or large, irregular calcifications (6). Less frequently, the lesion consists of a circumscribed, oil-filled, partly calcified cyst (7). Both patterns may coexist in a single lesion.

The initial histologic change in fat necrosis is disruption of fat cells and hemorrhage (Fig. 1). Evolution of the lesion is marked by the appearance of histiocytes, hemosiderin deposition, and a variable infiltrate of lymphocytes, plasma cells, and sometimes eosinophils (Fig. 2). A foreign-body giant-cell reaction may be elicited (Fig. 3). Fibrosis develops peripherally, demarcating the area of necrotic fat, cellular debris, and calcifications (Fig. 4). In late lesions, the reactive inflammatory components replaced by fibrosis contract into a scar. Loculated, necrotic fat with calcification may persist for months or years within such a scar (Fig. 5). Squamous metaplasia may develop in the epithelium of ducts and lobules in the vicinity of fat necrosis.

Biopsy is required in most instances because the clinical and radiologic features resemble those of carcinoma. When there is a history of trauma or prior surgery and the characteristic radiologic findings of a demarcated lesion with typical calcifications are present, excision may not be performed after the diagnosis has been established by needle core biopsy.

BREAST INFARCT

The most frequent form of breast infarct occurs during pregnancy or post partum. The lesion presents as a discrete mass that can suggest carcinoma clinically. Pain and tenderness are sometimes reported. The firm mass is produced by infarcted mammary parenchyma. Hemorrhage and ischemic degeneration with little or no inflammation characterize the histologic appearance of early lesions. Later stages feature fully developed coagulative necrosis with loss of nuclear detail, pallor, and retention of architectural integrity.

Infarction also occurs in fibroadenomas and benign proliferative lesions. Foci of necrosis may be found in florid sclerosing adenosis, usually during pregnancy, when the epithelium in sclerosing adenosis may also exhibit pronounced hyperplasia, cytologic atypia, and mitotic activity. Papillomas are susceptible to partial or complete infarction, especially in major lactiferous ducts. Infarction can occur in papillomas at any age, but it tends to be more frequent in postmenopausal women, and there is no association with pregnancy (8). Bloody nipple discharge is the most frequent symptom, with or without a mass.

Acutely infarcted regions in a papilloma exhibit ischemic coagulative necrosis microscopically. Structural integrity is usually maintained in such foci despite progressive loss of cytologic detail (Fig. 6). At a late stage, fragmentation of superficial portions of infarcted regions occurs. Occasionally, an infarcted papilloma is reduced to an inflammatory intraductal polyp consisting of granulation tissue with little or no epithelium. Chronic ischemia and healing of infarcts are marked by fibrosis, which can cause considerable distortion of residual entrapped epithelium and produce a pattern that may be mistaken for carcinoma (8). Squamous metaplasia sometimes develops in the reparative epithelium that proliferates after infarction, and calcification can form in the infarcted tissue (8,9). Infarcted carcinoma can be distinguished from infarction of a benign lesion if there is residual intact *in situ* or invasive carcinoma (10).

Excisional biopsy is usually necessary for the diagnosis of a mammary infarct, although the findings in a needle core biopsy may be suggestive. In most cases, recognition of the underlying condition hinges on finding a residual uninfarcted component. A reticulin stain is helpful for unmasking the architecture of infarcted tissue. Rarely, the diagnosis of a

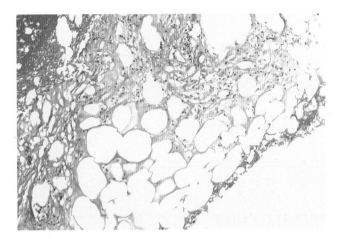

FIGURE 1. Fat necrosis. The needle core biopsy specimen obtained from a 1-cm stellate lesion comprises infarcted fat cells, hemorrhage, fibrin deposits, and reactive histiocytes. Note the loss of nuclear detail in the fat cells.

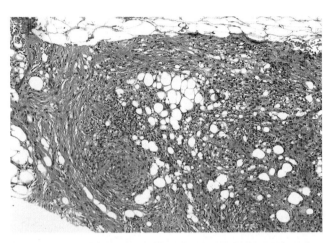

FIGURE 2. Fat necrosis. A needle core biopsy specimen from a mammographically detected mass at the site of a prior lumpectomy for intraductal carcinoma. Fibrosis and granulomatous reaction are evident in the fat necrosis. No foreign-body material was found.

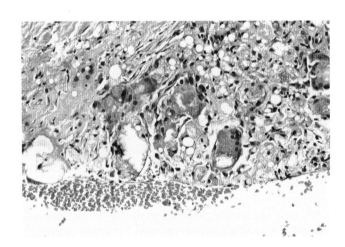

FIGURE 3. Fat necrosis. Multinucleated histiocytes with foreign-body material are shown in a needle core biopsy specimen from fat necrosis at a prior surgical site.

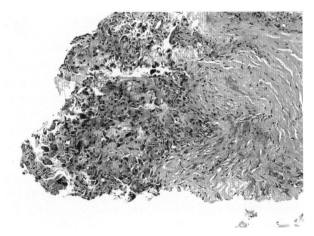

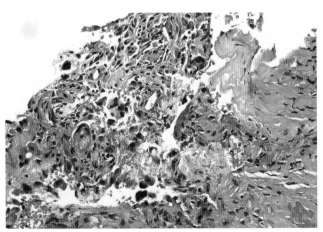

A   B

FIGURE 4. Fat necrosis. A,B: Fibrosis is evident around this focus of long-standing fat necrosis in a needle core biopsy specimen.

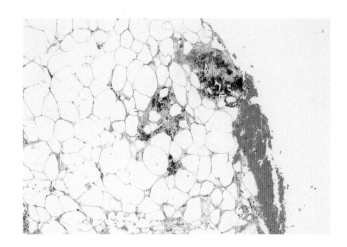

FIGURE 5. Fat necrosis. Infarcted fat with calcification in a needle core biopsy specimen. Nuclear detail is absent from the fat cells. This biopsy was obtained after nonpalpable calcifications were found on a routine mammogram.

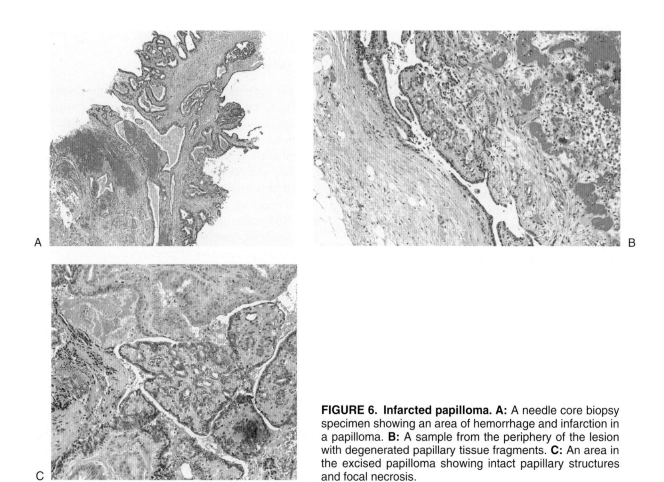

FIGURE 6. Infarcted papilloma. A: A needle core biopsy specimen showing an area of hemorrhage and infarction in a papilloma. **B:** A sample from the periphery of the lesion with degenerated papillary tissue fragments. **C:** An area in the excised papilloma showing intact papillary structures and focal necrosis.

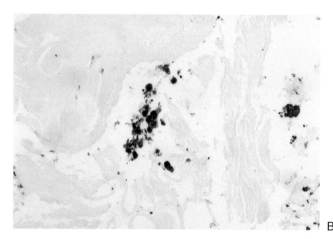

FIGURE 7. Infarct with atypical cells. A: This needle core biopsy specimen shows a totally infarcted lesion, possibly fat necrosis, and an attached fragment of tissue composed of atypical cells. **B:** The atypical cells proved to be epithelial rather than histiocytic with the CAM 5.2 cytokeratin immunostain (immunoperoxidase). Excisional biopsy revealed atypical duct hyperplasia near the fat necrosis.

totally infarcted lesion remains enigmatic (Fig. 7). If a papillary structure can be demonstrated in this circumstance, the lesion was probably a papilloma rather than a papillary carcinoma because infarction occurs considerably more often in benign papillary tumors than in papillary carcinomas.

GALACTOCELE

These lesions average about 2 cm in diameter, but galactoceles 5 cm or larger have been described (11). Mammography reveals a circumscribed density that in many instances has a characteristic appearance consisting of a hypodense upper area and a lower region with a density close to that of the surrounding tissue (12). The interface tends to remain horizontal as the patient changes position. The two zones consist of lighter, lipid-containing components located above the water-based constituents of the fluid. Comparable differences in echogenicity are observed on ultrasound examination.

The firm, usually painless tumor may suggest carcinoma clinically. Necrotic cells and nuclear debris, possibly accompanied by inflammatory cells, are seen in a fine-needle aspiration specimen (13). Cells with hyperchromatic, atypical-appearing nuclei may be present, but in this inflammatory background such changes should not be mistaken for carcinoma. Excisional biopsy is diagnostic and provides adequate therapy if the lesion does not resolve after aspiration of the cyst contents.

A galactocele is composed of cysts lined by smooth cuboidal epithelium. The cysts contain fluid contents resembling milk. Inspissated secretion may be present in the form of soft caseous material. Intact cysts are encompassed by a fibrous wall of varying thickness, with little or no inflammatory reaction. Leakage from a cyst elicits a chronic inflammatory reaction that may be accompanied by fat necrosis.

PLASMA CELL MASTITIS

In the early phase, patients experience the acute onset of mild pain, tenderness, redness, and nipple discharge that consists usually of thick secretion. After the inflammatory symptoms subside, the skin may be edematous over a firm-to-hard mass several centimeters in diameter remaining at the same site. Nipple discharge usually persists, and nipple retraction is observed in the majority of patients. Axillary lymph nodes are often enlarged. Plasma cell mastitis in its acute and mature phases is difficult to distinguish clinically from mammary carcinoma. The radiologic findings may be interpreted as indicative of carcinoma, especially when calcifications are present.

Plasma cell mastitis is a form of periductal mastitis characterized by variable hyperplasia of ductal epithelium and a marked, diffuse plasma cell infiltrate surrounding ducts as well as lobules (Fig. 8). A histiocytic reaction to the desquamated epithelium and lipid material in the ducts is responsible for areas that grossly appear to be xanthomatous and for the comedo-like character of the duct contents. Granulomatous features may be present microscopically, especially in areas of necrosis. Lymphocytes and neutrophils are variably present. Periductal fibrosis and obliterative intraductal proliferation of granulation tissue are not features of plasma cell mastitis. Hyperplastic epithelial cells, which may appear very atypical, can be mistaken for carcinoma in a needle core biopsy sample, leading to an erroneous diagnosis of comedocarcinoma.

MAMMARY DUCT ECTASIA

The earliest symptom is spontaneous, intermittent nipple discharge. In more advanced cases, subareolar induration progresses to the formation of a mass. The presence of nip-

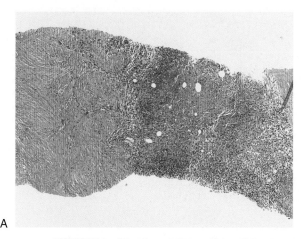
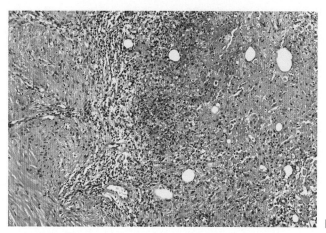

FIGURE 8. Plasma cell mastitis. A,B: A needle core biopsy specimen from a patient with a breast mass suspected to be carcinoma. Plasma cells are a prominent element in the reactive cellular infiltrate around the area of necrosis.

ple inversion is generally associated with periductal fibrosis and contracture. In some cases, squamous metaplasia of the terminal lactiferous duct epithelium results in obstruction that contributes to the development of duct ectasia and eventually to the formation of lactiferous duct fistulas (14,15). The mammographic abnormalities include microcalcifications, spiculated masses, and lobulated, partially smooth masses. In some instances, the mammographic findings suggest carcinoma (16).

The microscopic composition of the duct contents is variable. The most bland form consists of eosinophilic, granular or amorphous proteinaceous material. Usually, there is an admixture of lipid-containing histiocytic cells and desquamated duct epithelial cells. Cholesterol crystals and calcifications may be found in the intraductal debris (Fig. 9). Histiocytes that contain ceroid pigment, termed ochrocytes by Davies (17), and foam cells may be found within the epithe-

lial-myoepithelial layer of the duct, in periductal tissue, and in the lumen (Fig. 9). Neutrophils, lymphocytes, and plasma cells within the ducts are usually indicative of a more intense inflammatory reaction (Fig. 10). Disruption of ducts is accompanied by discharge of stasis material into the breast, causing periductal inflammation. Plasma cells and granulomas are not conspicuous features of the lesion in most cases.

Periductal fibrosis and hyperelastosis, often with a lamellar distribution, lead to mural thickening in the late phase of mammary duct ectasia (Fig. 11). The inflammatory reaction is less conspicuous, and the ducts are encased in a thick, laminated layer of hyaline fibrous and elastic tissue (18). The duct lumen may be patulous (Fig. 12). In some instances, the sclerotic process includes actively proliferating granulation tissue and hyperelastosis, which narrows and may totally occlude ducts (19). Remnants of persisting epithelium may proliferate to form secondary glands within the sclerotic

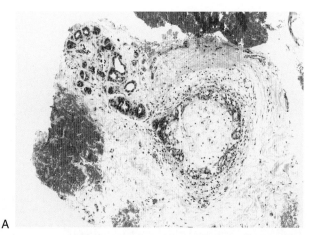
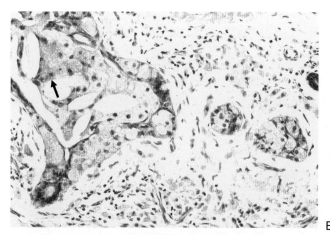

FIGURE 9. Duct ectasia. A: After calcifications were detected in a mammogram, this needle core biopsy specimen was obtained, which demonstrates dilated ducts with a histiocytic reaction. **B:** Histiocytes with finely granular, ceroid pigment (*arrow*), so-called ochrocytes, are present in the duct lumen, epithelium, and surrounding tissue.

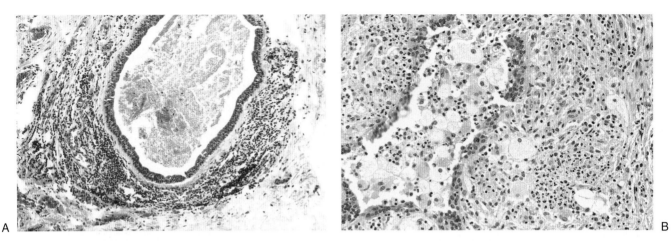

FIGURE 10. Duct ectasia and mastitis. A: The dilated duct with inspissated secretion is surrounded by lymphocytes. **B:** An intense inflammatory reaction composed of lymphocytes and neutrophils as well as histiocytes involves this duct. Note destruction of the epithelium.

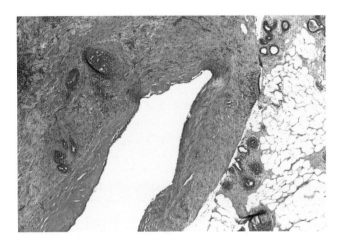

FIGURE 11. Duct ectasia. A late-stage lesion sampled by needle core biopsy. There is marked periductal fibrosis with minimal inflammation.

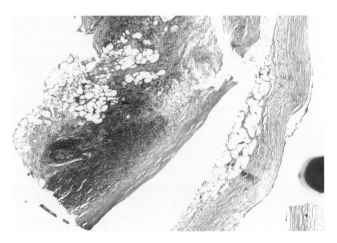

FIGURE 12. Duct ectasia. Portions of the walls of patulous, dilated ducts with chronic inflammation.

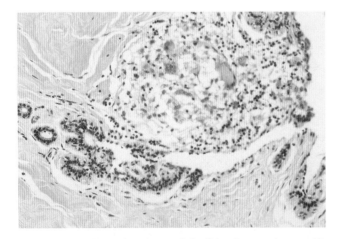

FIGURE 13. Granulomatous lobulitis. A granuloma with epithelioid giant cells in a lobule at the edge of a needle core biopsy specimen. No specific etiology was demonstrated in this patient.

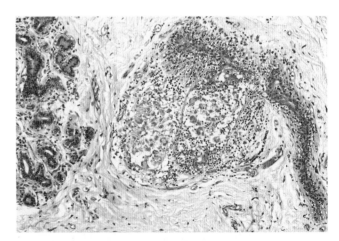

FIGURE 14. Sarcoidosis. The discrete granuloma adjacent to a duct does not involve the nearby lobule.

duct. When the epithelium is totally absent, the duct is reduced to fibrous scar.

GRANULOMATOUS MASTITIS

Numerous pathogenic processes responsible for granulomatous inflammation of the breast are included under the generic heading of granulomatous mastitis (20). The differential diagnosis of granulomatous mastitis includes many specific agents and conditions, such as tuberculosis, leprosy, brucellosis and other bacterial infections, fungi, parasitic infestations, and rheumatoid nodules (20,21). It is necessary to exclude the presence of acid-fast or other bacteria and fungi with cultures, histochemical stains, and appropriate clinical tests. Non-necrotizing, sarcoidlike granulomatous inflammation that develops in breast carcinomas is restricted to the tumor, immediately surrounding mammary parenchyma, and axillary lymph nodes (22).

Granulomatous lobular mastitis is a clinicopathologic condition characterized by perilobular granulomatous inflammation (23,24). This distribution suggests a cell-mediated reaction to one or more substances concentrated in the mammary secretion or lobular cells, but no specific antigen has been identified. The lesion usually appears at an average of 2 years after a pregnancy. The age at diagnosis ranges from 17 to 42 years, with a mean of about 33 years (24). Virtually all patients are parous. The distinct, firm-to-hard mass may involve any part of the breast but tends to spare the subareolar region. The breast tumors have reportedly measured from 1 cm to as much as 8 cm, averaging nearly 6 cm. The clinical findings often suggest carcinoma, and mammographic findings have been described as "suspicious" (20).

The primary pathologic change is a granulomatous lobulitis (Fig. 13). The granulomas are composed of epithelioid histiocytes and Langhans' giant cells accompanied by lymphocytes, plasma cells, and occasional eosinophils. Asteroid bodies are unusual, and Schaumann bodies have not been reported in the giant cells. Although not typically a conspicuous feature, fat necrosis and abscesses containing polymorphonuclear leukocytes are sometimes present, contributing to effacement of the lobulocentric distribution in confluent lesions. Squamous metaplasia of duct and lobular epithelium is unusual. Vasculitis is not seen. Results of stains and cultures for bacteria, acid-fast organisms, and fungi are negative.

Sarcoidosis tends to occur in women in their twenties and thirties, reflecting the overall age distribution of sarcoidosis (25,26). Mammary lesions usually are detected after the diagnosis has been established on the basis of the typical clinical manifestations of the disease. Only very rarely does sarcoidosis present as a primary breast tumor. The breast lesion caused by mammary sarcoidosis in some patients is a firm-to-hard mass that may be mistaken clinically for carcinoma. Occasionally, sarcoid granulomas are not apparent clinically, and they may be discovered when a biopsy is performed for an unrelated condition.

Microscopic examination reveals epithelioid granulomas in the mammary parenchyma among lobules and ducts (Fig. 14). Multinucleated Langhans' giant cells in the granulomas may contain asteroid or Schaumann bodies. The lesions do not exhibit caseous necrosis or calcification, and fat necrosis is not found in the surrounding breast. A lymphoplasmacytic reaction and fibrosis are present in varying amounts. Small, isolated granulomas with a sparse lymphocytic reaction may be found in surrounding breast tissue that appears grossly to be unaffected. These inconspicuous granulomatous foci tend to be associated with ducts or lobules.

INFLAMMATORY PSEUDOTUMOR

There is no well-characterized lesion of the breast that qualifies for this diagnosis. The diagnosis has been mistakenly used for metaplastic carcinoma, granulomatous mastitis, fibromatosis, and infarcts. In most cases, these lesions are probably the result of fat necrosis or duct ectasia with mastitis (Fig. 15). Localized nodular lesions in the breast consisting of fibrovascular stroma with a prominent infiltrate composed mainly of plasma cells and lymphocytes have been diagnosed as inflammatory pseudotumors (27,28). One patient had a unilateral lesion that did not recur after excision (28). In the other patient with bilateral tumors, recurrences developed in both breasts (27).

VASCULITIS

Inflammatory lesions of blood vessels are encountered in a variety of systemic disorders that are broadly grouped under the heading of collagen-vascular disease. The breasts may be affected as an isolated manifestation or as part of multiorgan involvement. The mammary lesions caused by vasculitis often resemble carcinoma clinically. Although there are differences in the histopathologic features of the

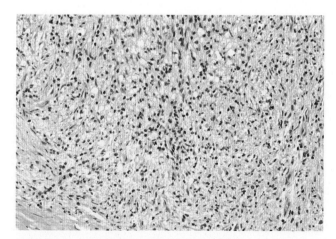

FIGURE 15. Inflammatory pseudotumor. The biopsy specimen was obtained from a 1-cm tumor that probably represents resolving fat necrosis. The lesion is composed of numerous histiocytes with scattered fibroblasts and lymphocytes.

vasculitides associated with various collagen-vascular diseases, the diagnosis of a specific condition is made on the basis of the clinical and pathologic findings. Some of these conditions may be manifested by a tumorous lesion or mammographically detected calcifications.

Giant-cell arteritis limited clinically to the breast has been reported in women 52 to 72 years of age who presented with one or more palpable breast tumors (29,30). The lesions were bilateral in nearly 50% of cases. The firm tumors have measured from less than 1 to 4 cm, and carcinoma was suspected in most cases. Axillary nodal enlargement has been noted in some cases (30). Systemic symptoms reported by patients with giant-cell arteritis of the breast include headache, muscle and joint pain, fever, and night sweats. Mild anemia and an elevated erythrocyte sedimentation rate are found in most cases.

Microscopically, transmural inflammation involves small and medium-size arteries throughout the affected tissue (Fig. 16). Veins and arterioles are largely spared. Fibrinoid necrosis is not a consistent feature, but fragmentation of the mural elastic fibers is demonstrable with an elastic tissue stain. Multinucleated giant cells tend to be oriented around the disrupted elastic fibers. The vascular lumen may be narrowed or occluded. The surrounding fibrofatty tissue exhibits fibrosis, edema, fat necrosis, and atrophy of glandular elements. The differential diagnosis includes other types of arteritis, phlebitis, infarction related to pregnancy or lactation, and traumatic fat necrosis.

Breast involvement has also been reported in patients with *Wegener's granulomatosis* (31), *polyarteritis* (32), *scleroderma* (33), *dermatomyositis* (34), and *lupus erythematosis* (35). In some instances, the lesions may be manifested by a mass with vascular calcifications. Biopsy reveals arterial necrosis and a transmural inflammatory reaction. Necrosis of surrounding breast parenchyma is often present.

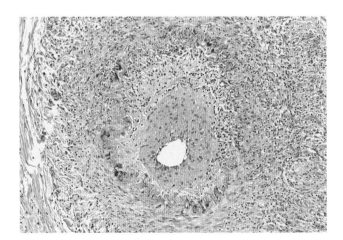

FIGURE 16. Giant cell arteritis. The patient presented with a mass, and biopsy revealed fat necrosis caused by diffuse arteritis. This artery is almost totally occluded by the inflammatory process. The elastica is fragmented. No giant cells are evident in this particular area.

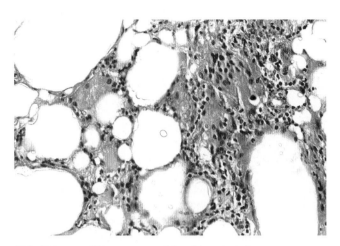

FIGURE 17. Silicone mastitis. Chronic inflammation surrounds vacuolar spaces that contain refractile silicone material.

SILICONE MASTITIS

The ability to detect carcinoma by mammography is impaired by mastitis caused by injected silicone or the reaction to a silicone-containing implant (36). Calcifications are generally irregular and coarse, but fine calcifications resembling those of carcinoma have been reported in silicone mastitis, and when present, biopsy specimens should be taken (37).

Silicone by itself or with adulterants causes fat necrosis and elicits a foreign-body giant-cell reaction (Fig. 17). The microscopic features of these processes are not specific for silicone injection. Silicone may also enter the lumina of ducts and lobular glands. During the processing of histologic sections, some of the silicone is lost from the tissue, leaving clear spaces of varying size. The presence of silicone can be confirmed by electron microscopy, infrared spectroscopy, atomic absorption spectrophotometry, and other procedures (38). The accompanying chronic inflammatory reaction and fibrosis vary in intensity.

DIABETIC MASTOPATHY

The occurrence of fibrous tumor-forming stromal proliferations in patients with diabetes mellitus is referred to as diabetic mastopathy (39). The pathologic changes are not entirely specific for insulin-dependent diabetes mellitus (40), and similar pathologic changes have been reported in patients who did not have diabetes (41).

With rare exceptions, diabetic mastopathy has been limited to female patients. Most patients were younger than 30 when type I insulin-dependent diabetes mellitus was diagnosed. Age at biopsy ranged from 19 to 63 years, with a mean of 34 to 47 years in six studies. The interval between the onset of diabetes and detection of the breast lesion has averaged about 20 years. Bilateral lesions have been present in nearly 50% of the cases. The majority of the patients have had complications of juvenile-onset diabetes, with severe diabetic retinopathy reported in many instances. The initial

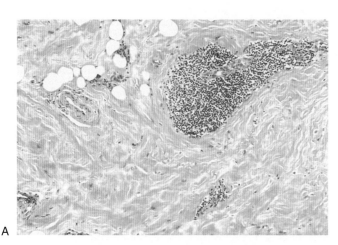 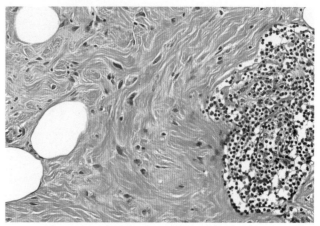

A   B

FIGURE 18. Diabetic mastopathy. A,B: Mature lymphocytes are clustered around a small blood vessel, and prominent myofibroblastic cells are evident in the stroma. The specimen was obtained from a young woman with juvenile-onset diabetes mellitus who presented with a unilateral breast mass.

clinical symptom is a palpable, firm-to-hard tumor that may suggest carcinoma. The mammogram reveals localized increased density, but no changes have been specifically associated with this condition. In some patients, the mammographic appearance of the mass resembles that of a carcinoma or a fibroadenoma (41,42).

The lesional tissue consists of collagenous stroma with keloidal features and a variably increased concentration of stromal cells in comparison with the surrounding breast tissue. Polygonal epithelioid cells are found dispersed in the collagen among the spindly stromal cells in most but not all cases. The stromal cells are myofibroblasts with variable fibroblastic and myoid differentiation (Fig. 18). Multinucleated stromal giant cells and mitotic activity are not part of this proliferative process. Mature lymphocytes are clustered around small blood vessels throughout the lesion as well as in and around lobules and ducts. Very few plasma cells or other leukocytes are present in the perivascular infiltrates. Germinal centers are rarely formed.

In most instances, diabetic mastopathy is associated with all the previously mentioned histologic features, but on occasion, one or more of the typical findings may be absent (43). Infarcts, fat necrosis, duct stasis, arteritis, and other inflammatory lesions are not a feature of diabetic mastopathy. Stromal collagen fibers may appear prominent, but they do not have a keloidal appearance. Proliferative epithelial changes may be present coincidentally, but they are not an integral component of diabetic mastopathy. The differential diagnosis of diabetic mastopathy includes nonspecific lymphocytic lobulitis (Fig. 19) and fibromatosis.

AMYLOID TUMOR

Amyloid deposits in the breast have been described in patients with predisposing systemic diseases such as primary amyloidosis, rheumatoid arthritis, and multiple myeloma. Primary amyloid tumors clinically limited to the breast are uncommon (44). Age at diagnosis ranges from 45 to 79 years

(median, 56 years). Bilateral involvement has been described. The tumors have usually been solitary. Clinical examination reveals a discrete, hard tumor that can mimic carcinoma and may contain calcifications on mammography (45,46).

Histologically, eosinophilic, amorphous, homogeneous deposits of amyloid are distributed in fat, fibrocollagenous stroma, and blood vessels (Fig. 20). Deposits of amyloid around ducts and in lobules are associated with atrophy and obliteration of these glandular components. In adipose tissue, thin ribbons of amyloid may be formed around individual fat cells. These so-called amyloid rings are accentuated when Congo red–stained sections are examined with polarized light (47). Varying numbers of plasma cells, lymphocytes, and multinucleated giant cells are usually present in association with the amyloid deposits, which can also have punctate or irregular calcifications. Amyloid is stained red-orange with alkaline Congo red, and it exhibits apple-green

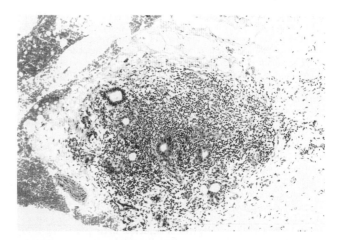

FIGURE 19. Lymphocytic lobulitis. A needle core biopsy was performed to assess a nonpalpable lesion without calcifications. The patient had no known systemic disease. One of several lobules infiltrated by mature lymphocytes is shown here.

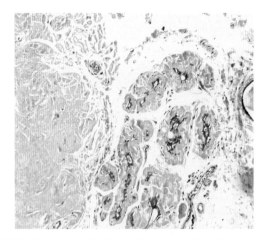

FIGURE 20. Amyloidosis. A thick layer of amyloid has been deposited in the basement membranes of the glands in a lobule next to a nodule of amyloid in the stroma on the left.

birefringence when the Congo red–stained section is examined with polarized light. Staining with crystal violet results in a strong metachromatic reaction.

REFERENCES

1. Clarke D, Curtis JL, Martinez A, Fajardo L, Goffinet D. Fat necrosis of the breast simulating recurrent carcinoma after primary radiotherapy in the management of early breast cancer. *Cancer* 1983;52:442–445.
2. Rostom AY, el-Sayed ME. Fat necrosis of the breast: an unusual complication of lumpectomy and radiotherapy in breast cancer. *Clin Radiol* 1987;38:31.
3. Girling AC, Hanby AM, Millis RR. Radiation and other pathological changes in breast tissue after conservation treatment for carcinoma. *J Clin Pathol* 1990;43:152–156.
4. Hogge JP, Robinson RE, Magnant CM, Zuurbier RA. The mammographic spectrum of fat necrosis of the breast. *Radiographics* 1995;15: 1347–1356.
5. Martin BF, Phillips JD. Gangrene of the female breast with anticoagulant therapy: report of two cases. *Am J Clin Pathol* 1970;53:622–626.
6. Isenberg JS, Tu Q, Rainey W. Mammary gangrene associated with warfarin ingestion. *Ann Plast Surg* 1996;37:553–555.
7. Bargum K, Moller Nielsen S. Case report: fat necrosis of the breast appearing as oil cysts with fat-fluid levels. *Br J Radiol* 1993;66:718–720.
8. Flint A, Oberman HA. Infarction and squamous metaplasia of intraductal papilloma: a benign breast lesion that may simulate carcinoma. *Hum Pathol* 1984;15:764–767.
9. Murad TM, Contesso G, Mouriesse H. Papillary tumors of large lactiferous ducts. *Cancer* 1981;48:122–133.
10. Jones EL, Codling BW, Oates GD. Necrotic intraduct breast carcinomas simulating inflammatory lesions. *J Pathol* 1973;110:101–103.
11. Golden GT, Wangensteen SL. Galactocele of the breast. *Am J Surg* 1972;123:271–273.
12. Salvador R, Salvador M, Jimenez JA, Martinez M, Casas L. Galactocele of the breast: radiologic and ultrasonographic findings. *Br J Radiol* 1990;63:140–142.
13. Novotny DB, Maygarden SJ, Shermer RW, Frable WJ. Fine needle aspiration of benign and malignant breast masses associated with pregnancy. *Acta Cytol* 1991;35:676–686.
14. Habif DV, Perzin KH, Lipton R, Lattes R. Subareolar abscess associated with squamous metaplasia of lactiferous ducts. *Am J Surg* 1970; 119:523–526.
15. Passaro ME, Broughan TA, Sebek BA, Esselstyn CB Jr. Lactiferous fistula. *J Am Coll Surg* 1994;178:29–32.
16. Sweeney DJ, Wylie EJ. Mammographic appearances of mammary duct ectasia that mimic carcinoma in a screening programme. *Australas Radiol* 1995;39:18–23.
17. Davies JD. Pigmented periductal cells (ochrocytes) in mammary dysplasias: their nature and significance. *J Pathol* 1974;114:205–216.
18. Davies JD. Inflammatory damage to ducts in mammary dysplasia: a cause of duct dilatation. *J Pathol* 1975;117:47–54.
19. Davies JD. Hyperelastosis, obliteration and fibrous plaques in major ducts of the human breast. *J Pathol* 1973;110:13–26.
20. Fitzgibbons PL. Granulomatous mastitis. *N Y State J Med* 1990;90:287.
21. Cooper NE. Rheumatoid nodule of the breast. *Histopathology* 1991;19: 193–194.
22. Bässler R, Birke F. Histopathology of tumour-associated sarcoid-like stromal reaction in breast cancer. An analysis of 5 cases with immunohistochemical investigations. *Virchows Arch [A]* 1988;412:231–239.
23. Fletcher A, Magrath IM, Riddell RH, Talbot IC. Granulomatous mastitis: a report of seven cases. *J Clin Pathol* 1982;35:941–945.
24. Going JJ, Anderson TJ, Wilkinson S, Chetty U. Granulomatous lobular mastitis. *J Clin Pathol* 1987;40:535–540.
25. Fitzgibbons PL, Smiley DF, Kern WH. Sarcoidosis presenting initially as breast mass: report of two cases. *Hum Pathol* 1985;16:851–852.
26. Banik S, Bishop PW, Ormerod LP, O'Brien TEB. Sarcoidosis of the breast. *J Clin Pathol* 1986;39:446–448.
27. Yip CH, Wong KT, Samuel D. Bilateral plasma cell granuloma (inflammatory pseudotumour) of the breast. *Aust N Z J Surg* 1997;67: 300–303.
28. Pettinato G, Manivel JC, Insabato L, De Chiara A, Petrella G. Plasma cell granuloma (inflammatory pseudotumour) of the breast. *Am J Clin Pathol* 1988;90:627–632.
29. Clement PB, Senges H, How AR. Giant cell arteritis of the breast: case report and literature review. *Hum Pathol* 1987;18:1186–1189.
30. Lau Y, Mak YF, Hui PK, Ahchong AK. Giant cell arteritis of the breast. *Aust N Z J Surg* 1996;66:259–261.
31. Jordan JM, Rowe TW, Allen NB. Wegener's granulomatosis involving the breast. Report of three cases and review of the literature. *Am J Med* 1987;83:159–164.
32. Yamashina M, Wilson TK. A mammographic finding in focal polyarteritis nodosa. *Br J Radiol* 1985;58:91–92.
33. Harrison GO, Elliott RL. Scleroderma of the breast: light and electron microscopy study. *Am Surg* 1987;53:526–531.
34. Gyves-Ray KM, Adler DD. Dermatomyositis: an unusual cause of breast calcifications. *Breast Dis* 1989;2:195–201.
35. Cernea SS, Kihara SM, Sotto MN, Vilela MAC. Lupus mastitis. *J Am Acad Dermatol* 1993;29:343–346.
36. Destouet JM, Monsees BS, Oser RF, Nemecek JR, Young VL, Pilgram TK. Screening mammography in 350 women with breast implants: prevalence and findings of implant complications. *AJR Am J Roentgenol* 1992;159:973–978.
37. Morgenstern L, Gleischman SH, Michel SL, Rosenberg JE, Knight I, Goodman D. Relation of free silicone to human breast carcinoma. *Arch Surg* 1986;120:573–577.
38. Travis WE, Balogh K, Abraham JL. Silicone granulomas: report of three cases and review of the literature. *Hum Pathol* 1985;16:19–27.
39. Tomaszewski JE, Brooks JSJ, Hicks D, LiVolsi VA. Diabetic mastopathy: a distinctive clinicopathologic entity. *Hum Pathol* 1992;23: 780–786.
40. Seidman JD, Schnaper LA, Phillips LE. Mastopathy in insulin-requiring diabetes mellitus. *Hum Pathol* 1994;25:819–824.
41. Ashton MA, Lefkowitz M, Tavassoli FA. Epithelioid stromal cells in lymphocytic mastitis—a source of confusion with invasive carcinoma. *Mod Pathol* 1994;7:49–54.
42. Byrd BF Jr, Hartmann WH, Graham LS, Hogle HH. Mastopathy in insulin-dependent diabetics. *Ann Surg* 1987;205:529–532.
43. Morgan MC, Weaver MG, Crowe JP, Abdul-Karim FW. Diabetic mastopathy: a clinicopathologic study of palpable and nonpalpable breast lesions. *Mod Pathol* 1995;8:349–354.
44. Silverman JF, Dabbs DJ, Norris HT, Pories WJ, Legier J, Kay S. Localized primary (AL) amyloid tumor of the breast. Cytologic, histologic, immunocytochemical and ultrastructural observations. *Am J Surg Pathol* 1986;10:539–545.
45. Hecht AH, Tan A, Shen JF. Case report: primary systemic amyloidosis presenting as breast masses, mammographically simulating carcinoma. *Clin Radiol* 1991;44:123–124.
46. Liaw Y-S, Kuo S-H, Yang P-C, Luh K-T. Nodular amyloidosis of the lung and the breast mimicking breast carcinoma with pulmonary metastasis. *Eur Respir J* 1995;5:871–873.
47. Libbey CA, Skinner M, Cohen AS. The abdominal fat aspirate for the diagnosis of systemic amyloid. *Arch Intern Med* 1983;143:1549–1552.

CHAPTER 3

Specific Infections

FUNGAL INFECTIONS

Actinomycotic infection of the breast typically presents as an abscess beneath or near the nipple and areola. Sinus tracts usually develop following incision and drainage when the specific diagnosis is not suspected clinically, or with progression of the untreated lesion. A chronic abscess may form, creating a hard mass that simulates carcinoma. Axillary nodal enlargement typically reflects reaction to the inflammatory process more often than spread of actinomycosis to the lymph nodes, but actinomycotic axillary lymphadenitis has been reported (1). In advanced cases, the infection can spread to the chest wall. Extension of pulmonary actinomycosis to the breast has also been reported (2). The diagnosis of mammary actinomycosis is made by demonstrating the gram-positive organism as filaments or colonies (sulfur granules). Treatment with penicillin has reportedly been effective (1), but recurrent or advanced infections may require mastectomy.

Infection with *Histoplasma capsulatum* is endemic in some regions of the United States and other nations. Calcified granulomas have not been described in the breast, and there have been rare instances of localized mammary *Histoplasma* infection presenting as a solitary unilateral mass that suggested a neoplasm clinically (3). Histologically, the lesions consist of confluent necrotizing granulomas in which *H. capsulatum* is demonstrated by a methenamine-silver reaction. The granulomatous reaction is histologically similar to that of nonspecific granulomatous lobular mastitis (4).

Rare instances of other fungal infections of the breast have been reported. These include infection with *Cryptococcus* (3), *Aspergillus* (5), *Coccidioides* (6), *Blastomyces* (7), and *Nocardia asteroides* (8).

PARASITIC INFECTIONS

Mammary *filariasis* caused most frequently by *Wuchereria bancrofti* has been reported from tropical and semitropical regions in South America, China, and the Indian subcontinent, where infection with this organism is endemic. Involvement of the breast occurs in the chronic phase of infection.

The patient usually presents with a solitary, nontender, painless, unilateral breast mass. Multiple lesions occur in a minority of cases. Many of the lesions involve subcutaneous tissue, and they may be fixed to the skin. The resultant hard mass with cutaneous attachment, sometimes accompanied by inflammatory changes including edema of the skin, appears to be clinically indistinguishable from carcinoma (9). In this setting, axillary nodal enlargement caused by filarial lymphadenitis further complicates the differential diagnosis. Viable microfilariae can be detected in the breast by ultrasound examination if they produce a distinctive pattern of movement referred to as the "filaria dance" sign (10). Mammographically detected calcifications attributed to *W. bancrofti* and *Loa loa* infection have been described as having a spiral or serpiginous configuration (11). Microscopic examination typically reveals adult filarial worms, which may be well preserved or in varying stages of degeneration (Fig. 1). Granulomatous reaction with eosinophilia is present in the surrounding tissue. Fully degenerated worms are likely to become calcified. Adult worms and microfilariae may also be found in axillary lymph nodes (12).

Several examples of mammary *cysticercosis*, an infection caused by the larvae of tapeworms, have been described. Most instances of mammary cysticercosis were caused by *Taenia solium* (13). The breast can also be the site of hydatid cyst formation caused by *Echinococcus granulosus*. The lesion typically presents as a firm, discrete, mobile mass. Mammography reveals a dense, well-circumscribed tumor within which internal ring structures representing air-fluid levels may be seen in an overly penetrated view. Air-fluid levels and multiple cysts are seen to better advantage by ultrasound (14). Mammary hydatid disease can be recognized by finding fragments of the adult worm, hydatid membranes, and hooklets in a biopsy specimen or in the aspirated cyst contents (15) (Fig. 2).

Calcified ova of *Schistosoma* can produce a radiologic appearance in mammograms suggestive of carcinoma (16).

TUBERCULOSIS

Tuberculosis of the breast is not an uncommon condition in some regions of the world (17). Tuberculous mastitis has been reported as a manifestation of AIDS, and this presentation may be encountered with increasing frequency in HIV-positive individuals (18).

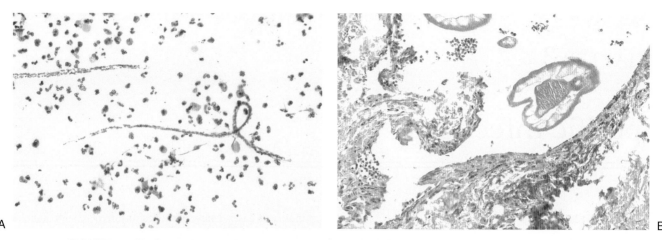

FIGURE 1. Filariasis. A: Microfilariae in a fine needle aspiration specimen with *Wuchereria bancrofti* infection. **B:** Biopsy specimen from a filarial abscess showing a microfilaria in cross section and fragments of the surrounding tissue. (Courtesy of Dr. Kusum Kapila.)

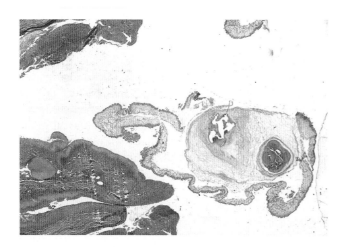

FIGURE 2. Cysticercosis. Part of hydatid cyst wall and a cross section of the larval tape worm. (Courtesy of Dr. Kusum Kapila.)

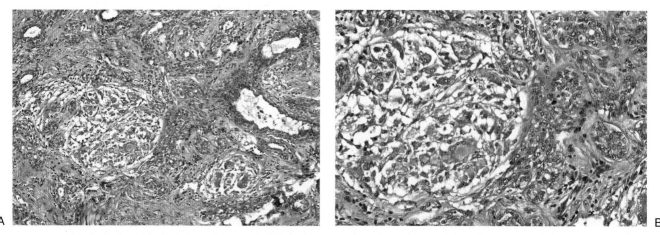

FIGURE 3. Tuberculous mastitis. A,B: Granulomatous inflammation in sclerosing adenosis in a patient with active pulmonary tuberculosis. The needle core biopsy was performed to evaluate a breast mass. No acid-fast bacteria were found with the Ziehl-Neelsen stain.

Mammary tuberculosis is primarily a disease of pre-menopausal women. It has a predilection for the lactating breast (19) but can affect the breast of a female adult of any age. Infection of the breast may be the primary manifestation of tuberculosis, but the breasts are probably infected secondarily in most patients, even when the primary, nonmammary focus remains clinically inapparent.

The diagnosis of tuberculous mastitis is difficult because the disease has multiple patterns of clinical presentation. The most common form is nodular mastitis, in which a slowly growing, solitary mass develops. The mammographic appearance of such lesions resembles that of carcinoma (20,21). Microcalcifications are typically absent. Advanced nodular lesions become fixed to the skin, and draining sinuses may develop (20). A diffuse type of tuberculous mastitis is characterized by the acute development of multiple painful nodules throughout the breast, producing a pattern that can be mistaken for inflammatory carcinoma clinically and mammographically (21). The third, sclerosing variety of infection occurs predominantly in elderly women and results in diffuse induration of the breast and diffuse areas of increased density on mammography. The clinical distinction between tuberculous mastitis and mammary carcinoma is complicated by the occasional coexistence of the lesions (22).

Microscopically, granulomatous lesions in tuberculous mastitis do not always exhibit caseous necrosis, and in chronic cases, fibrosis may be prominent. The granulomas are associated with ducts and lobules (Fig. 3). Acid-fast bacteria are not detected histologically in most cases. Neutrophils can obscure the granulomatous character of the process in specimens from patients with necrotizing abscesses or sinus tracts. Calcifications are uncommon.

REFERENCES

1. Jain BK, Sehgal VN, Jagdish S, Ratnakar C, Smile SR. Primary actinomycosis of the breast: a clinical review and a case report. *J Dermatol* 1994;21:497–500.

2. Pinto MM, Longstreth GB, Khoury GM. Fine needle aspiration of *Actinomyces* infection of the breast. A novel presentation of thoracopleural actinomycosis. *Acta Cytol* 1991;35:409–411.

3. Salfelder K, Schwarz J. Mycotic "pseudotumors" of the breast. *Arch Surg* 1975;110:751–754.

4. Osborne BM. Granulomatous mastitis caused by *Histoplasma* and mimicking inflammatory breast carcinoma. *Hum Pathol* 1989;20: 47–52.

5. Williams K, Walton RL, Bunkis I. *Aspergillus* colonization associated with bilateral silicone mammary implants. *J Surg Pathol* 1982;71: 260–261.

6. Bocian JJ, Fahmy RN, Michas CA. A rare case of "coccidioidoma" of the breast. *Arch Pathol Lab Med* 1991;115:1064–1067.

7. Propeck PA, Scanlan KA. Blastomycosis of the breast. *AJR Am J Roentgenol* 1996;166:726.

8. Simpson AJH, Jumaa PA, Das SS. Breast abscess caused by *Nocardia asteroides*. *J Infect* 1995;30:266–267.

9. Choudhury M. Bancroftian microfilaria in the breast clinically mimicking malignancy. *Cytopathology* 1995;6:132–133.

10. Dreyer G, Brandão AC, Amaral F, Medeiros Z, Addiss D. Detection by ultrasound of living adult *Wuchereria bancrofti* in the female breast. *Mem Inst Oswaldo Cruz* 1996;91:95–96.

11. Chow CK, McCarthy JS, Neafie R, et al. Mammography of lymphatic filariasis. *AJR Am J Roentgenol* 1996;167:1425–1426.

12. Chen YH, Qun X. Filarial granuloma of the female breast: a histopathologic study of 131 cases. *Am J Trop Med Hyg* 1981;30:1206–1210.

13. Kunkel JM, Hawksley CZ. Cysticercosis presenting as a solitary dominant breast mass. *Hum Pathol* 1987;18:1190–1191.

14. Vega A, Ortega E, Cavada A, Garijo F. Hydatid cyst of the breast: mammographic findings. *AJR Am J Roentgenol* 1994;162:825–826.

15. Sagin HB, Kiroglu Y, Aksoy F. Hydatid cyst of the breast diagnosed by fine needle aspiration biopsy. A case report. *Acta Cytol* 1994;38: 965–967.

16. Sloan BS, Rickman LS, Blau EM, Davis CE. Schistosomiasis masquerading as carcinoma of the breast. *South Med J* 1996;89:345–347.

17. Hale JA, Peters GN, Cheek JH. Tuberculosis of the breast: rare but still extant. *Am J Surg* 1985;150:620–624.

18. Hartstein M, Leaf HL. Tuberculosis of the breast as a presenting manifestation of AIDS. *Clin Infect Dis* 1992;15:692–693.

19. Alagaratnam TT, Ong GB. Tuberculosis of the breast. *Br J Surg* 1980; 67:125–126.

20. Makanjuola D, Murshid K, Sulaimani A, Al Saleh M. Mammographic features of breast tuberculosis: the skin bulge and sinus tract sign. *Clin Radiol* 1996;51:354–358.

21. Sopeña B, Arnillas E, Garcia-Vila LM, Climent A, Miramontes S. Tuberculosis of the breast: unusual clinical presentation of extrapulmonary tuberculosis. *Infection* 1996;24:57–58.

22. Rothman GM, Kolkov Z, Meroz A, Lewinski UH. Breast tuberculosis and carcinoma. *Israel J Med Sci* 1989;25:339–340.

CHAPTER 4

Benign Papillary Tumors

INTRADUCTAL PAPILLOMA

A papilloma is a discrete, benign papillary tumor that arises most often in the central part of the breast from a lactiferous duct, but it can occur in any quadrant. An *intracystic papilloma* is a papilloma in a cystically dilated duct. Solid, noncystic papillomas have been classified as *ductal adenomas* or *adenomyoepitheliomas*. Papillomas may be *solitary*, consisting of a single papillary tumor in one duct, or *multiple*, usually growing in contiguous branches of the ductal system. Intraductal papillomas should be distinguished from papillomatosis (epitheliosis), a term that describes microscopic duct hyperplasia. Papillomatosis may coexist with solitary or multiple papillomas.

A subareolar mass may be palpable in patients with a central solitary papilloma, and a palpable tumor can be the first clinical manifestation of a papilloma in one of the quadrants. Cystic papillary tumors may appear to be well circumscribed on mammography (1) (Fig. 1). The presence of a cystic component is best appreciated by ultrasonography or pneumocystography. Solitary papillomas occur at any age, from infancy to the ninth decade, but they are frequent in the sixth decade of life. Nipple discharge occurs in most patients with a central papilloma.

Multiple papillomas develop more often peripherally than centrally and typically present as a palpable lesion. These patients tend to be younger on average than women with solitary papillomas, often presenting in their forties and early fifties.

Part of the mass associated with a solitary papilloma may be the cyst formed by the dilated duct in which the papilloma arose. Some papillomas obliterate the cystic space. These lesions are well circumscribed and appear to be enclosed in a capsule formed by the duct wall and accompanying reactive changes. Solitary papillomas can occur as clinically symptomatic tumors 1 cm or less in diameter in a major lactiferous duct, or small, asymptomatic, peripheral papillomas may be detected by mammography, but the average size of palpable lesions is 2 to 3 cm. Cystic papillomas can be larger than 10 cm.

A series of 26 papillary tumors diagnosed by needle core biopsy included 19 papillomas (2). Ten were classified as atypical. Calcifications were detected more often in lesions classified as atypical than in papillomas without atypia, whereas a mass was less frequently the mammographic abnormality that led to biopsy of atypical papillomas. Intraductal carcinoma was found in excisional biopsy specimens in 3 of 10 (33%) atypical papillomas but not in 7 excised papillomas.

The most orderly form of papilloma consists of branching fronds of stroma supporting a layer of epithelium composed of cuboidal to columnar epithelial cells and myoepithelial cells (Fig. 2). The papillary stroma may arise from a single base or from several sites in the duct wall. The nonpapillary portion of the duct usually exhibits little or no epithelial hyperplasia in such lesions (Fig. 3).

Many benign papillomas have a more complex structure resulting from stromal overgrowth, hyperplasia of the epithelium, or both processes, which cause fusion of papillary fronds. Secondary microlumina are formed within the hyperplastic epithelium, and there may be micropapillary epithelial hyperplasia (Fig. 4). Proliferation of epithelium within the fibrovascular stroma results in a pattern resembling that of sclerosing adenosis (Figs. 5–7). The most florid form of epithelial hyperplasia is the solid intraductal papilloma, in which virtually all space between fibrovascular stalks is filled by proliferative duct epithelium (Fig. 8). In the conventional papilloma, apocrine metaplasia is usually cytologically bland (Fig. 9), but apocrine atypia manifested by nuclear pleomorphism and cytoplasmic clearing is likely to be encountered in sclerosing papillary tumors (3) (Figs. 10,11).

In many papillomas, the stroma is limited to a network of slender, inconspicuous bands consisting of thin-walled capillaries accompanied by sparse fibroblasts, collagen, and mononuclear cells. Collagenization of the fibrovascular stroma occurs in some papillomas. The papillary architecture is accentuated when sclerosis is limited to the intrinsic papillary structure. If myofibroblastic proliferation accompanies collagenization of the stroma, the papillary arrangement is likely to become distorted (Fig. 12). Epithelial elements entrapped in this stroma may simulate invasive carcinoma within the lesion or at the periphery (Fig. 13). Fibrous sclerosis can be so severe that it virtually obliterates the papilloma, reducing it to a nodular scar containing scattered, benign glandular elements that may be difficult to distinguish

Text continues on page 27

21

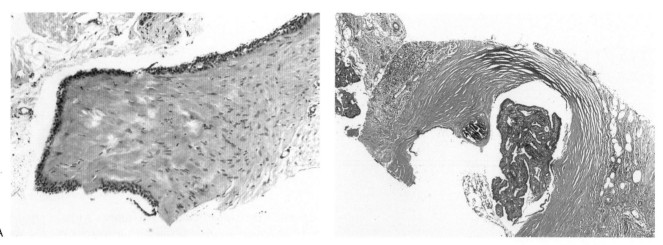

A

B

FIGURE 1. Cystic papilloma. A: A fragment of cyst wall around a cystic papilloma obtained in a needle core biopsy procedure. **B:** Part of an intracystic papilloma and the surrounding cyst wall. Note calcification in the cyst wall at the center of the picture.

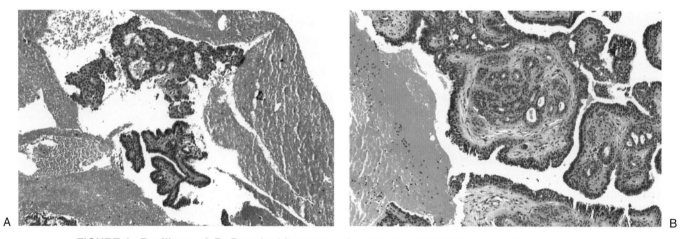

A

B

FIGURE 2. Papilloma. A,B: Detached fragments of papillary epithelium in a core biopsy specimen. Samples such as this are usually obtained from the superficial portions of cystic papillomas. Note the simple surface epithelium with minimal hyperplasia and inconspicuous myoepithelial cells, and the distinct fibrovascular cores.

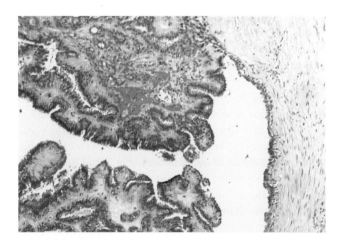

FIGURE 3. Cystic papilloma. This needle core biopsy sample shows a cyst wall and papillary fronds extending into the lumen. Epithelium lining the cyst between the papillary fronds is not hyperplastic.

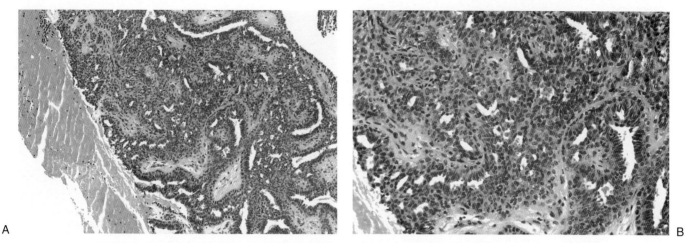

A
B

FIGURE 4. Papilloma with ductal hyperplasia. A,B: Hyperplasia in a needle core biopsy sample is manifested by increased thickness of the epithelial layer and bridging of epithelium across spaces between fronds, resulting in the formation of microlumina.

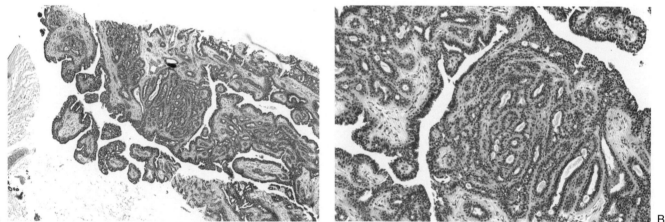

A
B

FIGURE 5. Papilloma with adenosis. A,B: Hyperplasia in this needle core sample takes the form of nodular adenosis within the fibrovascular stroma. The surface epithelium is not hyperplastic.

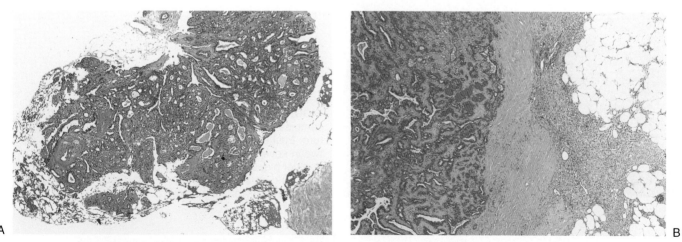

A
B

FIGURE 6. Papilloma with adenosis. A: A needle core biopsy sample from a mammographically detected circumscribed papillary tumor. The proliferation consists almost entirely of small, adenosis-type glands in the stroma. **B:** The excisional biopsy specimen is shown here. Scarring around the papilloma is due to the needle biopsy.

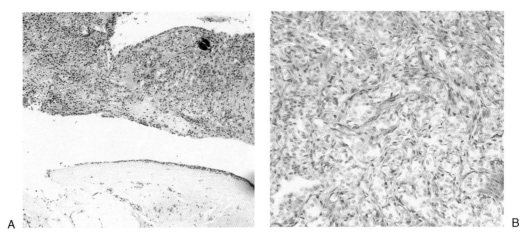

FIGURE 7. Cystic papilloma with florid adenosis. A: The needle core biopsy sample contains a compact proliferation of adenosis glands lacking lumina. A calcification is present. Part of the cyst wall is shown at the lower border of the picture. **B:** The immunohistochemical stain for actin highlights myoepithelial cells, which appear red-orange in this preparation (immunoperoxidase: smooth-muscle actin).

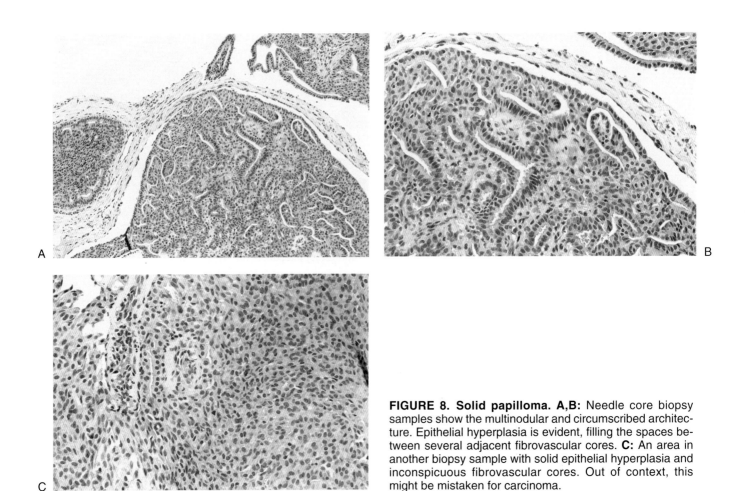

FIGURE 8. Solid papilloma. A,B: Needle core biopsy samples show the multinodular and circumscribed architecture. Epithelial hyperplasia is evident, filling the spaces between several adjacent fibrovascular cores. **C:** An area in another biopsy sample with solid epithelial hyperplasia and inconspicuous fibrovascular cores. Out of context, this might be mistaken for carcinoma.

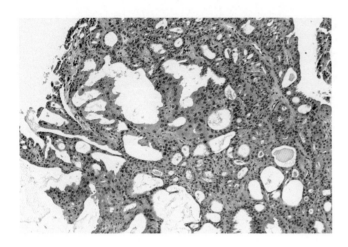

FIGURE 9. Papilloma with apocrine metaplasia. Apocrine metaplasia is shown in the hyperplastic epithelium of this needle core biopsy sample of a papilloma.

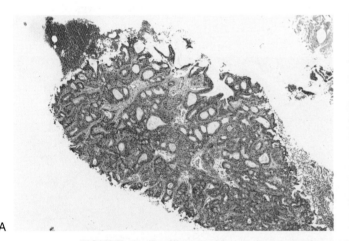

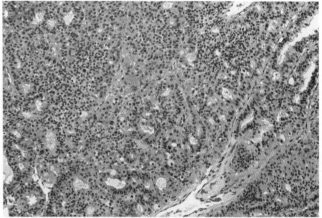

A   B

FIGURE 10. Papilloma with atypical apocrine metaplasia. A,B: The complex hyperplastic epithelium between fibrovascular cores has foci of apocrine metaplasia in which some cells have enlarged, hyperchromatic nuclei. Architectural atypia is manifested by the loss of cell polarity in some areas and the cribriform-like structure.

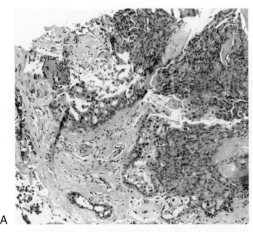

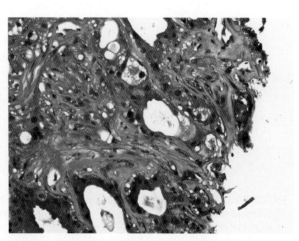

A   B

FIGURE 11. Papilloma with atypical apocrine metaplasia. A,B: Cytoplasmic vacuolization and clearing and nuclear hyperchromasia are atypical cytologic features in these needle core biopsy samples from two different papillomas.

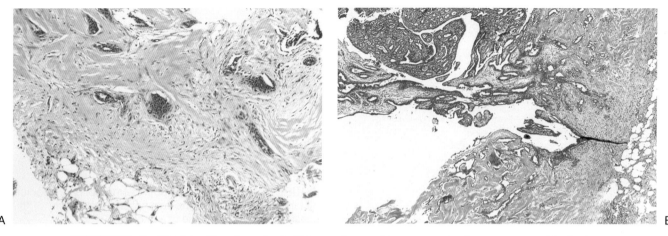

A

B

FIGURE 12. Papilloma with sclerosis. A: This needle core biopsy sample of a mammographically detected circumscribed mass shows small nests of epithelial cells in collagenized stroma with myofibroblastic proliferation. This pattern is easily mistaken for invasive carcinoma. **B:** Subsequent excisional biopsy revealed a partly cystic papilloma. Mural sclerosis with trapped glandular tissue shown here was the source of the material seen in (A).

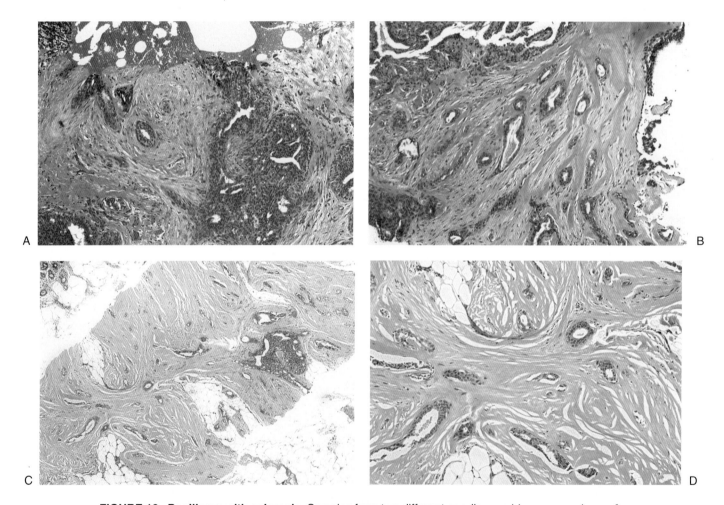

A

B

C

D

FIGURE 13. Papilloma with sclerosis. Samples from two different needle core biopsy procedures. **A:** This tissue has an area of papillary hyperplasia in sclerotic stroma. Note the epithelium cut tangentially as it protrudes into the stroma. This appearance should not be interpreted as invasive carcinoma. **B:** The cords of cells are distributed here largely in parallel arrays between bands of partly collagenized stroma. The glands with angular contours resemble tubular carcinoma. Myoepithelial cells are inconspicuous in this section stained with hematoxylin and eosin. **C,D:** These needle core biopsy samples from a severely sclerotic papillary lesion were mistakenly interpreted as tubular carcinoma. A myoepithelial layer is evident around some of the glandular structures in (D).

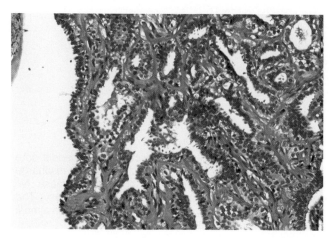

FIGURE 14. Papilloma with prominent myoepithelial cells. Myoepithelial cells with clear cytoplasm are shown outlining glands in this needle core biopsy sample from a papilloma.

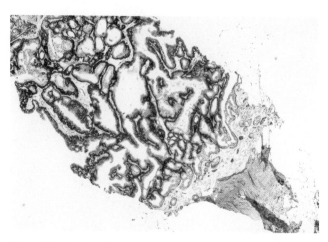

FIGURE 16. Papilloma with myoepithelial cell hyperplasia. An exaggerated myoepithelial cell zone is highlighted by an actin immunostain in this sample (immunoperoxidase: smooth-muscle actin).

from a fibroadenoma. The epithelial cells in papillomas typically exhibit strong nuclear immunoreactivity for estrogen receptor.

The epithelium of intraductal papillomas contains a myoepithelial cell layer. Myoepithelial cells are not equally apparent in all portions of a papilloma, and they may be focally absent. The nuclei of quiescent myoepithelial cells are usually inconspicuous and flattened along the basement membrane, whereas hyperplastic myoepithelial cells form a prominent layer of columnar or cuboidal cells that often have relatively clear cytoplasm (Fig. 14). Some papillomas have markedly hyperplastic myoepithelial cells that assume an epithelioid phenotype (Fig. 15). The myoepithelial cells are immunoreactive for S-100 and actin (4) (Fig. 16). Epithelioid myoepithelial cells may also be immunoreactive for cytokeratin.

Infarction can occur in a papilloma, usually without an apparent cause (Fig. 17). The presence of chronic inflammation and hemosiderin in and around many papillomas suggests that these lesions are prone to intermittent, transient bleeding. Rarely, the entire lesion is destroyed. The underlying architecture of an infarcted papilloma can be demonstrated with a reticulin stain, but there is no procedure for distinguishing between the infarcted epithelium of a papilloma and a papillary carcinoma. Cytologic atypia, manifested by nuclear hyperchromasia and pleomorphism, is commonly found in the partially degenerated epithelium of a papilloma in the vicinity of an infarct. These cytologic abnormalities may lead to an erroneous diagnosis of carcinoma in the needle core biopsy sample from a such a lesion.

Squamous metaplasia can occur in the epithelium of a papilloma with infarction or in the absence of infarction (5) (Fig. 18). Extension of squamous metaplasia to the epithelium of adjacent ducts is an uncommon finding (6). Entrapped metaplastic epithelium in the stromal reaction may simulate metaplastic or squamous carcinoma, and in some instances the distinction between these processes is very difficult (5).

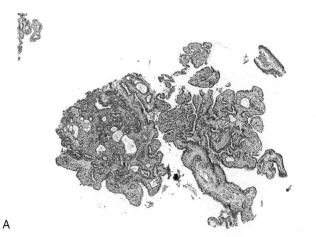

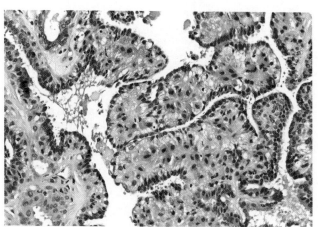

A   B

FIGURE 15. Papilloma with hyperplastic myoepithelial cells. A,B: Clusters of myoepithelial cells with epithelioid and myoid appearances fill the subepithelial stroma in this needle core biopsy sample.

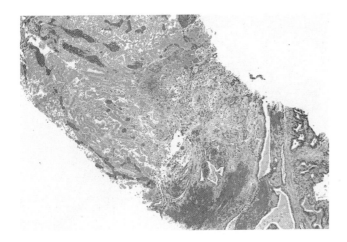

FIGURE 17. Papilloma with infarction. This needle core biopsy sample is from a patient with bloody nipple discharge and a mammographically detected nonpalpable mass. No needling procedure was performed before the biopsy. The ghost architecture of a papilloma is evident in this almost completely infarcted sample.

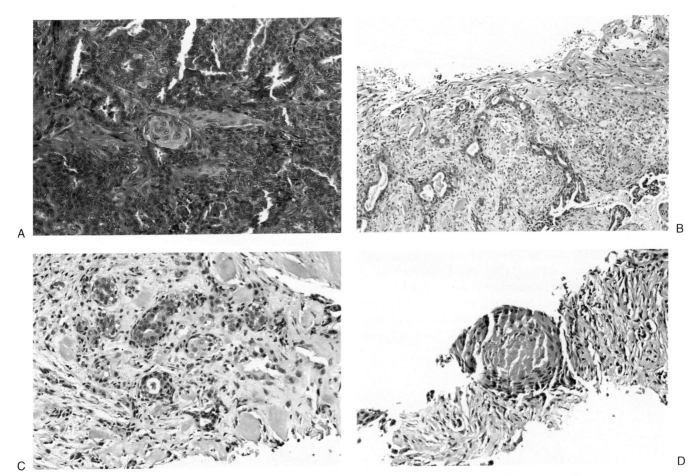

A

B

C

D

FIGURE 18. Papilloma with squamous metaplasia. A: A nest of squamous cells is present in the papillary glandular epithelium with florid hyperplasia. **B–D:** This needle core biopsy sample from a sclerosing papilloma had focal squamous metaplasia, illustrated in (D). The biopsy specimen was misinterpreted as infiltrating carcinoma with squamous differentiation.

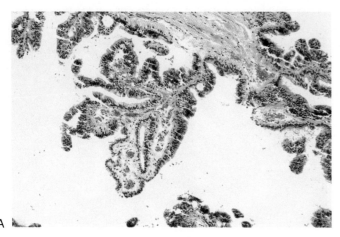 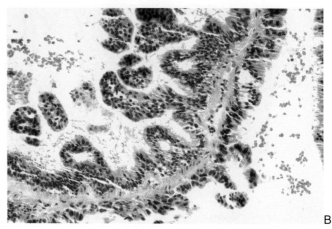

A
B

FIGURE 19. Papilloma with atypical hyperplasia. A: The epithelium of the papillary fronds in this part of the needle core biopsy sample is composed of an orderly layer of columnar cells. **B:** This frond from the same biopsy sample exhibits atypical micropapillary hyperplasia. Note nuclear condensation at the apical ends of the micropapillae and residual columnar epithelium of the duct between the micropapillae.

Surgical excision is recommended for most papillomas diagnosed by needle core biopsy, especially if the lesion exhibits atypia (Figs. 19,20). Most follow-up studies of papillomas confirm the low "precancerous" potential of these lesions after excision (7–9). The diagnosis of orderly papillary carcinoma can be complicated by associated areas of papilloma. This combination was observed in 7 of 41 papillary carcinomas studied by Papotti et al. (4). The reported frequency of carcinoma subsequent to the excision of a papilloma has been less than 5%. Nearly half of the subsequent cancers were detected in the opposite breast. A greater risk for subsequent carcinoma has been demonstrated in women with multiple papillomas (9–11).

COLLAGENOUS SPHERULOSIS

This form of duct hyperplasia occurs as an incidental microscopic finding in 1% to 2% of surgical biopsy specimens with hyperplastic duct lesions. In collagenous spherulosis, the hyperplastic epithelium forms glands, with intervening spherules composed of basement membrane components surrounded by myoepithelial cells creating an adenoid cystic configuration (12) (Figs. 21,22).

Collagenous spherulosis occurs in benign proliferative lesions, including papilloma, papillary duct hyperplasia, atypical duct hyperplasia, and sclerosing adenosis (13,14). Carcinoma may be present coincidentally in the same specimen,

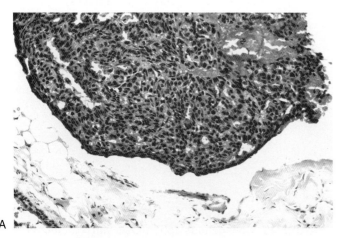 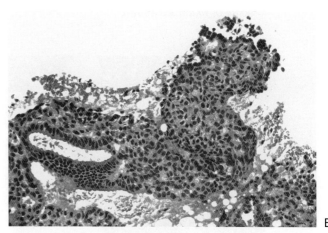

A
B

FIGURE 20. Papilloma with atypical hyperplasia. A,B: Detached epithelial fragments in a needle core biopsy specimen. Note the tendency of the cells to be oriented around microlumens.

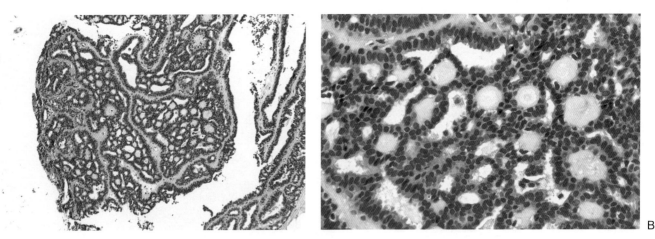

A

B

FIGURE 21. Collagenous spherulosis in a papilloma. A,B: The spherules are round, weakly eosinophilic bodies in the epithelium. Myoepithelial cells are for the most part inconspicuous, but they can be seen rimming a spherule in the lower right corner of (B). The true glandular lumina have irregular contours.

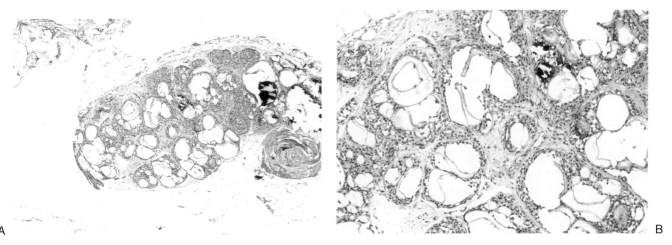

A

B

FIGURE 22. Collagenous spherulosis with degenerative changes. A,B: Degeneration in collagenous spherulosis with detachment of basement membranes that have collapsed into the degenerative cystic spaces. This appearance, shown in a needle core biopsy sample, can easily be mistaken for cribriform carcinoma. The biopsy was performed for mammographically detected nonpalpable calcifications, some of which are shown.

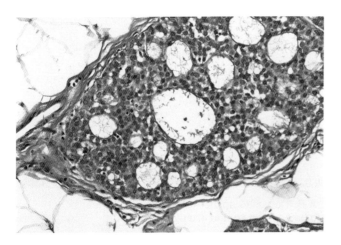

FIGURE 23. Collagenous spherulosis with carcinoma *in situ*. Lobular carcinoma *in situ* has expanded and filled the epithelium between edematous spherules. Note the fine stellate filamentous material in some spherules.

and rarely, carcinoma *in situ* replaces the benign epithelium of collagenous spherulosis (Fig. 23). There is no evidence to indicate that collagenous spherulosis is a precancerous lesion.

The stromal component of the lesion consists of spherules measuring 20 to 100 μm in diameter. The spherules have various staining patterns and may be eosinophilic, amphophilic, or nearly transparent. In some spherules, it is possible to see stellate fibrils radiating from a central nidus toward the periphery. Degenerative changes in spherules can result in loss of the radial structure and an empty space or calcification. Constituents in spherules include components of basement membrane: elastin, polysaccharides positive for periodic acid–Schiff (PAS), and type IV collagen (12,15).

RADIAL SCLEROSING LESIONS

Radial sclerosing lesions (RSLs) have been described by a variety of names, but the term most widely employed in the diagnosis of these lesions is derived from Hamperl's phrase, *strahlige Narben* ("radial scar") (16). Use of the word scar implies that there is a reparative process in the stroma because the stellate configuration has a cicatrix-like appearance, but it is equally likely that the stromal change is an integral part of the overall proliferative lesion rather than a reactive process. The term radial sclerosing lesion is preferable because it describes the mammographic and histopathologic appearance of the process without suggesting histogenesis, and it is sufficiently nonspecific to encompass the many histologic variants included in this category.

Most RSLs are microscopic in size and not detectable by palpation. Multiple microscopic RSLs are not uncommon in one breast, and both breasts can be affected (17,18). RSLs have been detected in 1.7% (19) to 28% (20) of benign breast specimens. RSLs are uncommon before age 30 and are most frequent in patients between 40 and 60 years of age.

Clinically apparent RSLs are usually found by mammography. Radiologically, they form stellate or spiculated structures with a central dense or lucent core measuring less than 2 cm (21). Microcalcifications are detected in most mammograms of RSLs (22,23). Although some mammographic features may favor the radiologic diagnosis of a benign RSL rather than a stellate carcinoma, these are not distinct enough to be the basis for a specific diagnosis (21,23,24).

The proliferative components that most commonly contribute in differing proportions to an RSL are sclerosing adenosis, duct hyperplasia, and cysts. The central nidus is a relatively sclerotic zone composed of fibrosis and elastosis (Fig. 24). Elastin in the walls of ducts and in the stroma forms dense, sometimes granular eosinophilic deposits that

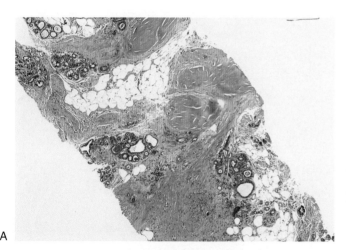

A

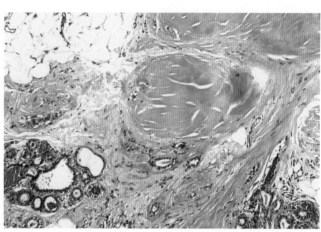

B

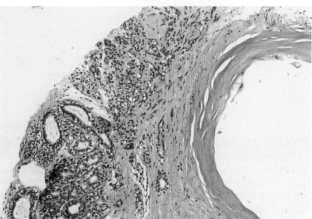

C

FIGURE 24. Radial sclerosing lesion. A,B: A needle core biopsy sample shows the central sclerotic zone consisting of dense collagenous tissue and adenosis with calcifications. **C:** A peripheral portion of the same lesion with prominent sclerosing adenosis and a cyst devoid of epithelium. Portions of the adenosis are attenuated and resemble infiltrating lobular carcinoma.

can be highlighted by an elastic tissue stain. In an early phase of development, an RSL is composed centrally of branching ductal structures that are surrounded by relatively cellular spindle-cell stroma extending along radiating fibrous bands toward the periphery (Fig. 25). Many of the stromal cells are myofibroblasts (25). In later stages, the stromal cells are less conspicuous as the tissue becomes more collagenized (Fig. 26).

A "corona" of ducts, lobules, and cysts is often present at the periphery of the lesion between the bands of radiating sclerotic tissue (see Fig. 25). This peripheral zone is not seen around every RSL, and when present it can appear to be incomplete. The variability is the result of the intrinsic asymmetry of lesions, or it may be a consequence of asymmetric sectioning. In some lesions, the corona consists predominately of cysts.

Apocrine metaplasia is frequently observed in RSLs, especially when a component of sclerosing adenosis is present. Clear-cell change and nuclear atypia are not uncommon in this apocrine epithelium. Squamous metaplasia is relatively infrequent in RSLs. Focal necrosis occurs in the proliferative duct epithelium of about 10% of RSLs, more often at the periphery than in the center of the lesion. The epithelium associated with these comedo-like foci is usually indistinguishable from the epithelium in hyperplastic ducts lacking

necrosis in the same RSL. Entrapped nerves are apparently incorporated into RSLs by the same mechanism that is responsible for this phenomenon in other sclerosing lesions (26). Atypical epithelial hyperplasia may be present in RSLs. Often, the significant proliferative foci are distributed in multiple tissue fragments in a needle core biopsy specimen. Care should be taken to avoid an erroneous diagnosis of intraductal carcinoma in this setting (Figs. 27 and 28).

A major consideration in the differential diagnosis of RSLs is tubular carcinoma. The epithelium in tubular carcinoma lacks the myoepithelial layer characteristically present in the hyperplastic component in RSLs. The glands in tubular carcinoma have round or distinctive angular shapes not ordinarily found in RSLs. The cystic component of RSLs is absent from most tubular carcinomas.

The presence of carcinoma in RSLs has been well documented. In one series, 28% of mammographically detected RSLs larger than 1 cm had foci of carcinoma (27). Carcinoma is more frequently found in RSLs larger than 2 cm and occurs most often in RSLs from women older than 50 years (28). The most common form of carcinoma arising in an RSL is lobular carcinoma *in situ* (Fig. 29). Intraductal carcinoma and tubular carcinoma are very infrequent.

Stereotactic needle core biopsy provides a tissue sample that is a more reliable basis for the specific diagnosis of a

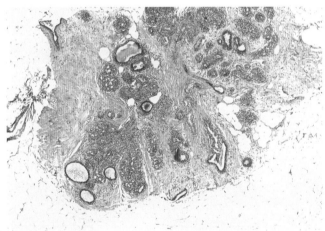

A

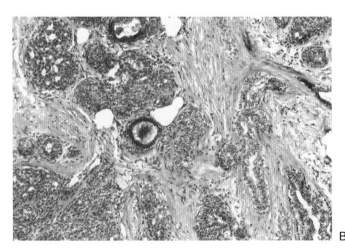

B

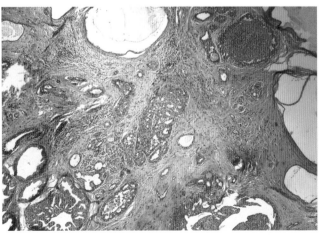

C

FIGURE 25. Radial sclerosing lesion. A,B: An early stage in the development of a radial sclerosing lesion with solid and papillary intraductal proliferation in an asymmetric distribution. The radial lesion is composed almost entirely of duct hyperplasia with slight stromal proliferation. **C:** Cysts and papillary apocrine metaplasia form a corona at the periphery of this radial sclerosing lesion.

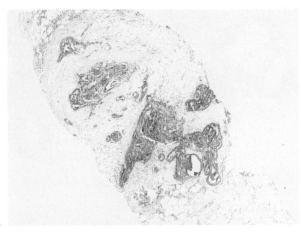

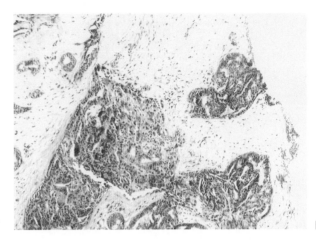

A

B

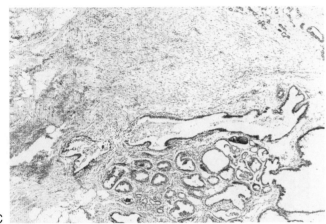

C

FIGURE 26. Radial sclerosing lesion. A,B: The papillary structure of this lesion is distorted by sclerotic stroma. **C:** The subsequent excisional biopsy showed an area of scar representing the core biopsy site and sclerosing adenosis. The needle core biopsy had been performed for mammographically detected calcifications.

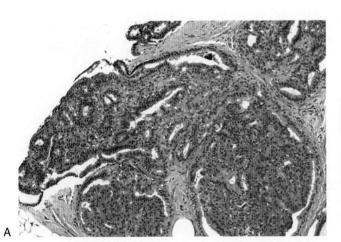

A

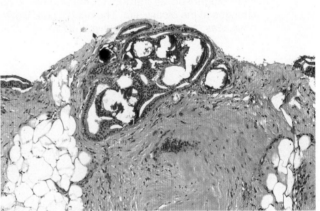

B

FIGURE 27. Radial sclerosing lesion. These needle core biopsy samples were obtained from a patient with a mammographically detected nonpalpable stellate lesion containing calcifications. **A:** Florid duct hyperplasia. **B:** Calcifications in a hyperplastic duct next to a sclerotic stromal nodule.

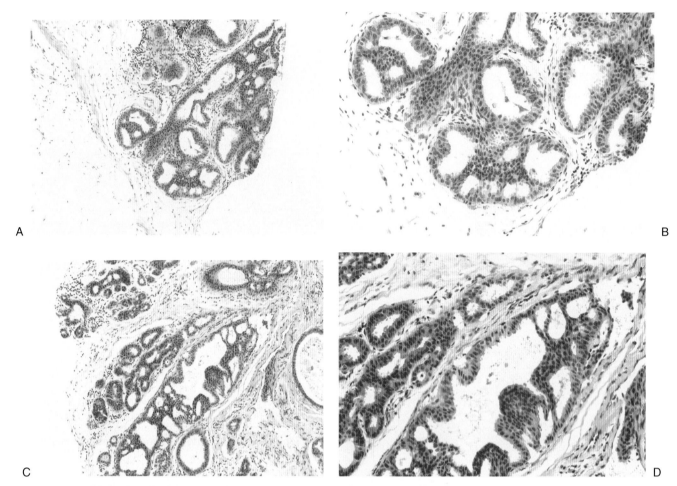

FIGURE 28. Radial sclerosing lesion with atypical duct hyperplasia. A–D: Two foci of atypical micropapillary hyperplasia in peripheral portions of a radial sclerosing lesion are seen in these needle core biopsy samples. Note the radial pattern and microcyst at the right border in (C). These findings were initially diagnosed as intraductal carcinoma. A subsequent excisional biopsy showed only reactive changes at the biopsy site. The needle core biopsy sample was reviewed in consultation, and the diagnosis was revised to atypical hyperplasia.

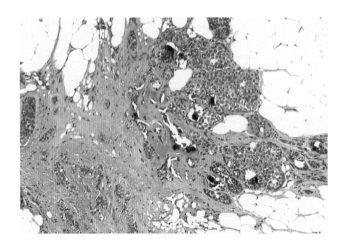

FIGURE 29. Radial sclerosing lesion with carcinoma. A mammographically detected nonpalpable stellate lesion with calcifications led to needle core biopsy. In the sample shown here, lobular carcinoma *in situ* fills glands with an adenosis pattern in sclerotic tissue in the upper right portion of the lesion.

RSL than does fine-needle aspiration cytology, but ultimately, complete excision is necessary to evaluate these lesions fully for focal carcinoma. Specimen radiography should be performed on the excisional biopsy specimen to confirm the excision of an RSL detected by mammography.

Follow-up studies of patients after excision of RSL have failed to disclose an increased risk for subsequent development of carcinoma. Andersen and Gram (19) reported one patient with subsequent carcinoma among 32 women followed for a mean of 19.5 years.

SUBAREOLAR SCLEROSING DUCT HYPERPLASIA

Sclerosing duct hyperplasia can produce a tumor of the central or subareolar breast parenchyma without involving the substance of the nipple. The term subareolar sclerosing duct hyperplasia (29) should be reserved for these lesions, which constitute a clinicopathologic entity distinct from florid papillomatosis of the nipple. The age at diagnosis ranges from 26 to 73 years, averaging about 50 years. The presenting symptom is a mass located beneath the nipple and/or areola or in the breast close to the areola. None of the lesions has been within the nipple. Erosion or ulceration of the nipple surface is absent. Nipple retraction may occur, and some patients have had bloody discharge. The mammographic findings have not been specific for this lesion and may suggest carcinoma.

The histologic structure of subareolar sclerosing duct hyperplasia is similar to that of radial sclerosing papillary lesions in other parts of the breast. Sclerosis and elastosis are more pronounced toward the center of the tumor, whereas duct hyperplasia is prominent at the periphery (Fig. 30). Cartilaginous metaplasia, a rare occurrence in these lesions, typically occurs in the sclerotic core. Much of the tumor has a rounded margin created by the nodular expansion of conflu-

ent large ducts with florid epithelial hyperplasia. Scattered mitotic figures may be encountered in the epithelium or in hyperplastic myoepithelial cells throughout the lesion. Rarely, focal comedo necrosis is found in the hyperplastic duct epithelium. In contrast to radial sclerosing proliferative lesions elsewhere in the breast, subareolar sclerosing duct hyperplasia generally lacks cysts, cystic and papillary apocrine change, and squamous metaplasia. Carcinoma may arise in subareolar sclerosing duct hyperplasia.

CYSTIC AND PAPILLARY APOCRINE METAPLASIA

Embryologically, the breasts develop from the anlage that give rise to apocrine glands, but apocrine differentiation is not a constituent of the normal microscopic anatomy of the mammary gland. Any benign proliferative lesion may contain cells with apocrine cytologic features. In their most banal form, these metaplastic apocrine cells are indistinguishable from the cells that comprise normal apocrine glands. Mitoses are almost never seen in ordinary apocrine metaplasia, and a low proportion of cells are in S-phase (30). There are no clinical features specifically attributable to cystic and papillary apocrine metaplasia.

Microscopic apocrine metaplasia is common in the female breast after age 30, with the highest frequency in the fifth decade (31,32), probably reflecting physiologic alterations associated with the menopause. Apocrine cysts and hyperplasia with apocrine metaplasia were more common in the breasts of American women in New York than in Japanese women from Tokyo (33). Haagensen et al. (34) reported finding apocrine metaplasia in 78% of 1,169 specimens from biopsies performed for gross cystic disease.

There is not a significant difference in the frequency of apocrine metaplasia when breasts with and without carcinoma are compared (35–37). Some follow-up studies have sug-

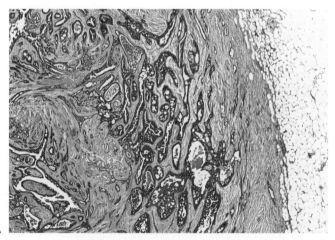

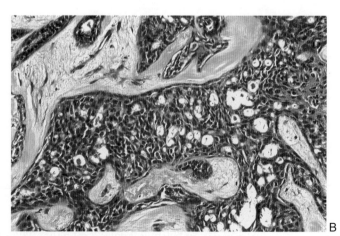

A B

FIGURE 30. Subareolar sclerosing duct hyperplasia. A: The border is usually well circumscribed, as shown here. A minority of the lesions have a stellate configuration. **B:** Florid duct hyperplasia with a fenestrated pattern. The hyperplastic ductal cells have a streaming pattern around microlumina that contain wisps of secretion.

gested that apocrine metaplasia is a predictor for the subsequent development of carcinoma. Haagensen et al. (34) reported a 10-fold greater frequency of carcinoma in women who had apocrine metaplasia in a prior biopsy specimen than in women in whom apocrine change was absent (34). When compared with a control population, patients with apocrine metaplasia had 3.5 times the expected frequency of carcinoma, whereas the risk was only 0.3 times that expected when apocrine metaplasia was absent. A slight increase in the number of subsequent carcinomas was observed by Page et al. (38) in women with papillary apocrine change in an antecedent benign biopsy specimen in comparison with the expected number of carcinomas based on a study of age-matched controls in the Third National Cancer Survey. The difference was statistically significant only in women who were older than 45 when the apocrine lesion was detected. Florid apocrine metaplasia with atypia often coexists with apocrine carcinoma (39). Short-term follow-up of patients with atypical apocrine lesions has not revealed a predisposition to the early onset of carcinoma of apocrine or nonapocrine type (40).

Cystic apocrine metaplasia is composed of flat and cuboidal cells that may form a single layer or blunt papillae (Fig. 31). The evenly spaced cells have round nuclei with homogeneous, moderately dense chromatin and a single central small nucleolus. A myoepithelial cell layer is present in cystic and papillary apocrine epithelium, but it may be inconspicuous. Florid papillary proliferation produces more elaborate patterns of hyperplasia that have a micropapillary or a branching, papillary architecture. Cellular crowding results in a thickened epithelium more than one cell in depth and the formation of a papilloma composed entirely of apocrine epithelium (Fig. 32). Calcifications associated with cystic and papillary apocrine metaplasia may be coarse, basophilic, easily fractured particles or birefringent calcium oxalate crystals (Fig. 33).

Atypical changes may be encountered in apocrine metaplasia in virtually any proliferative configuration (40). Architectural atypia consists of irregular papillary fronds with little or no stromal support in which the apocrine cells are arranged in a disordered fashion. Epithelial bridges and cribriform areas may be present (Fig. 34). Apocrine cells with mild cytologic atypia retain abundant, finely granular, eosinophilic cytoplasm. Small, clear cytoplasmic vacuoles may be found. The nuclei in apocrine atypia are not spaced at regular intervals, and they may not all be basally oriented. Nucleoli are less uniform and may be eccentric, and an occasional nucleus has more than one nucleolus. The cytoplasm of individual cells becomes vacuolated or clear (Fig. 35). Nuclear pleomorphism and hyperchromasia may become striking. Prominent pleomorphic nucleoli characterize the most atypical lesions. The cells generally retain relatively abundant cytoplasm in comparison with with those of nonapocrine epithelium.

When atypical apocrine metaplasia is present, the severity of the change is usually not uniform in a given lesion. Cysts and papillary duct hyperplasia partly or entirely occupied by bland metaplastic apocrine epithelium are commonly found in the vicinity of atypical apocrine metaplasia. The distinction between atypical apocrine metaplasia and apocrine carcinoma is ordinarily not difficult, but this may be a challenging diagnostic problem when marked atypia is not present. In the latter situation, cytologic features are less important than the growth pattern, especially in sclerosing lesions. In this setting, a diagnosis of carcinoma is warranted when the apocrine proliferation has the configuration of one of the conventional forms of intraductal carcinoma (3).

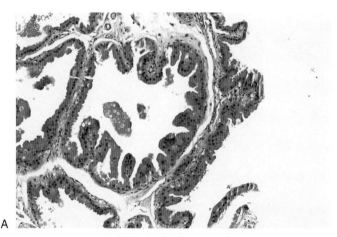

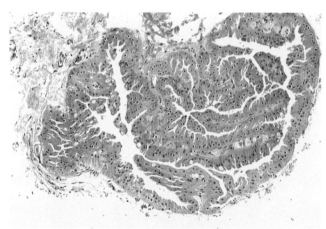

A

B

FIGURE 31. Cystic and papillary apocrine metaplasia. A: Apocrine metaplasia is present in multiple cysts. Note the evenly spaced, basally oriented distribution of the nuclei and blunt papillae. **B:** The partially collapsed cyst shown in this needle core biopsy sample contains papillary fronds of metaplastic apocrine epithelium.

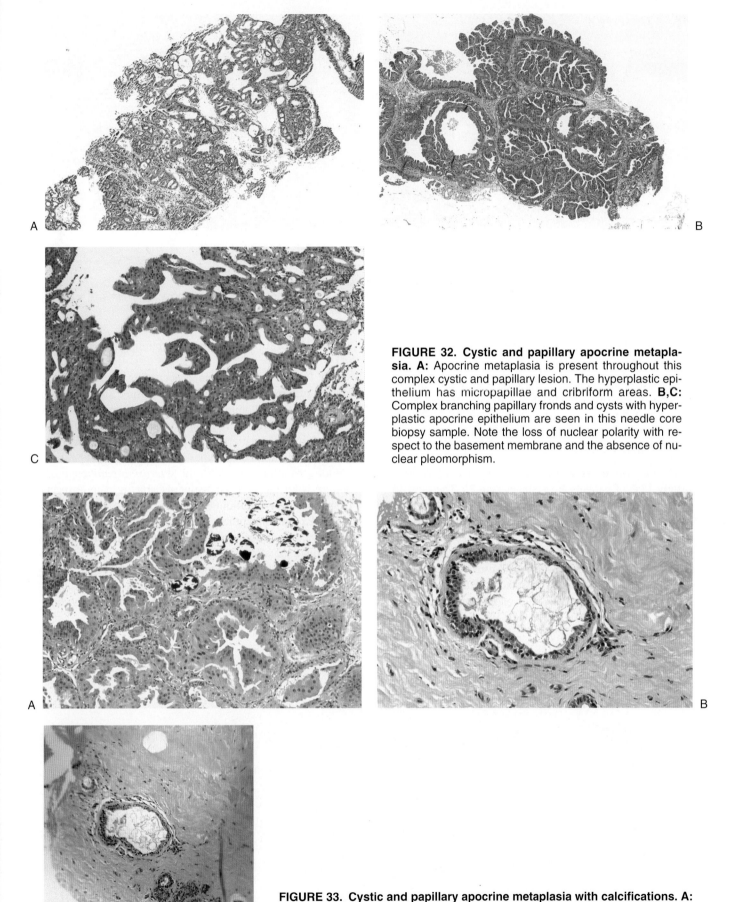

FIGURE 32. Cystic and papillary apocrine metaplasia. A: Apocrine metaplasia is present throughout this complex cystic and papillary lesion. The hyperplastic epithelium has micropapillae and cribriform areas. **B,C:** Complex branching papillary fronds and cysts with hyperplastic apocrine epithelium are seen in this needle core biopsy sample. Note the loss of nuclear polarity with respect to the basement membrane and the absence of nuclear pleomorphism.

FIGURE 33. Cystic and papillary apocrine metaplasia with calcifications. A: Round basophilic calcifications in a lesion composed of papillary apocrine epithelium. **B,C:** Platelike transparent calcium oxalate crystals are illuminated with polarized light in a small apocrine cyst in this needle core biopsy sample.

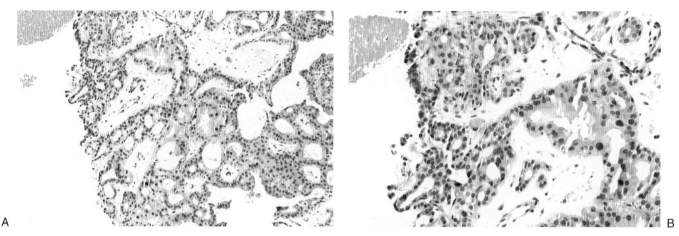

FIGURE 34. Cystic and papillary apocrine metaplasia with atypia. A,B: The epithelium has focal cribriform microlumina and isolated, hyperchromatic, enlarged nuclei in these needle core biopsy specimens.

FLORID PAPILLOMATOSIS AND SYRINGOMATOUS ADENOMA OF THE NIPPLE

Because of their superficial location in the nipple, these lesions are ordinarily not subjected to stereotactic needle core biopsy. A brief discussion of each is provided for reference.

Florid Papillomatosis

The majority of patients are 40 to 50 years old. Approximately 15% of patients are younger than 35. The most frequent presenting symptom is discharge that is often bloody. Pain and itching or burning sensations are not unusual (41). In many instances, the nipple appears enlarged, and a mass can be palpated. The surface of the nipple may appear granular, ulcerated, reddened, warty, or crusted. The symptoms and clinical findings can be mistaken for those of Paget's disease. The mammographic and sonographic findings may suggest carcinoma (42). Fewer than 5% of the reported examples of florid papillomatosis of the nipple were in men (41).

The lesions can be grouped according to microscopic growth pattern into four categories. In three subtypes, one structural feature dominates the lesion or is present exclusively, whereas the fourth group consists of tumors with two or three of these patterns. No prognostic significance has been attached to these subtypes.

Florid papillomatosis with the *sclerosing papillomatosis pattern* is histologically indistinguishable in many respects from sclerosing papillomas encountered elsewhere in the breast. Exuberant papillary hyperplasia of ductal epithelium is distorted by an accompanying stromal proliferation within and around the affected ducts (Fig. 36). Focal comedo-type necrosis may be found in the hyperplastic duct epithelium, sometimes associated with scattered mitoses in epithelial cells. Squamous cysts are commonly formed in the terminal portions of lactiferous ducts.

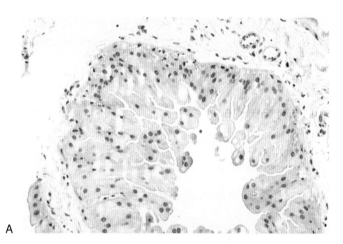
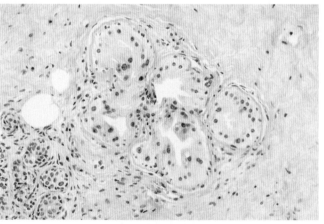

FIGURE 35. Papillary apocrine metaplasia with atypia. A: The small, round nuclei are distributed in a disorderly fashion in these fused papillary fronds. The abundant cytoplasm is vacuolated in some cells. **B:** Apocrine cells with pale cytoplasm and pleomorphic nuclei are shown. Note the presence of large nuclei near the tips of papillary fronds.

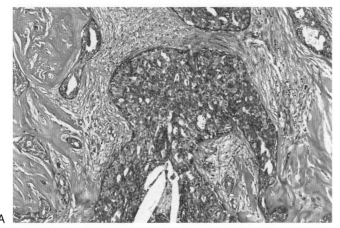

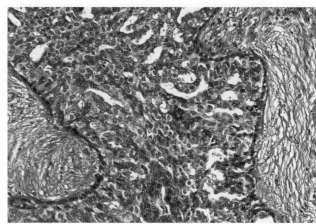

A

B

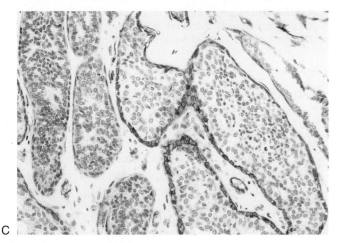

C

FIGURE 36. Florid papillomatosis of the nipple. A: Hyperplastic epithelium with a fenestrated pattern in sclerotic stroma is commonly present in the sclerosing type of florid papillomatosis shown here. **B:** Myoepithelial cells outline the hyperplastic epithelium. **C:** Myoepithelial cells are accentuated around some ducts by the immunostain for actin (immunoperoxidase: smooth-muscle actin).

Lesions with the *papillomatosis pattern* consist of florid papillary hyperplasia of ductal epithelium causing expansion and crowding of the affected ducts (Fig. 37). Focal epithelial necrosis and scattered mitotic figures may be found. These tumors lack the sclerosing stromal proliferation that characterizes the sclerosing papillomatosis type of lesion. Hyperplastic glandular tissue may replace the overlying squamous epithelium in part or all of the apical skin surface of the nipple. Squamous cell–lined cysts and apocrine metaplasia are not prominent in these lesions.

Florid papillomatosis with the *adenosis pattern* is composed of crowded, glandular structures arranged in a pattern indistinguishable from that of florid sclerosing adenosis. Myoepithelial hyperplasia accompanies the epithelial proliferation. Prominent apocrine metaplasia, hyperplasia of the squamous epithelium, and superficial squamous cysts may be encountered. Mitotic figures and focal necrosis are uncommon.

The *mixed proliferative type of florid papillomatosis* consists of varying combinations of the other three patterns. Prominent features in most cases include squamous metaplasia of ducts with cysts, apocrine metaplasia, and acanthosis of the overlying epithelium. Cystic dilation of ducts is not uncommon near the deep margin of the lesion. Focal necrosis may be found in the duct epithelium. Mitotic activity is minimal. Adenosis occurs in about one third of these lesions.

It can be difficult to detect carcinoma arising in florid papillomatosis of the nipple (43). Hyperplastic areas in the lesions often exhibit atypical features, which may include foci with necrosis as well as cribriform and micropapillary growth patterns, mitoses, and cytologic atypia. In the absence of definitive evidence of invasion, Paget's disease of

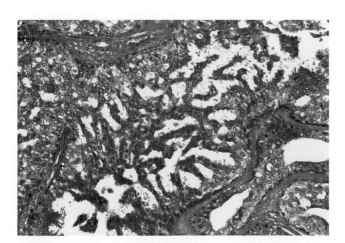

FIGURE 37. Florid papillomatosis of the nipple. Micropapillary hyperplasia in a papillomatosis-type lesion.

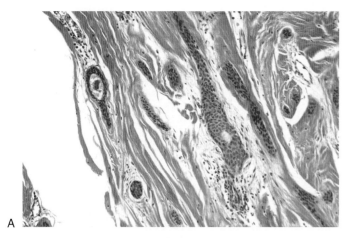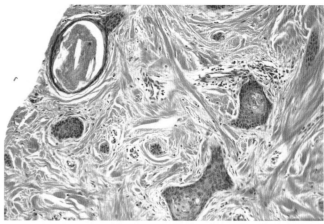

A

B

FIGURE 38. Syringomatous adenoma of the nipple. A: This area of a needle core biopsy specimen shows elongated, ductlike structures, one of which has an open lumen with secretion. Squamoid differentiation is shown in the center. **B:** An area with cystic dilatation and prominent squamous differentiation.

the nipple epidermis is the most reliable evidence for a diagnosis of carcinoma arising in florid papillomatosis. The CAM5.2 and CK7 immunostains for cytokeratin are helpful for detecting Paget's cells, which are immunoreactive for these markers in the epidermis. If Paget's disease or invasive carcinoma is not detected, a diagnosis of carcinoma arising in florid papillomatosis is extremely difficult to substantiate with routine sections.

Incisional biopsy or needle core biopsy is not satisfactory to exclude the possibility of carcinoma arising in florid papillomatosis. Complete excision, which is recommended as definitive treatment, usually requires removal of the nipple. Local recurrence of florid papillomatosis may follow subtotal excision, but a substantial number of patients have reportedly remained asymptomatic after incomplete excision.

Syringomatous Adenoma

This benign, locally infiltrating neoplasm of the nipple has a close histopathologic resemblance to syringomatous tumors that commonly arise in the skin of the face and other anatomic sites (44,45). The patients range in age from 11 to 74 years at diagnosis, with a median age of 36 years. The initial symptom is a unilateral mass in the nipple and/or subareolar region. The tumors have measured 1.0 to 3.5 cm. Pain, tenderness, redness, itching, discharge, or nipple inversion has been noted in isolated cases. Mammography reveals a dense stellate tumor (46).

The lesion consists of tubules, ductules, and strands of small, uniform, generally basophilic cells infiltrating the dermis of the skin and the stroma of the nipple. Invasion into the smooth-muscle bundles of the nipple is very common, and occasionally perineural invasion is observed. The neoplastic glands sometimes appear to be connected with the basal layer of the epidermis. Paget's disease is not present in this lesion.

The ducts, formed by one or more layers of cells, have "teardrop," "comma," and branching shapes, with lumina that are usually open and round (Fig. 38). Some cells may exhibit cytoplasmic clearing. A distinct layer of myoepithelial cells is not apparent. Mitoses are virtually absent, and nuclei lack prominent nucleoli and pleomorphism. The lumina are empty or contain deeply eosinophilic, retracted secretion. Flattening of cells around the lumina is early evidence of squamous differentiation, which in a fully developed form results in keratotic cysts. A foreign-body giant-cell reaction may be elicited in the vicinity of ruptured squamous cysts. Calcification is rarely seen in the keratinized epithelium. Secretion in tubular lumina is PAS-positive and weakly mucicarmine-positive (44). The differential diagnosis of syringomatous adenoma of the nipple includes florid papillomatosis, tubular carcinoma, and low-grade adenosquamous carcinoma (47).

REFERENCES

1. Cardenosa G, Eklund GW. Benign papillary neoplasms of the breast: mammographic findings. *Radiology* 1991;181:751–755.
2. Liberman L, Bracero N, Vuolo M, et al. Percutaneous large core biopsy of papillary breast lesions *Am J Roentgenology* (*in press*).
3. Carter DJ, Rosen PP. Atypical apocrine metaplasia in sclerosing lesions of the breast. A study of 51 patients. *Mod Pathol* 1991;4:1–5.
4. Papotti M, Gugliotta P, Eusebi V, Bussolati G. Immunohistochemical analysis of benign and malignant papillary lesions of the breast. *Am J Surg Pathol* 1983;7:451–461.
5. Flint A, Oberman HA. Infarction and squamous metaplasia of intraductal papilloma: a benign breast lesion that may simulate carcinoma. *Hum Pathol* 1984;15:764–767.
6. Soderstrom KO, Toikkanen S. Extensive squamous metaplasia simulating squamous cell carcinoma in benign breast papillomatosis. *Hum Pathol* 1983;14:1081–1082.
7. Kilgore AR, Fleming R, Ramos N. The incidence of cancer with nipple discharge and the risk of cancer in the presence of papillary disease of the breast. *Surg Gynecol Obstet* 1953;96:649–660.
8. Kraus FT, Neubecker RD. The differential diagnosis of papillary tumors of the breast. *Cancer* 1962;15:444–455.
9. Carter D. Intraductal papillary tumors of the breast. A study of 76 cases. *Cancer* 1977;39:1689–1692.

10. Estabrook A. Are patients with solitary or multiple intraductal papillomas at a higher risk of developing breast cancer? *Surg Oncol Clin North Am* 1993;2:45–56.
11. Haagensen CD, Bodian C, Haagensen DE. *Breast carcinoma: risk and detection.* Philadelphia: WB Saunders, 1981:146–237.
12. Clement PB, Young RH, Azzopardi JG. Collagenous spherulosis of the breast. *Am J Surg Pathol* 1987;11:411–417.
13. Guarino M, Tricomi P, Cristofori E. Collagenous spherulosis of the breast with atypical epithelial hyperplasia. *Pathologica* 1993;85:123–127.
14. Stephenson TJ, Hird PM, Laing RW, Davies JD. Nodular basement membrane deposits in breast carcinoma and atypical ductal hyperplasia: mimics of collagenous spherulosis. *Pathologica* 1994;86:234–239.
15. Grignon DJ, Ro JY, MacKay BN, Ordonez NG, Ayala AG. Collagenous spherulosis of the breast. Immunohistochemical and ultrastructural studies. *Am J Clin Pathol* 1989;91:386–392.
16. Hamperl H. Strahlige Narben und obliterierende Mastopathie Beitrage zur pathologischen histologie der Mamma. *Virchows Arch [A]* 1975;369:55–68.
17. Linell F, Ljungberg O, Anderson I. Breast carcinoma: aspects of early stage, progression and related problems. *Acta Pathol Microbiol Scand (Suppl)* 1980;272:1–233.
18. Nielsen M, Jensen J, Andersen JA. An autopsy study of radial scar in the female breast. *Histopathology* 1985;9:287–295.
19. Andersen JA, Gram JB. Radial scar in the female breast: a long-term follow-up study of 32 cases. *Cancer* 1984;53:2557–2560.
20. Nielsen M, Christensen L, Andersen J. Radial scars in women with breast cancer. *Cancer* 1987;59:1019–1025.
21. Adler DD, Helvie MA, Oberman HA, Ikeda DM, Bhan AO. Radial sclerosing lesion of the breast: mammographic features. *Radiology* 1990;176:737–740.
22. Ciatto S, Morrone D, Catarzi S, et al. Radial scars of the breast: review of 38 consecutive mammographic diagnoses. *Radiology* 1993;187:757–760.
23. Orel SG, Evers K, Yeh IT, Troupin RH. Radial scar with microcalcification: radiologic-pathologic correlation. *Radiology* 1992;183:479–484.
24. Mitnick JS, Vazquez MF, Harris MN, Roses DF. Differentiation of radial scar from scirrhous carcinoma of the breast: mammographic-pathologic correlation. *Radiology* 1989;173:697–700.
25. Battersby S, Anderson TJ. Myofibroblast activity of radial scars. *J Pathol* 1985;147:33–40.
26. Taylor HB, Norris HJ. Epithelial invasion of nerves in benign diseases of the breast. *Cancer* 1967;20:2245–2249.
27. Caneva A, Bonetti F, Manfrin E, et al. Is radial scar of the breast a premalignant lesion? *Mod Pathol* 1997;10:17A.
28. Sloane JP, Mayers MM. Carcinoma and atypical hyperplasia in radial scars and complex sclerosing lesions: importance of lesion size and patient age. *Histopathology* 1993;23:225–231.
29. Rosen PP. Subareolar sclerosing duct hyperplasia of the breast. *Cancer* 1987;59:1927–1930.
30. Bussolati G, Cattani MG, Gugliotta P, Patriarca E, Eusebi V. Morphologic and functional aspects of apocrine metaplasia in dysplastic and neoplastic breast tissue. *Ann N Y Acad Sci* 1986;464:262–274.
31. Benigni G, Squartini F. Uneven distribution and significant concentration of apocrine metaplasia in lower breast quadrants. *Tumori* 1986;72:179–182.
32. Wellings SR, Alpers CE. Apocrine cystic metaplasia: subgross pathology and prevalence in cancer-associated versus random autopsy breasts. *Hum Pathol* 1987;18:381–386.
33. Schuerch C III, Rosen PP, Hirota T, et al. A pathologic study of benign breast diseases in Tokyo and New York. *Cancer* 1982;50:1899–1903.
34. Haagensen CD, Bodian C, Haagensen DE Jr. Apocrine epithelium. In: *Breast carcinoma. Risk and detection.* Philadelphia: WB Saunders, 1981:83–105.
35. Foote FW Jr, Stewart FW. Comparative studies of cancerous versus non-cancerous breasts. *Ann Surg* 1945;12:6–79.
36. McCarty KS Jr, Kesterson GHD, Wilkinson WE, Georigiade N. Histopathologic study of subcutaneous mastectomy specimens from patients with carcinoma of the contralateral breast. *Surg Gynecol Obstet* 1978;147:682–688.
37. Nielsen M, Thomsen JL, Primdahl L, Dyreborg U, Andersen JA. Breast cancer and atypia among young and middle-aged women: a study of 110 medicolegal autopsies. *Br J Cancer* 1987;56:814–819.
38. Page DL, Van der Zwaag R, Rogers LW, Williams LT, Walker WE, Hartmann WH. Relation between component parts of fibrocystic disease complex and breast cancer. *J Natl Cancer Inst* 1978;61:1055–1063.
39. Abati AD, Kimmel M, Rosen PP. Apocrine mammary carcinoma: a clinicopathologic study of 72 cases. *Am J Clin Pathol* 1990;94:371–377.
40. Carter D, Rosen PP. Atypical apocrine metaplasia in sclerosing lesions of the breast: a study of 31 patients. *Mod Pathol* 1991;4:1–5.
41. Rosen PP, Caicco J. Florid papillomatosis of the nipple: a study of 51 patients including nine having mammary carcinoma. *Am J Surg Pathol* 1986;10:87–101.
42. Fornage BD, Faroux MJ, Pluot M, Bogomoletz W. Nipple adenoma simulating carcinoma. Misleading clinical, mammographic, sonographic and cytologic findings. *J Ultrasound Med* 1991;10:55–57.
43. Diaz NM, Palmer JO, Wick MR. Erosive adenomatosis of the nipple: histology, immunohistology, and differential diagnosis. *Mod Pathol* 1992;179–184.
44. Rosen PP. Syringomatous adenoma of the nipple. *Am J Surg Pathol* 1983;7:739–745.
45. Ward BE, Cooper PH, Subramony C. Syringomatous tumor of the nipple. *Am J Clin Pathol* 1989;92:692–696.
46. Slaughter MS, Pomerantz RA, Murad T, Hines JR. Infiltrating syringomatous adenoma of the nipple. *Surgery* 1992;111:711–713.
47. Rosen PP, Ernsberger D. Low grade adenosquamous carcinoma. A variant of metaplastic mammary carcinoma. *Am J Surg Pathol* 1987;11:351–358.

CHAPTER 5

Myoepithelial Neoplasms

Myoepithelial cells comprise part of the normal microscopic anatomy of lobules and ducts (1). They participate in many benign proliferative processes, most notably sclerosing adenosis and papillary proliferative lesions of ducts (2,3). Benign tumors composed of myoepithelial cells are termed myoepitheliomas. If epithelial and myoepithelial cells participate in the proliferation, the term adenomyoepithelioma is appropriate. Malignant neoplasms formed by myoepithelial cells may have an epithelial phenotype (myoepithelial carcinoma), a myoid phenotype (leiomyosarcoma), or both appearances (malignant adenomyoepithelioma) (4–6).

ADENOMYOEPITHELIOMA

All patients have been women ranging in age from 26 to 82 years (average, about 60 years) who presented with a solitary, unilateral, painless mass. Nipple discharge, pain, and tenderness are infrequent. The mammographic findings may be interpreted as suspect in some patients (6). Nonpalpable adenomyoepitheliomas measuring 2 cm or less have been described as mammographically well-circumscribed mass lesions (7). Calcifications are rarely present, and one malignant adenomyoepithelioma appeared to be cystic on mammography (8). Results of estrogen receptor analysis are positive in about 50% of cases. Progesterone receptors are usually absent.

The majority of adenomyoepitheliomas are variants of intraductal papilloma, but a small number of these tumors appear to arise from a lobular proliferation. Adenomyoepithelioma is closely related to ductal adenoma (9,10) and pleomorphic adenoma (mixed tumor) (11). Foci of adenomyoepithelioma can frequently be detected in tubular adenomas and in mammary pleomorphic adenomas.

Microscopically, adenomyoepitheliomas are circumscribed and composed of aggregated nodules (Fig. 1). Some nodules consist of a compact proliferation of epithelial and myoepithelial cells, but most lesions have one or more nodules in which there is at least a focal papillary growth pattern. Sometimes, the papillary intraductal component extends into ducts outside the gross tumorous lesion. This characteristic may be responsible for recurrence after seemingly adequate excision.

The basic microscopic structural unit of the adenomyoepithelioma is a small glandular lumen encompassed by cuboidal epithelial cells. Surrounding the glands are polygonal or spindle-shaped myoepithelial cells with eosinophilic or clear cytoplasm and a basement membrane (Fig. 2). The most common microscopic pattern, sometimes referred to as the tubular type of adenomyoepithelioma, is a proliferation of tubular glandular elements separated by islands and bands of polygonal myoepithelial cells that have clear cytoplasm. In some lesions, myoepithelial cells proliferate between glands in broad bands and trabeculae and are separated by strands of basement membrane and stroma (Figs. 3 and 4). The contrast between the darkly staining cytoplasm of glandular cells and the pale cytoplasm of myoepithelial cells is striking. Fragments of adenomyoepithelioma in needle core biopsy samples can be mistaken for infiltrating carcinoma (Fig. 5).

Apocrine metaplasia may be encountered in the glandular epithelium, particularly in papillary areas, and it can be cytologically atypical. Foci of sebaceous and squamous metaplasia are variably present (Fig. 6). Calcifications are occasionally formed in glandular spaces. In some tumors, central fibrosis or necrosis develops. A cystic papillary type of adenomyoepithelioma is uncommon.

Some adenomyoepitheliomas have foci of myoid growth composed of a mixture of spindle and polygonal cells (Fig. 7). Palisading of spindle cells and alveolar clustering of polygonal myoepithelial cells are common myoid patterns. The glandular elements may be intermixed with myoid areas, or they may be largely overgrown by the myoepithelial proliferation (Fig. 8). Atypical features include scattered mitotic figures, nuclear pleomorphism and hyperchromasia, and occasional multinucleated cells. Myoid hyperplasia may give rise to areas with leiomyomatous features, and rarely, this process produces leiomyosarcoma (3,12).

Origin of a malignant neoplasm in an adenomyoepithelioma has only very rarely been documented. Some lesions were reported to have an associated high mitotic rate and local recurrence (5,13), whereas others have resulted in metastases and a fatal outcome (14,15). Malignant adenomyoepitheliomas may have a biphasic growth pattern at the primary site and in metastases. Myoepithelial carcinoma with an epithelial phenotype can arise in an adenomyoepithelioma. Features indicative of myoepithelial carcinoma in this setting are overgrowth by epithelioid myoepithelial cells with nuclear pleomorphism, mitotic activity, and necrosis (Fig. 9).

Text continues on page 47

43

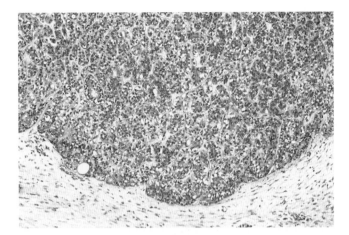

FIGURE 1. Adenomyoepithelioma. The lesion has a well-circumscribed border. Darkly stained epithelial cells and myoepithelial cells with clear cytoplasm are apparent.

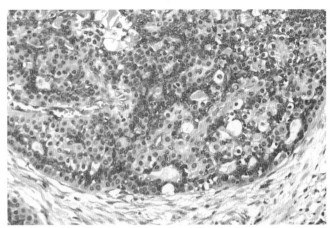

FIGURE 2. Adenomyoepithelioma. Glandular elements composed of darkly stained epithelial cells are compressed by myoepithelial cells with an epithelioid phenotype and eosinophilic cytoplasm. There are a few small, glandular lumina containing secretion.

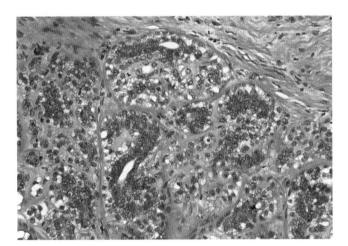

FIGURE 3. Adenomyoepithelioma. This lesion has prominent myoepithelial cells with clear cytoplasm that provide a striking contrast to the epithelial cells.

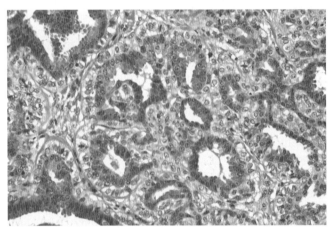

FIGURE 4. Adenomyoepithelioma. Epithelioid myoepithelial cells form bands between glands composed of hyperplastic cells. Slender strands of basement membrane and fibrovascular stroma are evident.

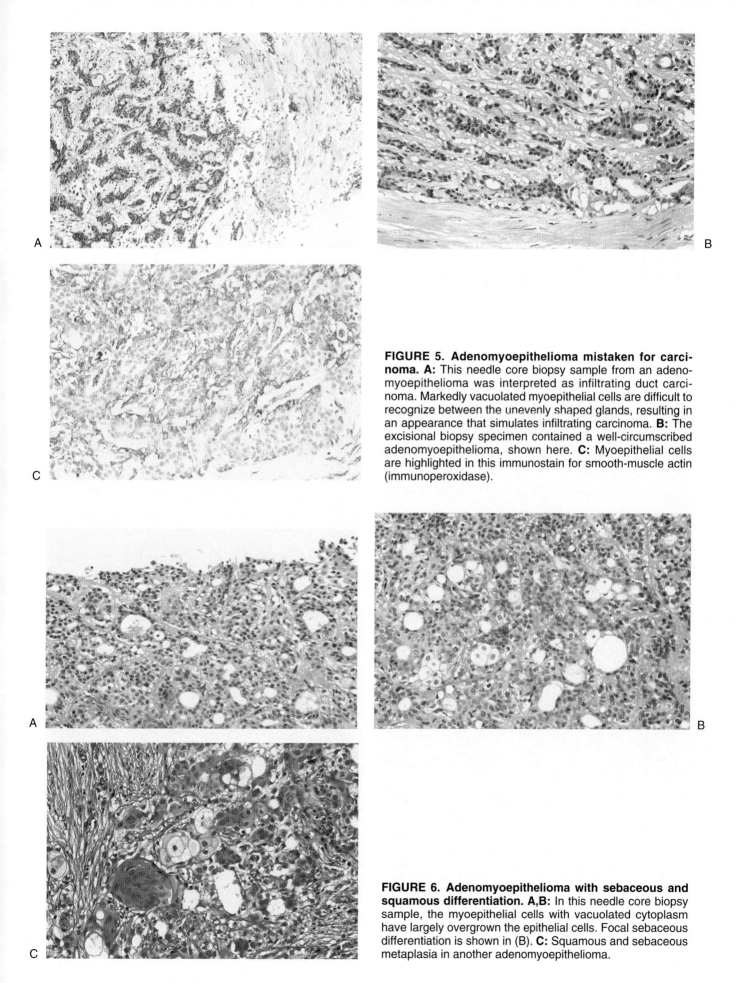

FIGURE 5. Adenomyoepithelioma mistaken for carcinoma. A: This needle core biopsy sample from an adenomyoepithelioma was interpreted as infiltrating duct carcinoma. Markedly vacuolated myoepithelial cells are difficult to recognize between the unevenly shaped glands, resulting in an appearance that simulates infiltrating carcinoma. **B:** The excisional biopsy specimen contained a well-circumscribed adenomyoepithelioma, shown here. **C:** Myoepithelial cells are highlighted in this immunostain for smooth-muscle actin (immunoperoxidase).

FIGURE 6. Adenomyoepithelioma with sebaceous and squamous differentiation. A,B: In this needle core biopsy sample, the myoepithelial cells with vacuolated cytoplasm have largely overgrown the epithelial cells. Focal sebaceous differentiation is shown in (B). **C:** Squamous and sebaceous metaplasia in another adenomyoepithelioma.

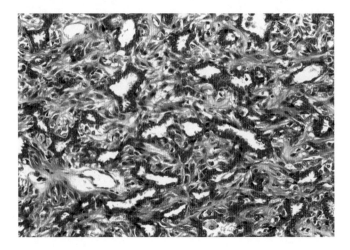

FIGURE 7. Adenomyoepithelioma with myoid differentiation. The spindly myoepithelial cells in this lesion have a myoid phenotype characterized by eosinophilic cytoplasm.

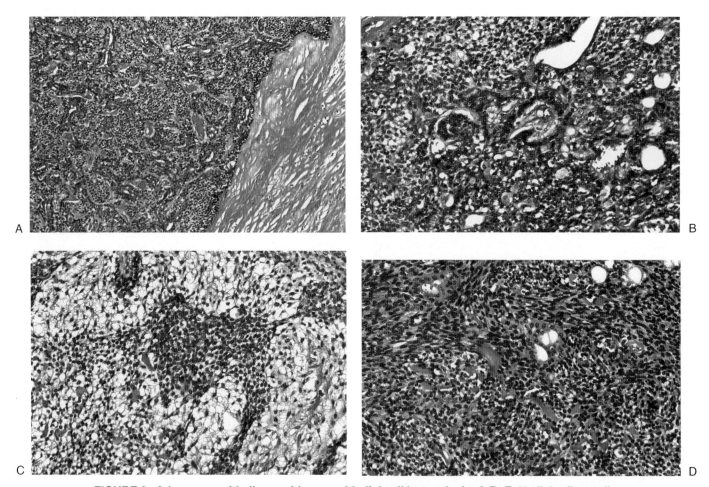

FIGURE 8. Adenomyoepithelioma with myoepithelial cell hyperplasia. A,B: Epithelial cells are distributed in bands and nests with inconspicuous glandular lumina. The myoepithelial cells, which have small, punctate nuclei and sparse clear cytoplasm, tend to aggregate in poorly defined alveolar groups. **C:** This part of the tumor shown in (A) is composed entirely of myoepithelial cells. The combination of small, compact cells and cells with extremely vacuolated cytoplasm resembles a pattern seen in cellular pleomorphic adenoma (mixed tumor) of salivary gland origin. **D:** Spindle-cell myoid differentiation of myoepithelial cells is shown surrounding inconspicuous glands.

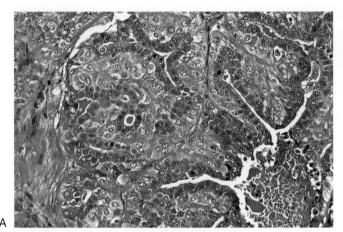

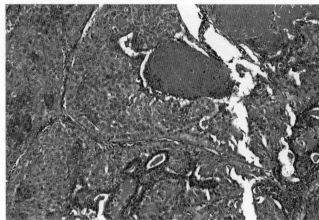

A

B

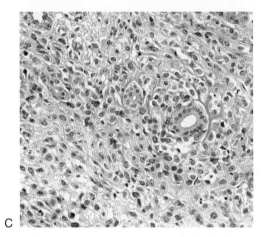

C

FIGURE 9. Myoepithelial carcinoma arising in an adenomyoepithelioma. A: Epithelioid myoepithelial cells with large vesicular nuclei are indicative of an atypical proliferation in this adenomyoepithelioma. The epithelial cells are also hyperplastic. Mitoses are present in epithelial and myoepithelial cells. Focal necrosis is apparent in the lower right corner. **B:** Neoplastic myoepithelial cells surround a focus of comedo-type necrosis. Residual glands are present. **C:** Infiltrating myoepithelial carcinoma surrounds two non-neoplastic glands. The tumor cells have eosinophilic or vacuolated cytoplasm, and nucleoli are seen in some nuclei.

Glands may contain secretion positive for periodic acid–Schiff (PAS) or mucicarmine, but intracytoplasmic secretion is absent. The cytoplasm of glandular cells is strongly reactive with antibodies to cytokeratin, and the luminal surfaces of these cells are positive for epithelial membrane antigen (Fig. 10). Most epithelial cells are negative for S-100, but small groups may be strongly reactive for this antigen.

Polygonal and spindle myoepithelial cells are not reactive for epithelial membrane antigen and variably reactive for low-molecular-weight cytokeratin. Actin staining tends to be more conspicuous in spindle than in clear polygonal myoepithelial cells, and no reactivity is seen in epithelial cells (see Fig. 10). A subset of myoepithelial cells is positive for S-100 in virtually all tumors, but the intensity and uniformity of reactivity vary considerably. Because S-100 reactivity is expressed by glandular and myoepithelial cells, it is not a specific marker for the latter cell type (16).

Adenomyoepithelioma is usually a benign tumor that can be treated by local excision (6). Local recurrence has been reported, usually more than 2 years after the initial excision (5,6). The multinodular character of the lesion and peripheral intraductal extension contribute to local recurrence. Excision may be repeated when the tumor is incompletely excised, especially in the case of multinodular lesions with peripheral intraductal extension. Mastectomy, breast irradiation, and axillary dissection are not appropriate treatment for benign adenomyoepitheliomas but may be considered in exceptional patients who have malignant tumors.

MYOEPITHELIOMA

Myoid transformation of myoepithelial cells is sometimes present in foci of sclerosing adenosis, and it may occasionally dominate the process, leading to a leiomyomatous appearance. Myoepithelial neoplasms of the breast are extremely uncommon, and reports are limited to case studies. Hamperl's review of the subject in 1970 (3) described lesions composed of epithelioid and spindle-shaped myoepithelial cells. Leiomyomatous proliferation in these neoplasms may be coordinated with glandular components, so that adenomyoepitheliomatous features are retained.

Spindle-cell neoplasms composed entirely of myoepithelial cells consist of interlacing bundles of cells, sometimes arranged in a storiform pattern. The cytoplasm is more often eosinophilic than clear. An infiltrative growth pattern may be present. The spindle cells are immunoreactive for actin. Tumors with few or no mitotic figures have had a benign clinical course after relatively short follow-up (17,18), whereas those with multiple mitoses are likely to result in metastases.

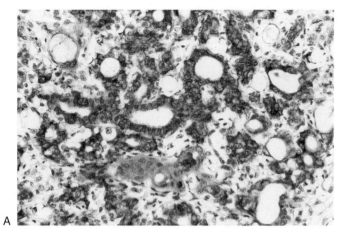

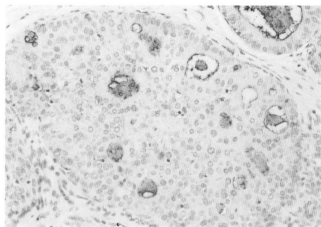

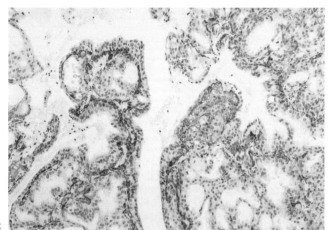

FIGURE 10. Adenomyoepithelioma immunohistochemistry. A: Epithelial cells are highlighted in this cytokeratin immunohistochemical preparation. A focus of squamous metaplasia is apparent in the lower center. Myoepithelial cells with clear cytoplasm are not stained (immunoperoxidase: AE1/AE3). **B:** The luminal borders of epithelial cells are highlighted by the immunostain for epithelial membrane antigen (immunoperoxidase: epithelial membrane antigen). **C:** Myoepithelial cells are shown with an immunostain for actin (immunoperoxidase: smooth-muscle actin).

Myoepithelial carcinomas composed entirely of epithelioid polygonal cells have received less attention than spindle-cell myoepithelial tumors. This is remarkable, as myoepithelial cells frequently have an epithelial configuration within adenomyoepithelial neoplasms of the breast. Pure myoepithelial carcinomas are extremely unusual and difficult to recognize. Most myoepithelial carcinomas arise in and have remnants of an underlying adenomyoepithelioma (see Fig. 9). Myoepithelial carcinomas typically have an alveolar growth pattern, and most are probably misclassified as examples of clear-cell, apocrine, secretory, or signet-ring cell carcinoma. Two examples of intralobular myoepithelial carcinoma have been described (19).

REFERENCES

1. Gusterson BA, Warburton MJ, Mitchell D, Ellison M, Neville AM, Rudland PS. Distribution of myoepithelial cells and basement membrane proteins in the normal breast and in benign and malignant breast diseases. *Cancer Res* 1982;42:763–770.
2. Ahmed A. The myoepithelium in human breast carcinoma. *J Pathol* 1974;112:129–135.
3. Hamperl H. The myoepithelia (myoepithelial cells): normal state; regressive changes; hyperplasia; tumors. *Curr Top Pathol* 1970;53:161–213.
4. Cameron NM, Hamperl H, Warambo W. Leiomyosarcoma of the breast originating from myoepithelium (myoepithelioma). *J Pathol* 1974;114:89–92.
5. Loose JH, Patchefsky AS, Hollander IJ, Lavin LS, Cooper HS, Katz SM. Adenomyoepithelioma of the breast. A spectrum of biologic behavior. *Am J Surg Pathol* 1992;16:868–876.
6. Rosen PP. Adenomyoepithelioma of the breast. *Hum Pathol* 1987;18:1232–1237.
7. Weidner N, Levine JD. Spindle-cell adenomyoepithelioma of the breast. A microscopic ultrastructural and immunocytochemical study. *Cancer* 1988;62:1561–1567.
8. Trojani M, Guiu M, Trouette H, DeMascarel I, Cocquet M. Malignant adenomyoepithelioma of the breast. An immunohistochemical, cytophotometric and ultrastructural study of a case with lung metastases. *Am J Clin Pathol* 1992;98:598–602.
9. Gusterson BA, Sloane JP, Middwood C, et al. Ductal adenoma of the breast—a lesion exhibiting a myoepithelial/epithelial phenotype. *Histopathology* 1987;11:103–110.
10. Guarino M, Reale D, Squillaci S, Micoli G. Ductal adenoma of the breast. An immunohistochemical study of five cases. *Pathol Res Pract* 1993;189:515–520.
11. Diaz NM, McDivitt RW, Wick MR. Pleomorphic adenoma of the breast: a clinicopathologic and immunohistochemical study of 10 cases. *Hum Pathol* 1991;22:1206–1214.
12. Zarbo RJ, Oberman HA. Cellular adenomyoepithelioma of the breast. *Am J Surg Pathol* 1983;7:863–870.
13. Pauwels C, de Potter C. Adenomyoepithelioma of the breast with features of malignancy. *Histopathology* 1994;24:94–96.
14. Chen PC, Chen C-K, Nicastri AD, Wait RB. Myoepithelial carcinoma of the breast with distant metastasis and accompanied by adenomyoepitheliomas. *Histopathology* 1994;24:543–548.

15. Michal M, Baumruk L, Burger J, Manhalova M. Adenomyoepithelioma of the breast with undifferentiated carcinoma component. *Histopathology* 1994;24:274–276.
16. Gilett CE, Bobrow LG, Millis RR. S-100 protein in human mammary tissue—immunoreactivity in breast carcinoma including Paget's disease of the nipple, and value as a marker of myoepithelial cells. *J Pathol* 1990;160:19–24.
17. Erlandson RA, Rosen PP. Infiltrating myoepithelioma of the breast. *Am J Surg Pathol* 1982;6:785–793.
18. Bigotti G, DiGiorgio G. Myoepithelioma of the breast: histologic, immunologic and electron microscopic appearance. *J Surg Oncol* 1986;32:58–64.
19. Soares J, Tomasic G, Bucciarelli M, Eusebi V. Intralobular growth of myoepithelial cell carcinoma of the breast. *Virchows Arch [A]* 1994; 425:205–210.

CHAPTER 6

Adenosis and Microglandular Adenosis

ADENOSIS

Adenosis is a proliferative lesion largely derived from the terminal duct-lobular unit. Epithelial and myoepithelial cells participate in adenosis, which is characteristically a lobulocentric lesion (Fig. 1). Adenosis usually occurs as part of a spectrum of proliferative abnormalities commonly referred to as fibrocystic changes. The entire complex may produce a palpable mass that is usually not attributable only to the adenosis component. When limited to isolated lobules that are not part of fibrocystic change, adenosis is a microscopic lesion that comes to attention clinically if it contains calcifications that are detected by mammography.

A palpable mass formed largely or completely by adenosis develops when the affected lobules fuse to form an *adenosis tumor* (Fig. 2). Patients with an adenosis tumor are almost always premenopausal, averaging about 30 years of age at diagnosis (1). The tumor is usually smaller than 2 cm and easily mistaken for a fibroadenoma (1,2). Nonpalpable adenosis tumors that contain calcifications may be detected by mammography.

Adenosis tends to have a more prominent glandular pattern in premenopausal women, whereas sclerosis and loss of gland formation are conspicuous after the menopause. In some patients, there is very little variability in the spectrum of adenosis, but others exhibit diverse patterns.

Florid adenosis, the most cellular type of adenosis, is the growth pattern usually present in adenosis tumors. Proliferation of ductules and lobular glands severely distorts and usually effaces the architecture of the underlying lobules. The hyperplastic structures elongate and become tortuous and entwined, so that many more ductular cross sections are present than in an anatomically normal lobule (Fig. 3). In the plane of section, the complex proliferative structure has a swirling pattern, punctuated by glands cut transversely that have round, open lumina. The majority of the ductular structures cut tangentially or longitudinally have elongated lumina, sometimes with angular contours.

Epithelial cells lining the tubules and glands are flattened, cuboidal, or slightly columnar and are arranged in one or two layers surrounded by myoepithelial cells. Increases in cell size and nuclear pleomorphism are found in florid adenosis, especially during pregnancy or lactation. Intracytoplasmic mucin vacuoles and signet-ring cells are not present in the benign glandular epithelium of florid adenosis. Luminal se-

cretion may undergo calcification, but this is less common and less extensive than in sclerosing adenosis. Hyperplastic change in the epithelial component of florid adenosis is mirrored in hyperplasia of the myoepithelium. Mitoses in epithelial and myoepithelial cells are very infrequent, but they may be more evident during pregnancy (Fig. 4). Apocrine metaplasia occurs in florid adenosis. Florid adenosis may surround nerves in adjacent breast parenchyma.

In *sclerosing adenosis*, there is preferential preservation of myoepithelial cells, with variable atrophy of epithelial cells accompanied by lobular fibrosis (Fig. 5). The swirling lobulocentric pattern encountered in adenosis is retained, but epithelial cells are less conspicuous and the tubular structures more attenuated. Some examples of sclerosing adenosis are not limited to a lobulocentric pattern. When this occurs, the proliferating benign glands produce an infiltrative pattern in the stroma (Fig. 6) and fat (Fig. 7) that can be mistaken for invasive carcinoma (Fig. 8). Epithelial cells may be markedly reduced in number or even absent, leaving compressed, elongated myoepithelial cells. The persisting myoepithelial cells with a pronounced spindle shape or myoid phenotype are strongly immunoreactive with markers of smooth-muscle differentiation (Fig. 9). Calcifications become more numerous, with increasing sclerosis and thickening of basement membranes (Fig. 10).

Apocrine metaplasia is relatively common in adenosis, a configuration that has been referred to as apocrine adenosis (2,3) (Fig. 11). The cytologic appearance of apocrine metaplasia in adenosis is quite varied (4). In some cases, the cells have conventional pink, finely granular apocrine cytoplasm and round, regular nuclei. Atypical features include clearing or vacuolization of the cytoplasm and nuclear pleomorphism (Fig. 12). Hyperchromasia of nuclei and prominent nucleoli are found in the most extreme examples of apocrine atypia (Fig. 13). Mitotic figures are very uncommon in atypical apocrine metaplasia in sclerosing adenosis.

Perineural invasion has been found in 1% to 2% of breast specimens exhibiting benign proliferative changes, including sclerosing adenosis (5,6). Sclerosing adenosis can penetrate into and focally through the perineurium. Myoepithelial cells are evident in most, but not all, foci of perineural invasion by sclerosing adenosis.

Tubular adenosis is composed of ductules arranged so that

Text continues on page 57

51

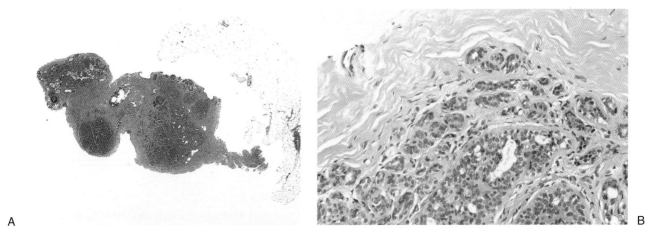

A

B

FIGURE 1. Adenosis. A,B: Multiple nodules of adenosis are shown in this needle core biopsy specimen. Smaller, lobulocentric foci are present near the upper edge in the center of (A). Larger nodules are the result of coalescent lobules, such as the one shown in (B).

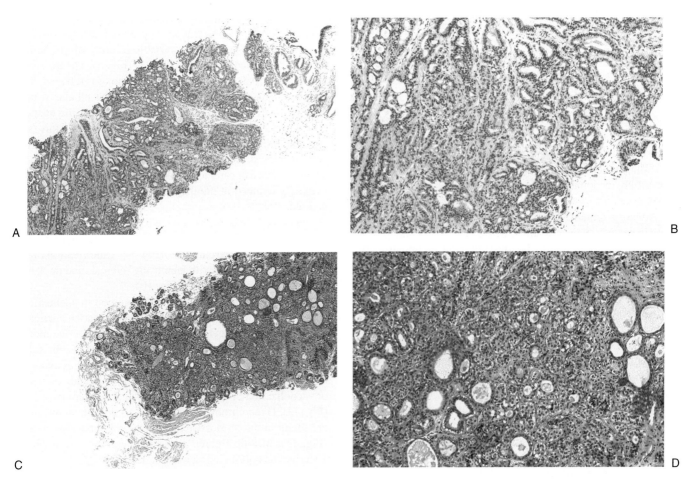

A

B

C

D

FIGURE 2. Adenosis tumor. A,B: Traces of the underlying lobular structure are visible in this needle core biopsy sample. The nonpalpable lesion has a sharply defined border. The adenosis glands vary in size, and some are elongated or tubular. **C,D:** A very dense proliferation of hyperplastic epithelial and myoepithelial cells characterizes this lesion. Note the distinct border on the left in (C) and numerous microcysts.

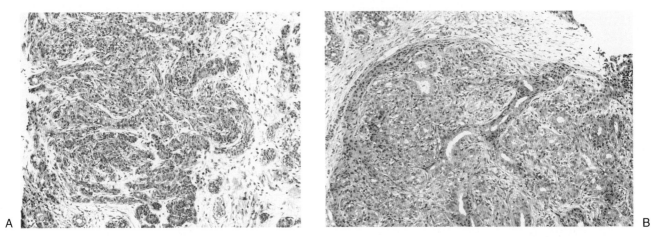

FIGURE 3. Florid adenosis. A,B: Elongated, hyperplastic, entwined adenosis glands are shown in a needle core biopsy specimen. The epithelium in (B) has areas with a trace of apocrine metaplasia where glandular lumina are formed.

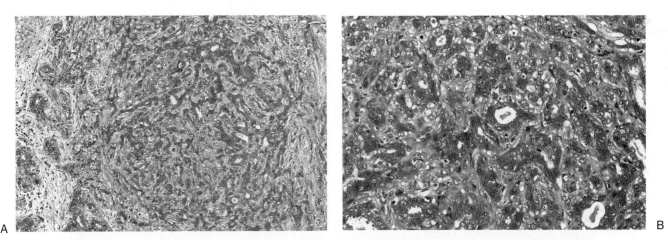

FIGURE 4. Florid adenosis in pregnancy. This needle core biopsy sample was obtained from a palpable tumor in a 35-year-old woman who was 9 weeks pregnant. **A,B:** There is marked hyperplasia of epithelial and myoepithelial cells in this example of florid adenosis. Mitoses are present in both cell types.

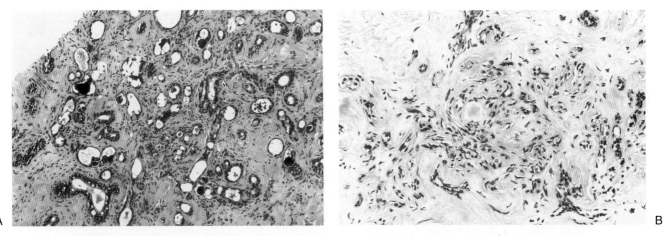

FIGURE 5. Sclerosing adenosis. A: The characteristic features are stromal fibrosis, relative atrophy of epithelial cells with predominance of spindly myoepithelial cells, microcystic dilatation of glands, and numerous calcifications. **B:** Almost complete atrophy of glandular cells, leaving swirling, elongated myoepithelial cells, characterizes this lesion.

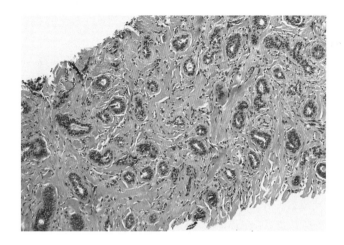

FIGURE 6. Adenosis with a dispersed pattern. Glands with round, angular, and tubular shapes are dispersed in collagenous stroma, which exhibits pseudoangiomatous hyperplasia. This type of adenosis bears a superficial resemblance to tubular carcinoma. Note the thick basement membranes around some glands.

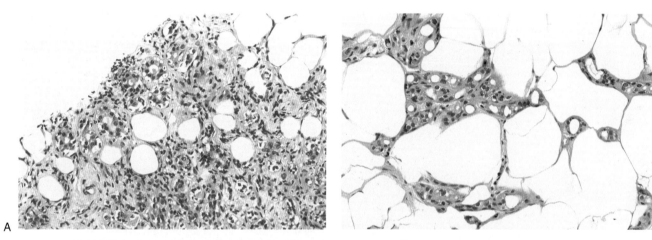

A   B

FIGURE 7. Sclerosing adenosis with an invasive pattern. A: Sclerosing adenosis in this needle core biopsy specimen extends into fat in a pattern resembling that of invasive carcinoma. Spindly and epithelioid myoepithelial cells with clear cytoplasm are present. **B:** In another needle core biopsy sample, fat cells are surrounded by sclerosing adenosis and isolated glands are shown in the fat.

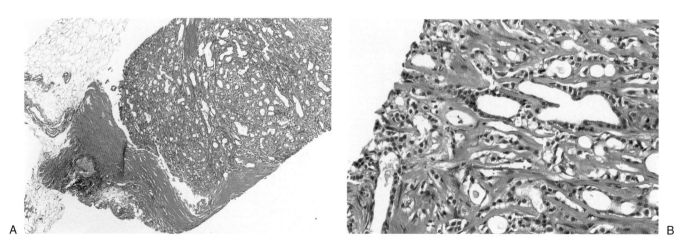

A   B

FIGURE 8. Sclerosing adenosis mistaken for carcinoma. A,B: This needle core biopsy sample of a palpable adenosis tumor was interpreted as invasive well-differentiated duct carcinoma. The lesion has a well-circumscribed border and lacks a lobulocentric architecture. Myoepithelial cells with clear cytoplasm are evident at high magnification. *Figure continues*

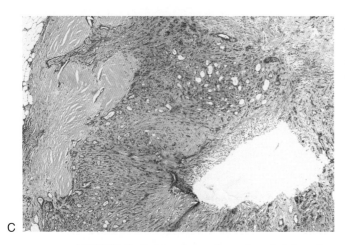

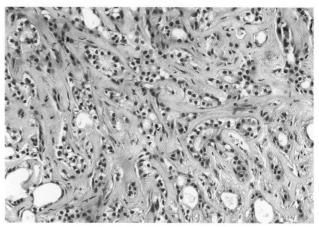

FIGURE 8. Sclerosing adenosis mistaken for carcinoma. *Continued* **C,D:** The subsequent excisional biopsy specimen revealed a circumscribed focus of sclerosing adenosis with a defect in the center at the site of the previous needle core biopsy. The glands are outlined by thin basement membranes.

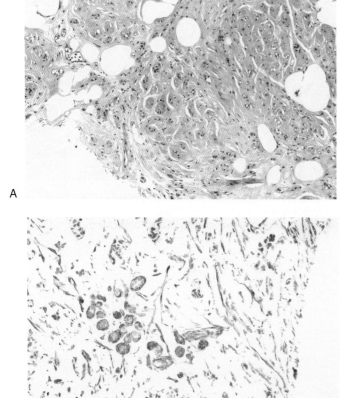

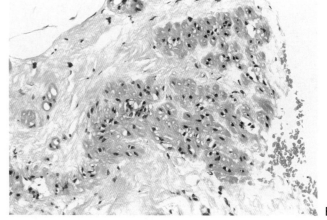

FIGURE 9. Sclerosing adenosis with myoid metaplasia. A,B: Well-developed myoid metaplasia of myoepithelial cells is apparent in this needle core biopsy specimen. Epithelial cells are almost entirely absent, and the myoepithelial cells have the eosinophilic cytoplasm of smooth muscle. **C:** An immunostain for actin confirms myoid differentiation in cells surrounding a cluster of glands (immunoperoxidase: smooth-muscle actin).

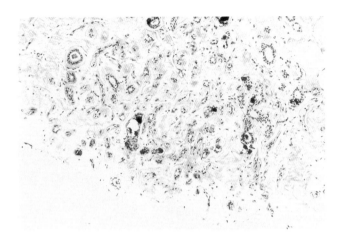

FIGURE 10. Sclerosing adenosis. Thickened basement membranes, glandular atrophy, and calcifications characterize well-developed sclerosing adenosis in this lobule.

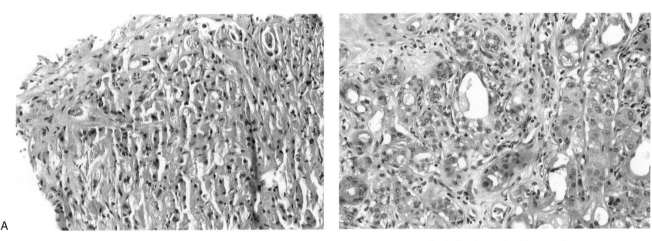

A

B

FIGURE 11. Adenosis with apocrine metaplasia. A: Apocrine metaplasia is shown in this needle core biopsy fragment. Preservation of the tissue structure is suboptimal, and myoepithelial cells are difficult to detect. **B:** Another area from the same biopsy specimen with apocrine metaplasia in adenosis glands.

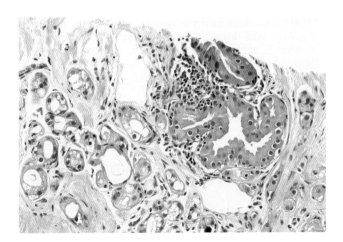

FIGURE 12. Adenosis with atypical apocrine metaplasia. Enlarged adenosis glands formed by cells with abundant eosinophilic or clear cytoplasm and pleomorphic, unevenly distributed nuclei in a needle core biopsy sample. Myoepithelial cells with elongated nuclei are apparent in some glands.

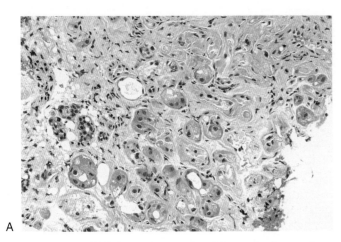

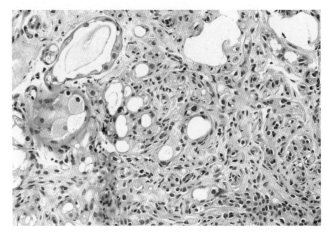

A   B

FIGURE 13. Adenosis with atypical apocrine metaplasia. A,B: Some of the adenosis glands in this needle core biopsy sample are expanded by apocrine metaplasia composed of cells with deeply eosinophilic cytoplasm and pleomorphic nuclei.

the majority are cut longitudinally in the plane of section (Fig. 14). The proliferation lacks the lobulocentric distribution of florid or sclerosing adenosis, and the ductules extend in a seemingly haphazard pattern into fibrous mammary stroma and fat. In some instances, there is a dense proliferation of tubular structures that appear to be entwined or interdigitated. Secretion that may calcify is variably present in the ductules. Virtually all the tubular structures have basement membranes and an outer myoepithelial cell layer (7). These features are important in the distinction between tubular carcinoma and tubular adenosis.

Atypical hyperplasia (Fig. 15) and carcinoma *in situ* occur in sclerosing adenosis and tubular adenosis. The majority of carcinomas that develop in adenosis are of the lobular type

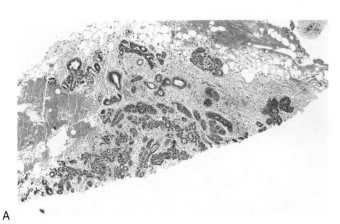

A

FIGURE 14. Tubular adenosis. A,B: Elongated adenosis glands that resemble tubules with epithelial hyperplasia and thick basement membranes are present in this needle core biopsy sample from a premenopausal woman. **C:** Epithelial atrophy, calcifications, and stromal fibrosis in a biopsy specimen from a postmenopausal patient.

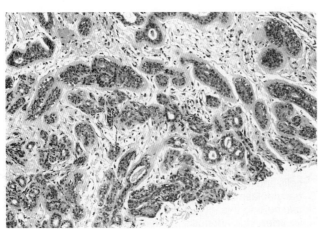

B

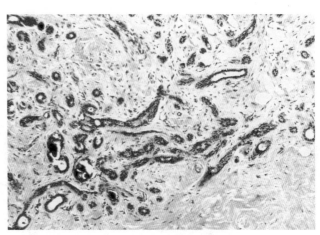

C

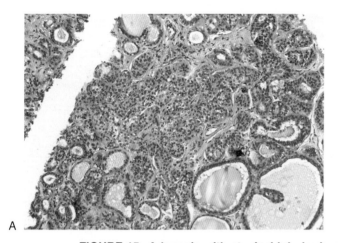

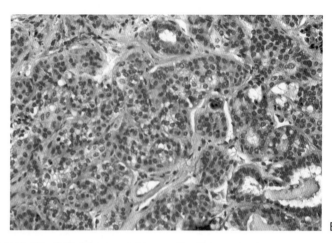

FIGURE 15. Adenosis with atypical lobular hyperplasia. A,B: Monomorphic small cells are apparent in some adenosis glands in this needle core biopsy specimen. The biopsy was performed for mammographically detected nonpalpable calcifications. Note the microcystic dilatation of some glands and a small calcification.

(8) (Fig. 16). Lobular carcinoma *in situ* causes expansion of the epithelial component in adenosis, but in some foci of sclerosing adenosis, the neoplastic process is manifested by sparsely distributed, poorly cohesive pagetoid cells (9). Lobular carcinoma *in situ* in adenosis often has signet-ring cells (Fig. 17). Signet-ring cells and stainable intracytoplasmic mucin are not a feature of benign epithelium in adenosis. It is not unusual to find lobular carcinoma *in situ* in other lobules, unaffected by sclerosing adenosis, in the same specimen.

Intraductal carcinoma arises less often in adenosis than does lobular carcinoma *in situ* (Fig. 18). Intraductal carcinoma can be identified in adenosis when comedo necrosis is

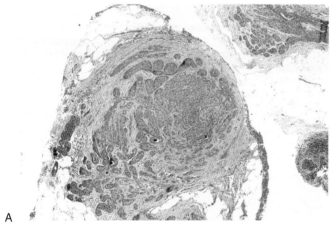

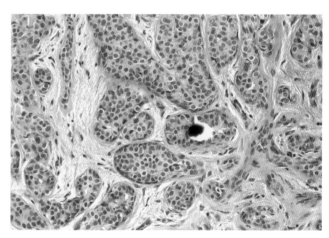

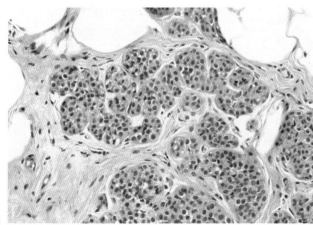

FIGURE 16. Tubular adenosis with lobular carcinoma *in situ*. A,B: Swirling tubular adenosis glands are expanded by lobular carcinoma *in situ*. The needle core biopsy was performed for mammographically detected microcalcifications. Myoepithelial cells are represented by hyperchromatic, elongated nuclei between the carcinoma cells and the basement membranes in some glands. **C:** Intracytoplasmic vacuoles are present in some carcinoma *in situ* cells in this lobule, which is not appreciably distorted by sclerosing adenosis in the same biopsy.

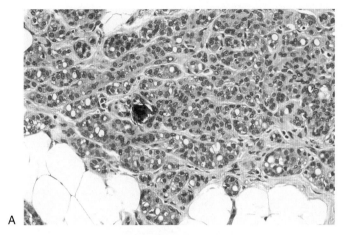

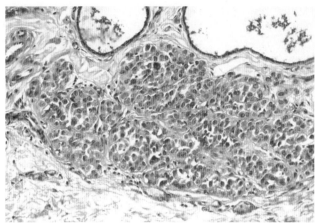

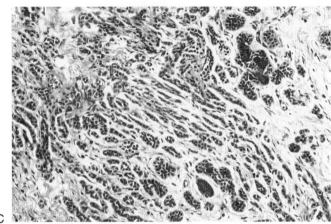

FIGURE 17. Sclerosing adenosis with lobular carcinoma *in situ*. Three patterns of involvement are shown. **A,B:** Signet-ring cell carcinoma *in situ* with intracytoplasmic mucin demonstrated in virtually all cells with the mucicarmine stain in (B). **C:** Lobular carcinoma *in situ* manifested by cellular discohesion in a severely sclerotic lesion (hematoxylin-phloxine-eosin stain).

present if the proliferation is solid, cribriform, or papillary, and when substantial cytologic atypia is present in an expanded epithelial component (2). Apocrine intraductal carcinoma is a relatively frequent type of intraductal carcinoma in adenosis. Despite considerable cytologic atypia, apocrine metaplasia in adenosis should not be interpreted as carcinoma until epithelial proliferation is sufficient to form one of the conventional structural patterns of intraductal carcinoma (4,10) (Fig. 19).

The underlying architecture of adenosis is preserved when *in situ* lobular and intraductal carcinoma arise in this setting. The integrity of individual glands, sometimes difficult to ascertain in these complex proliferative lesions, may be confirmed with a reticulin stain and immunohistochemical studies for basement membrane or myoepithelial cells (7,11). Even when basement membranes and a myoepithelial layer appear discontinuous, it is usually not possible to diagnose invasion with confidence in adenosis. The most convincing evidence for a diagnosis of invasive carcinoma arising in adenosis is the finding of invasive foci extending beyond the adenosis lesion. The glands or cells interpreted as invasive carcinoma should not be accompanied by myoepithelial cells. Basement membrane is largely or completely absent, and the invasive elements should have a growth pattern different from that of the adjacent adenosis. Double immunolabeling for cytokeratin and actin can detect isolated invasive carcinoma cells in areas of sclerosing adenosis that are involved by carcinoma (Fig. 20).

When adenosis is diagnosed in a stereotactic needle core biopsy, surgical excision of the lesional area is recommended to rule out an associated carcinoma, especially if the lesion has florid or atypical epithelial hyperplasia. When car-

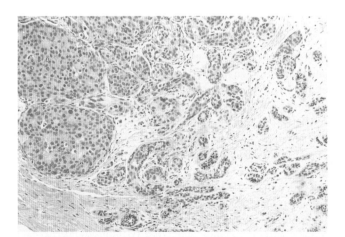

FIGURE 18. Sclerosing adenosis with intraductal carcinoma. The glands on the left are markedly enlarged by intraductal carcinoma that has a solid growth pattern and is composed of cells with pale-to-clear cytoplasm. Remnants of adenosis are evident on the right.

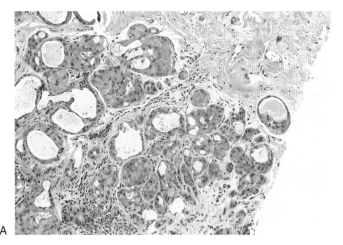
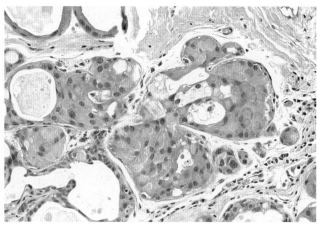

A   B

FIGURE 19. Sclerosing adenosis with apocrine intraductal carcinoma. A,B: The adenosis glands in this needle core biopsy specimen are expanded by apocrine carcinoma composed of cells with abundant eosinophilic or clear cytoplasm and pleomorphic nuclei with prominent nucleoli.

cinoma is present, it is often in breast tissue outside the area of adenosis (8,9). Some investigators have reported an increased risk for subsequent carcinoma after previously diagnosed sclerosing adenosis. The overall relative risk in comparison with control populations for subsequent development of carcinoma in women with adenosis ranges from 2.1 (12) to 2.5 (12–14).

MICROGLANDULAR ADENOSIS

Microglandular adenosis is a proliferative glandular lesion that mimics carcinoma clinically and pathologically (15–17). All reported patients with microglandular adenosis

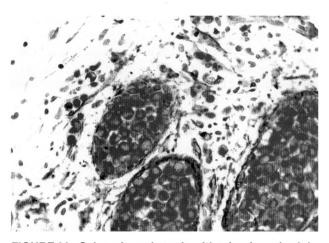

FIGURE 20. Sclerosing adenosis with microinvasive lobular carcinoma. Double immunolabeling has been used to detect microinvasive lobular carcinoma in this specimen, in which *in situ* lobular carcinoma has involved sclerosing adenosis. Epithelial cells stained crimson are evident in the stroma outside glands bounded by myoepithelial cells stained brown (immunoperoxidase: AE1/AE3; alkaline phosphatase: smooth-muscle actin). (Courtesy of Dr. Syed Hoda.)

have been women. They ranged in age from 28 to 82 years, with the majority 45 to 55 years old. The presenting symptom in most instances was a mass or "thickening" in the breast. Mammography may reveal increased density, and findings are sometimes "suspicious," but there are no specific radiologic changes. The tumor usually has measured 3 to 4 cm, but lesions as large as 20 cm have been described.

Microglandular adenosis is an infiltrative proliferation of small glands in fibrous or fatty mammary stroma. Most often, the distribution seems disorderly. The round glands are lined by a single layer of flat-to-cuboidal epithelial cells (Fig. 21). Each cell has a single round nucleus with an inconspicuous or absent nucleolus. The cytoplasm tends to be clear or amphophilic, but pronounced eosinophilia may be encountered. Inspissated secretion forms distinct, deeply stained globules in the glands. This material is usually positive for periodic acid–Schiff (PAS) and mucicarmine, and it may calcify.

Cells forming microglandular adenosis are strongly immunoreactive for cytokeratin, S-100 protein, and cathepsin D. They have proved to be negative for nuclear estrogen and progesterone receptors, nuclear p53 oncogene expression, and for HER2/neu membrane immunoreactivity (18). Eusebi et al. (19) reported that microglandular adenosis lacks immunoreactivity for gross cystic disease fluid protein (GCDFP-15) and for epithelial membrane antigen (EMA). The absence of EMA is helpful in distinguishing microglandular adenosis from tubular carcinoma, which is often EMA-positive.

Myoepithelial cells are not evident in sections stained with hematoxylin and eosin or with immunohistochemical stains for actin. A basement membrane is demonstrable by immunoreactivity for laminin and type IV collagen (18,19), and the glands are typically invested by a reticulin ring that can be highlighted by silver impregnation and PAS stains. In some instances, the glands are surrounded by a thick collar of collagen and reticulin.

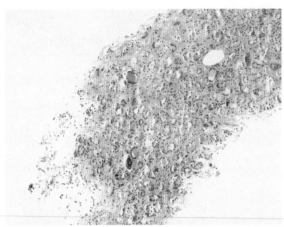

FIGURE 21. Microglandular adenosis. A–C: This needle core biopsy specimen shows small, haphazardly distributed glands in fibrous stroma. Many of the gland-forming cells have clear cytoplasm. A few glands contain secretion. The secretion and basement membranes are highlighted with the periodic acid–Schiff (PAS) reaction in (C). Note the cytoplasmic clearing (PAS without diastase). **D:** In this sample from a surgical biopsy performed 5 years later, microglandular adenosis was present in the same breast as the lesion shown in (A–C). **E:** Microglandular adenosis in fat shown here could be mistaken for infiltrating carcinoma.

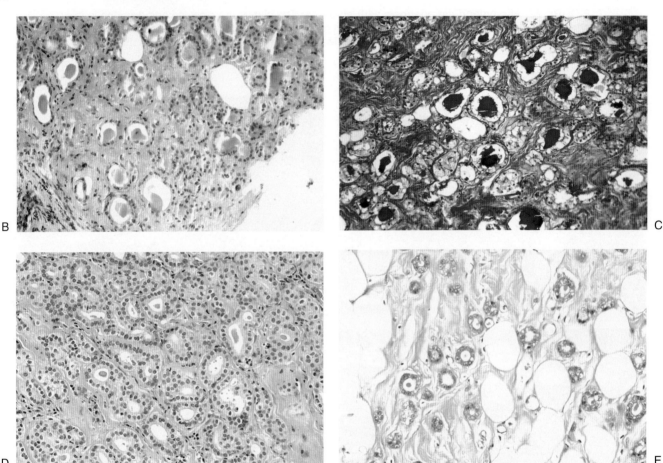

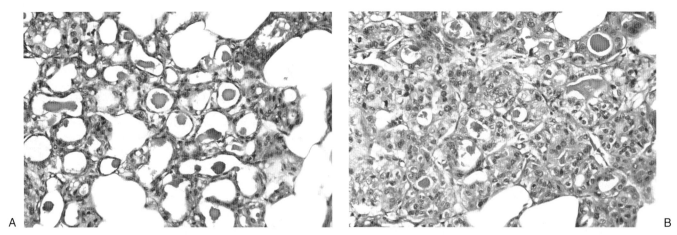

FIGURE 22. Microglandular adenosis with atypia. A: The glands are crowded and distorted in this otherwise ordinary example of microglandular adenosis. **B:** Marked cellular crowding and overgrowth have obscured most of the glands in this atypical lesion.

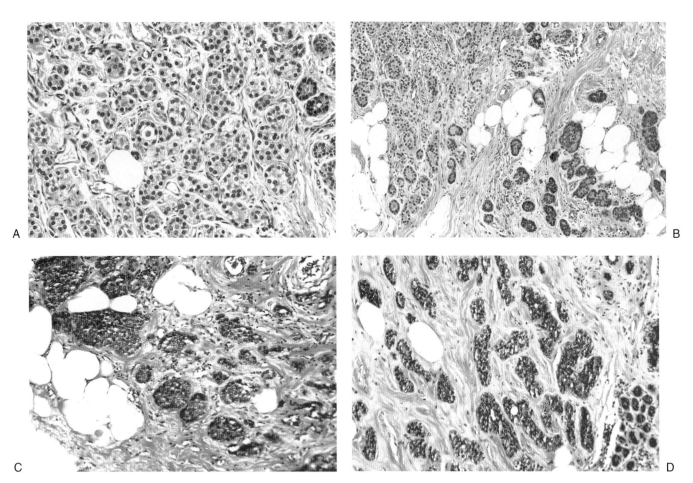

FIGURE 23. Microglandular adenosis with carcinoma. A: Most of this focus is composed of glands with increased cellularity, representing mild atypia. **B:** Atypical glands are shown on the right, with transitions to *in situ* carcinoma on the left grouped around fat lobules. **C,D:** Solid masses of poorly differentiated cells that fill the enlarged glands in this biopsy specimen from another patient illustrate the appearance of intraductal carcinoma in microglandular adenosis. This distorted glandular pattern resembles invasive carcinoma.

Substantial variation in the growth pattern and cytologic appearance of the glands can be encountered in microglandular adenosis. In some lesions, the cells lining the glands tend to be pleomorphic, with varying amounts of cytoplasm that is clear or exhibits eosinophilia (see Fig. 21). Prominent, coarse, deeply eosinophilic cytoplasmic granules are present in a minority of cases. Lesions classified as "atypical" microglandular adenosis have elements of microglandular adenosis in its uncomplicated form as well as foci with a more complex structure and cytologic atypia (20). Atypical lesions have a pleomorphic mixture of connected microacini and larger glands. Ordinary microglandular adenosis may have crowded, "back-to-back" glands, but each acinus remains separate. The more florid epithelial proliferation of the atypical lesion produces interconnected, budding glandular units with microcribriform nests (Fig. 22). When luminal bridging occurs, the monolayered epithelium is replaced by a stratified proliferation that evolves into solid nests of cells.

When carcinoma arises in microglandular adenosis, transitions from atypical microglandular adenosis to carcinoma are usually observed (20). Duct-forming carcinomatous areas have the acinar budding pattern of atypical microglandular adenosis, but they exhibit a high mitotic rate, substantial cytologic abnormalities, necrosis, and a desmoplastic stromal reaction. A chronic inflammatory infiltrate often accompanies the development of carcinoma. Chondromyxoid metaplasia has been described in a minority of cases (20).

Many carcinomas arising in microglandular adenosis have an alveolar growth pattern (Fig. 23). The fully developed lesion is usually composed of malignant cells growing in solid nests. The carcinomas may have some clear cells, and a few tumors are entirely composed of such cells or of cells with prominent cytoplasmic granularity.

The histologic differential diagnosis of microglandular adenosis includes tubular carcinoma and sclerosing adenosis. Tubular carcinoma is usually composed of angular glands of varying size, and the lesion often has a stellate or radial configuration with central sclerosis. Intraductal carcinoma is present in most tubular carcinomas, typically with micropapillary or cribriform patterns. Myoepithelial cells and a basement membrane are absent. Occasionally, the glands in tubular carcinoma are rounded and the cells have clear or apocrine cytoplasm, making it difficult to distinguish them from microglandular adenosis, especially in the limited sample of a needle core biopsy. A thorough search for intraductal carcinoma is necessary in this situation. Sclerosing adenosis features myoepithelial proliferation that often has a spindle-cell configuration. The process is commonly lobulocentric, and the compressed glands tend to be arranged in a whorled or laminated fashion within the lobular nodules.

Excisional biopsy is necessary if microglandular adenosis is diagnosed in a needle core biopsy. Repeated excision should be considered if the margins of a lumpectomy are found to be microscopically involved, as little is known about the long-term course of incompletely excised lesions.

REFERENCES

1. Urban JA, Adair FE. Sclerosing adenosis. *Cancer* 1949;2:625–634.
2. Nielsen BB. Adenosis tumour of the breast—a clinicopathological investigation of 27 cases. *Histopathology* 1987;11:1259–1275.
3. Simpson JF, Page DL, Dupont WD. Apocrine adenosis—a mimic of mammary carcinoma. *Surg Pathol* 1990;3:289–299.
4. Carter DJ, Rosen PP. Atypical apocrine metaplasia in sclerosing lesions of the breast. A study of 51 patients. *Mod Pathol* 1991;4:1–5.
5. Taylor HB, Norris HJ. Epithelial invasion of nerves in benign diseases of the breast. *Cancer* 1967;20:2245–2249.
6. Davies JD. Neural invasion in benign mammary dysplasia. *J Pathol* 1973;109:225–231.
7. Lee K-C, Chan JKC, Gwi E. Tubular adenosis of the breast. A distinctive benign lesion mimicking invasive carcinoma. *Am J Surg Pathol* 1996;20:46–54.
8. Oberman HA, Markey BA. Non-invasive carcinoma of the breast presenting in adenosis. *Mod Pathol* 1991;4:31–35.
9. Fechner RE. Lobular carcinoma *in situ* in sclerosing adenosis. A potential source of confusion with invasive carcinoma. *Am J Surg Pathol* 1981;5:233–239.
10. Abati AD, Kimmel M, Rosen PP. Apocrine mammary carcinoma: a clinicopathologic study of 72 cases. *Am J Clin Pathol* 1990;94: 371–377.
11. Eusebi V, Collina G, Bussolati G. Carcinoma *in situ* in sclerosing adenosis of the breast: an immunocytochemical study. *Semin Diagn Pathol* 1989;6:146–152.
12. Jensen RA, Page DL, DuPont WD, Rogers LW. Invasive breast cancer risk in women with sclerosing adenosis. *Cancer* 1989;64:1977–1983.
13. Bodian CA, Perzin KH, Lattes R, Huffman P, Abernathy TG. Prognostic significance of benign proliferative breast disease. *Cancer* 1993;71: 3896–3907.
14. Krieger N, Hiatt RA. Risk of breast cancer after benign breast diseases: variation by histologic type, degree of atypia, age at biopsy, and length of follow-up. *Am J Epidemiol* 1992;136:619–631.
15. Clement PB, Azzopardi JG. Microglandular adenosis of the breast. A lesion simulating tubular carcinoma. *Histopathology* 1983;7:169–180.
16. Rosen PP. Microglandular adenosis. *Am J Surg Pathol* 1983;7: 137–144.
17. Tavassoli FA, Norris HJ. Microglandular adenosis of the breast. *Am J Surg Pathol* 1983;7:731–737.
18. James BA, Cranor ML, Rosen PP. Carcinoma of the breast arising in microglandular adenosis. *Am J Clin Pathol* 1993;100:507–513.
19. Eusebi V, Faschini MP, Betts CM, et al. Microglandular adenosis, apocrine adenosis and tubular carcinoma of the breast. An immunohistochemical comparison. *Am J Surg Pathol* 1993;17:99–109.
20. Rosenblum MK, Purrazzella R, Rosen PP. Is microglandular adenosis a precancerous disease? A study of carcinoma arising therein. *Am J Surg Pathol* 1986;10:237–245.

CHAPTER 7

Fibroepithelial Neoplasms

FIBROADENOMATOID MASTOPATHY (SCLEROSING LOBULAR HYPERPLASIA)

This benign proliferative lesion usually presents as a localized tumor with a mean diameter of 4 cm, but asymptomatic lesions have been detected by mammography (1,2). The most frequent mammographic finding is a well-defined mass. Microcalcifications are not commonly present. The imaging characteristics are not sufficiently specific to distinguish sclerosing lobular hyperplasia from a fibroadenoma. Patients range in age from 14 to 46 years, with a mean age of about 32 years (1,2).

Microscopic examination reveals enlarged lobules composed of an increased number of intralobular glands (Fig. 1). The intralobular stroma is collagenized, and there is variable sclerosis of the interlobular stroma. Individual lobules and groups of lobules sometimes have the appearance of miniature fibroadenomas with a prominent glandular component (Fig. 2). Secretory activity is variably present or absent, and calcifications are not formed. Sclerosing lobular hyperplasia or fibroadenomatoid mastopathy is found in breast tissue surrounding about 50% of fibroadenomas (1). Because the fibroadenoma produces a dominant tumor, associated sclerosing lobular hyperplasia may be overlooked.

FIBROADENOMA

These benign tumors arise from the epithelium and stroma of the terminal duct-lobular unit. They account for about one fifth of all benign masses and approximately 10% of breast lesions in postmenopausal patients. The relative risk for subsequent carcinoma may be higher for patients with a concurrent fibroadenoma and benign proliferative changes (3). Dupont et al. (3) found that the increased breast carcinoma risk was dependent on the presence of proliferative changes in the fibroadenoma itself or in the surrounding breast, and a family history of breast carcinoma.

The age distribution ranges from childhood to more than 70 years, with a mean age of about 30 and a median around 25 years (4). The most frequent presenting symptom is a self-detected painless, firm, well-circumscribed solitary tumor. A growing proportion of fibroadenomas are nonpalpable tumors that are detected by mammography. Multiple fibroadenomas occur in about 15% of patients, with equal proportions found synchronously and metachronously in the same or opposite breast. An uncommon syndrome occurring in adolescence is the metachronous and synchronous development of multiple fibroadenomas, usually in both breasts (5). The intervening breast tissue often manifests extensive fibroadenomatoid hyperplasia.

Coarse calcifications are not uncommon in fibroadenomas after the menopause (Fig. 3). In one series, only 10% of fibroadenomas measured more than 4.0 cm (4). Tumors larger than 4 cm are significantly more frequent in patients 20 years or younger than in older patients (4). Fibroadenomas that involve most or all of the breast, often referred to as adolescent giant fibroadenomas, develop as solitary or multiple tumors shortly after puberty (5).

More than 90% of fibroadenomas are of the adult type, with the remainder fulfilling criteria for a diagnosis of juvenile fibroadenoma or other unusual types of fibroadenoma. *Tubular adenoma* (6) is a variant of fibroadenoma composed of closely approximated round or oval glandular structures consisting of a single layer of epithelium supported by myoepithelial cells. Foci with the tubular adenoma pattern can be encountered within an otherwise ordinary fibroadenoma. Other so-called adenomas are unrelated to the fibroadenoma category. *Apocrine adenoma* is a localized nodular focus of prominent papillary and cystic apocrine metaplasia (7) (see Chapter 4). Nodular foci of sclerosing adenosis with apocrine metaplasia have been variously termed apocrine adenoma and apocrine adenosis. *Ductal adenoma* (8) and *pleomorphic adenoma* (9) are variants of intraductal papilloma or adenomyoepithelioma.

The histologic hallmark of a fibroadenoma is concurrent proliferation of glandular and stromal elements. The majority of adult fibroadenomas have growth patterns that have been referred to as intracanalicular and pericanalicular (Fig. 4). The former pattern is produced when the stroma compresses ducts into elongated linear branching structures with slitlike lumina. When the ducts are not compressed by the stroma, the architecture is described as having a pericanalicular pattern. These structural features are of no known prognostic or clinical significance, and many tumors have both components. Fibroadenomas with a prominent intracanalicular pattern may be mistaken for benign cystosarcomas, especially in a needle core biopsy specimen.

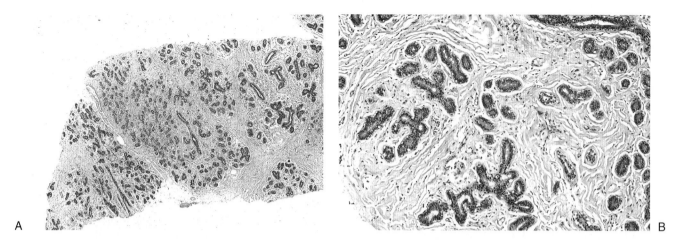

FIGURE 1. Fibroadenomatoid mastopathy. A,B: This needle core biopsy sample was obtained from one of multiple bilateral breast nodules in a 16-year-old girl. The specimen consists of enlarged lobules with sclerotic stroma.

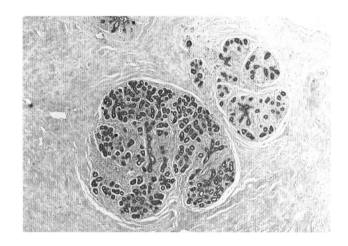

FIGURE 2. Fibroadenomatoid mastopathy. The lobules resemble small fibroadenomas.

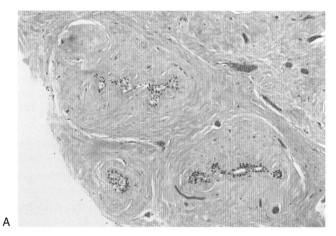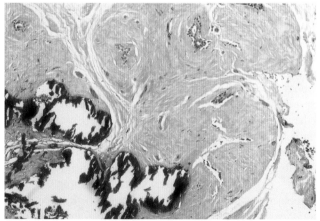

FIGURE 3. Fibroadenoma with sclerosis and calcification. A,B: This needle core biopsy specimen is from a nonpalpable calcified lesion in a 74-year-old woman.

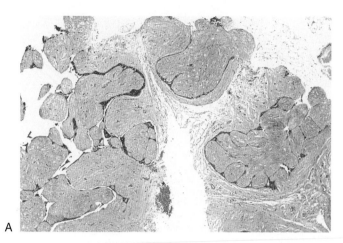
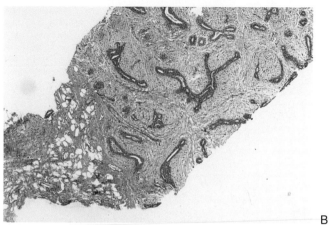

FIGURE 4. Fibroadenoma growth patterns. A: The intracanalicular growth pattern is formed by compressed epithelial lined spaces in myxoid stroma. **B:** A pericanalicular lesion in which the stroma is arranged in a circumferential nodular pattern around ductules with focal epithelial hyperplasia.

The appearance of the stroma varies from one fibroadenoma to another, but it is relatively homogeneous in any given lesion. The average fibroadenoma in adults has evenly distributed similar proportions of epithelium and stroma throughout the tumor. The density of stromal cellularity is not related to tumor size. Fibroadenomas from women less than 20 years of age tend to have more proliferative epithelium and more cellular stroma as a group than tumors from older women (Fig. 5). Mitotic figures are extremely unusual in fibroadenomatous stroma.

Uncommon types of stroma encountered in fibroadenomas exhibit smooth-muscle metaplasia, usually derived from myoid metaplasia of myoepithelial cells in sclerosing adenosis or myofibroblasts in the fibroadenoma (10), and adipose differentiation (11). Giant cells, sometimes with multiple hyperchromatic nuclei, are found in the stroma of fibroadenomas as well as in cystosarcomas (12). These cells do not influence the clinical course of the lesion. A tumor that has the

structural features of a fibroadenoma should not be classified as a cystosarcoma solely because it contains multinucleated stromal giant cells. Osteochondroid metaplasia is very uncommon and almost always occurs in a fibroadenoma from a postmenopausal woman (13). The stroma of a fibroadenoma can undergo marked myxoid change, and in extreme cases the needle core biopsy specimen from such a tumor could be mistaken for mucinous carcinoma (Fig. 6).

Squamous metaplasia, cysts, duct hyperplasia, adenosis, and apocrine metaplasia (Fig. 7) can develop in the epithelial component of fibroadenomas. Sclerosing adenosis in a fibroadenoma can be mistaken for infiltrating carcinoma (Fig. 8) and can develop calcifications (Fig. 9). Fibroadenomas with adenosis, papillary apocrine hyperplasia, cysts, or epithelial calcifications have been designated "complex" (3). Marked epithelial hyperplasia can be encountered in a complex fibroadenoma (Fig. 10). These proliferative changes are not dependent on exposure to exogenous hormones (14). Im-

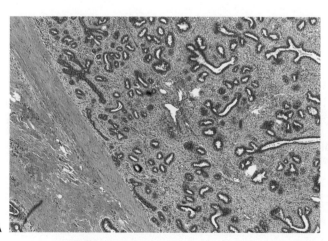
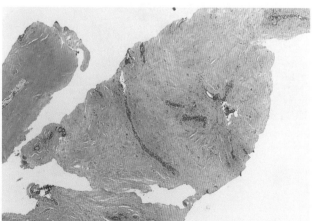

FIGURE 5. Fibroadenomas in young and elderly women. A: Well-formed lobular glands and evenly distributed cellular stroma are present in this tumor from a 23-year-old woman. **B:** This needle core biopsy specimen from a nonpalpable lesion in a 71-year-old woman shows marked fibrosis and sparse atrophic epithelial elements.

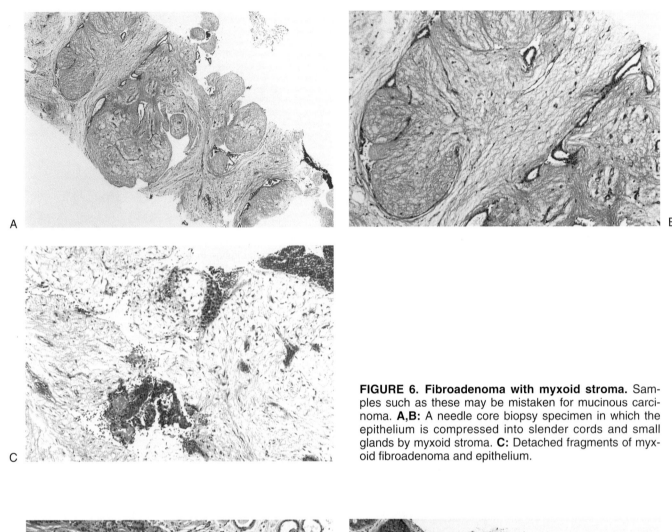

A

B

C

FIGURE 6. Fibroadenoma with myxoid stroma. Samples such as these may be mistaken for mucinous carcinoma. **A,B:** A needle core biopsy specimen in which the epithelium is compressed into slender cords and small glands by myxoid stroma. **C:** Detached fragments of myxoid fibroadenoma and epithelium.

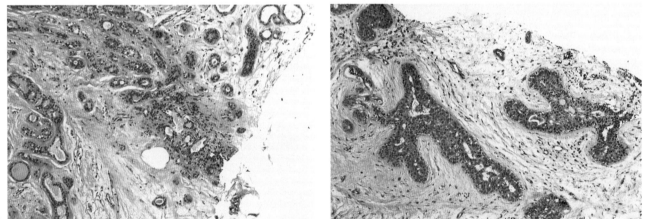

A

B

FIGURE 7. Fibroadenoma with benign proliferative changes. A: This needle core biopsy specimen reveals sclerosing adenosis and cysts. **B:** A focus of duct hyperplasia in another fibroadenoma.

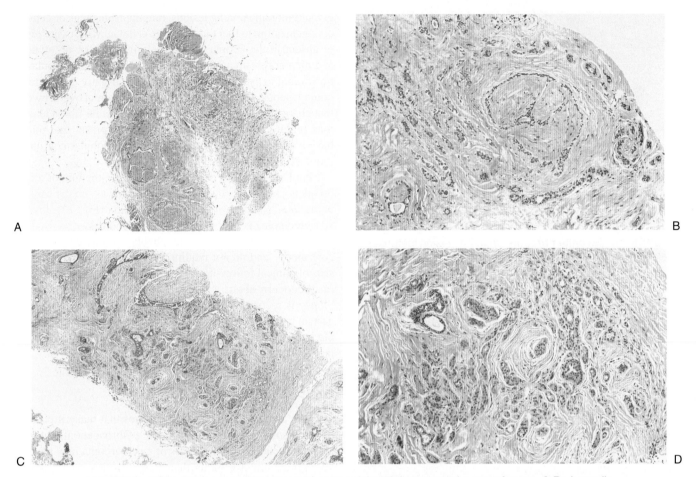

FIGURE 8. Fibroadenomas with sclerosing adenosis misinterpreted as carcinoma. A,B: A needle core biopsy specimen of sclerosing adenosis in a fibroadenoma. This specimen was erroneously interpreted as infiltrating lobular carcinoma. **C,D:** In this needle core biopsy specimen, sclerosing adenosis in a fibroadenoma was interpreted as showing invasive tubular carcinoma.

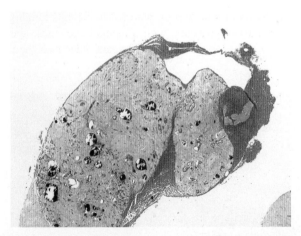

FIGURE 9. Fibroadenoma with sclerosing adenosis and calcifications. The needle core biopsy specimen contained this tissue fragment. The excised tumor was a very sclerotic fibroadenoma.

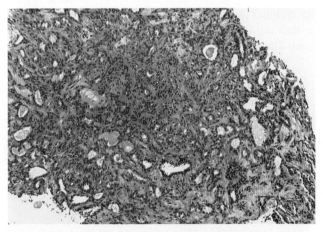

FIGURE 10. Fibroadenoma with florid sclerosing adenosis. This needle core biopsy specimen reveals a dense glandular proliferation characteristically found in an adenosis tumor. The pattern shown here could be mistaken for infiltrating carcinoma.

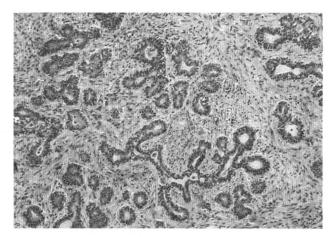

FIGURE 11. Juvenile fibroadenoma. The lesion features a balanced proliferation of glands and stroma.

munohistochemistry shows estrogen receptor activity to be largely in the epithelium of fibroadenomas, whereas progesterone receptor is reportedly localized in the stroma as well as the epithelium (15,16). Secretory hyperplasia sometimes occurs diffusely in fibroadenomas during pregnancy. Fibroadenomas with secretory hyperplasia should be distinguished from the tumor commonly referred to as *lactating adenoma*, which is a compact aggregate of lobules exhibiting secretory hyperplasia. Ultrasonography of lactating adenomas reveals one or more hypoechoic, well-defined masses (17).

Juvenile fibroadenomas account for less than 4% of all fibroadenomas, with the majority of the patients under 20 years of age (18). Tumors with the histologic features of juvenile fibroadenoma have been found in adult women as old as 72 years (19). Juvenile fibroadenomas are characterized microscopically by stromal cellularity and epithelial hyperplasia (Fig. 11). The architecture is more often pericanalicular than intracanalicular or exhibits a mixture of these patterns. The cellular density of the stroma is variable in any given tumor and among lesions, ranging from areas of dense collagenization to foci that are quite cellular. Mitoses are few or absent in the stroma and epithelium. Little or no atypia and pleomorphism are encountered in the bipolar fibroblastic stromal cells. Epithelial elements are usually distributed homogeneously in the tumor without the stromal overgrowth that characterizes cystosarcomas. Most juvenile fibroadenomas feature conspicuous epithelial hyperplasia that may have a ductal, lobular, or combined ductal-lobular configuration (19).

Neoplastic changes can develop in the epithelium of a fibroadenoma. This is more often manifested as lobular carcinoma *in situ* than as intraductal carcinoma (Fig. 12). Invasive carcinoma is uncommon in fibroadenomas.

Many fibroadenomas can be reliably diagnosed by needle core biopsy and do not require excision. Management consists of clinical follow-up. When the sample has features that raise concern about a possible cystosarcoma, excisional biopsy is recommended (Fig. 13). Abnormalities that suggest an indeterminate diagnosis in a needle core biopsy sample include an ill-defined border, noteworthy stromal cellularity, and mitoses and atypia of stromal cells (Fig. 14).

CYSTOSARCOMA PHYLLODES

There are no specific clinical features that make it possible to distinguish reliably between a fibroadenoma and a cystosarcoma (20). A diagnosis of cystosarcoma may be favored if the tumor is larger than 4 cm or if there is a history of rapid growth. Cystosarcomas usually occur as solitary unilateral tumors. Rarely, multifocal cystosarcomas have been detected in a single breast, or both breasts may be affected (21). Coexistent fibroadenomas, which are found histologically in nearly 40% of cases, are not always apparent clinically (21).

Cystosarcomas have been reported in patients ranging in age from 10 to 86 years, with a median and mean age of about 45 years, approximately 20 years older than the me-

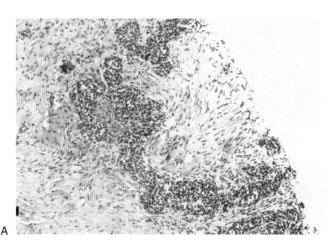

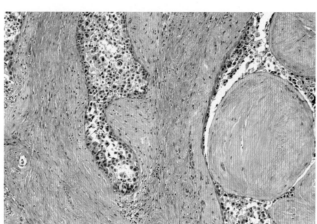

A   B

FIGURE 12. Fibroadenoma with carcinoma. A: A needle core biopsy specimen with lobular carcinoma *in situ* in a fibroadenoma. **B:** Intraductal carcinoma is present in this sclerotic fibroadenoma.

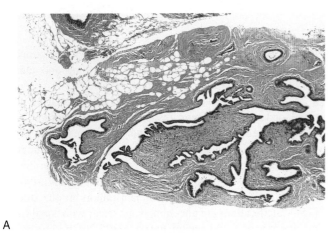

A

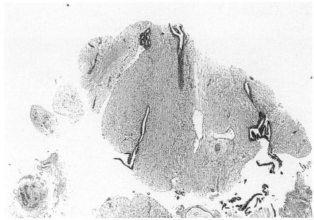

B

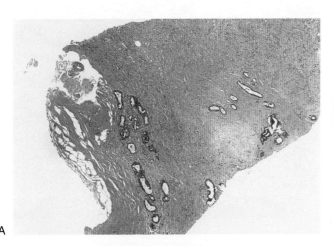

C

FIGURE 13. Fibroadenoma versus cystosarcoma. A:
This needle core biopsy specimen shows a fibroadenoma
with an exaggerated intracanalicular growth pattern suggestive of a cystosarcoma. **B,C:** This needle core biopsy
sample is from a lesion that proved to be a benign cystosarcoma, a diagnosis suggested by the moderately cellular stroma and epithelium-lined clefts.

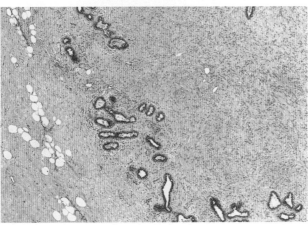

A

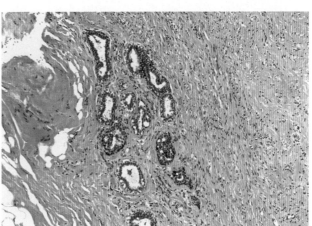

B

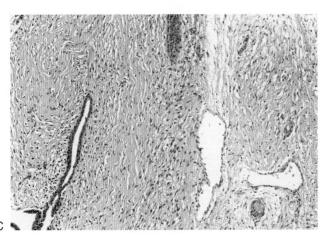

C

FIGURE 14. Fibroadenoma versus cystosarcoma.
A,B: This needle core biopsy specimen reveals stromal
overgrowth and an ill-defined junction with the adjacent
breast tissue. **C:** The excisional biopsy specimen shown
here duplicates the findings in the needle biopsy specimen
and is diagnostic of a benign cystosarcoma. The stroma of
the tumor consists of uniform spindle cells with an interlacing pattern.

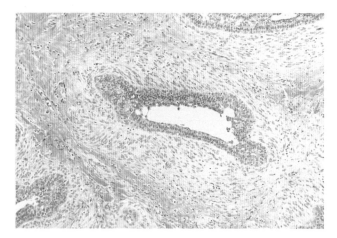

FIGURE 15. Cystosarcoma, benign. The stroma is characterized by greater cellularity in the subepithelial region.

dian age of patients with fibroadenomas. Cystosarcoma occurs rarely in children and female adolescents (22). The majority have been classified as benign, but a few examples of malignant cystosarcomas have been described in this age group (22). The reported average size of cystosarcomas is 4 to 5 cm (20,21,23). Although malignant cystosarcomas tend

to be larger than benign variants, there have been exceptional high-grade malignant lesions smaller than 2 cm and some very large histologically benign tumors.

Mammography reveals a round or lobulated, sharply defined, opaque mass in most instances. Indistinct borders are seen in a minority of cases. The tumor also appears to be well circumscribed with ultrasound, but it may be inhomogeneous because of the presence of cysts and epithelium-lined clefts (24). Cystic components were evident by ultrasound slightly more frequently in malignant tumors in one study (25). Calcifications are uncommon and occur with equal frequency in benign and malignant lesions (25,26). It is not possible to distinguish reliably between benign and malignant cystosarcomas by mammography or ultrasonography (24–26).

The tumors arise from periductal rather than intralobular stroma and usually contain sparse lobular elements. Most cystosarcomas are characterized by expansion and increased cellularity of the stromal component. In some tumors, cellularity is more dense in the periductal stroma (Fig. 15), but a substantial number of cystosarcomas have little or no zonal stromal distribution (Fig. 16). The presence of epithelium-lined clefts is associated with cystosarcomas (Fig. 17). Marked expansion of these spaces can result in a cystosar-

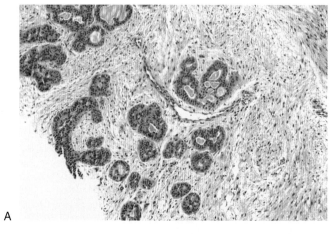

A

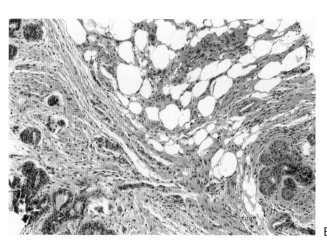

B

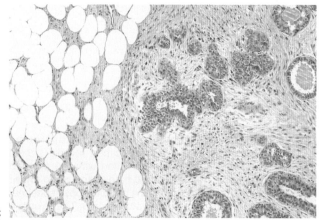

C

FIGURE 16. Cystosarcoma, benign. A,B: A needle core biopsy specimen showing invasive stroma at the periphery of the tumor in (B). There is no subepithelial concentration of stromal cells, and the epithelial proliferation has an adenosis-like appearance. **C:** Excisional biopsy specimen of the lesion shown in (A) and (B).

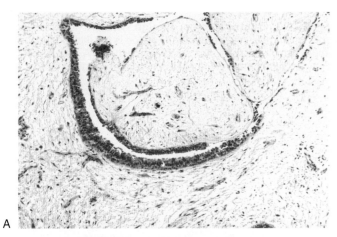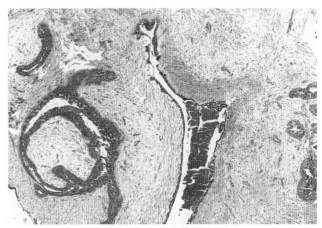

A   B

FIGURE 17. Cystosarcoma. A: Epithelium-lined spaces in a benign tumor are apparent in this needle core biopsy specimen. **B:** The excisional biopsy specimen shown here has epithelium-lined spaces and focal hemorrhage caused by the needle core biopsy.

coma that has a papillary structure (Fig. 18). The intracanalicular architecture of some fibroadenomas bears a superficial resemblance to the clefted structure of benign cystosarcomas, and occasionally the distinction between the two tumor types may be difficult in a needle core biopsy sample.

The stroma in many cystosarcomas is heterogeneous. Foci indistinguishable from a fibroadenoma may abut sharply on much more cellular regions. This structural variability can create substantial difficulty in the accurate classification of lesions sampled by needle core biopsy. Reported instances of malignant clinical behavior or metastases from a "benign" cystosarcoma are probably a reflection of inaccurate classification of the tumor because of incomplete sampling. Ultimately, excisional biopsy is required to grade a cystosarcoma, a determination based on stromal cellularity, mitotic activity, and the microscopic character of the tumor border.

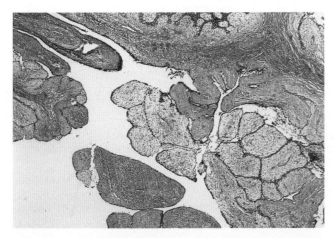

FIGURE 18. Cystosarcoma, papillary. Exaggerated spaces outlined by epithelium create a cystic papillary appearance in this benign tumor.

A benign cystosarcoma is characterized by few or no stromal mitoses, rarely more than one per 10 high-power fields (HPF), and modest stromal cellular overgrowth (Fig. 19). Epithelial hyperplasia is not conspicuous in the average benign cystosarcoma. The border of the tumor is more often circumscribed than invasive. Sometimes, invasion takes the form of secondary peripheral fibroepithelial nodules (Fig. 20). Adipose (Fig. 21) and osseous metaplasia can occur in the stroma of a benign cystosarcoma, and stromal cells with multiple hyperchromatic nuclei may be present (Fig. 22). Pseudoangiomatous hyperplasia of the stroma occurs in a small percentage of cystosarcomas (Fig. 23).

A high-grade malignant cystosarcoma is characterized by marked hypercellular stromal overgrowth that results in substantial separation of epithelial elements, proliferative activity in the stroma (typically exceeding five mitoses per 10 HPF), and usually an invasive tumor border (Fig. 24). Stromal cellular pleomorphism is common in these lesions. Rarely, the stroma contains heterologous sarcomatous elements, such as angiosarcoma, liposarcoma, or myosarcoma (27,28).

A low-grade malignant or "borderline" cystosarcoma usually has a microscopically invasive border, two to five mitoses per 10 HPF, and moderate stromal cellularity that is often heterogeneously distributed in the midst of hypocellular areas. The spindle-cell stroma in most of these lesions resembles low-grade fibrosarcoma (Fig. 25). Infrequent instances of cartilaginous, osseous, and lipomatous differentiation have been reported in low-grade malignant cystosarcomas.

Many cystosarcomas have foci of epithelial hyperplasia (Fig. 26). There is a general tendency for the severity of epithelial hyperplasia to parallel the intensity of stromal proliferation, but many exceptions to this rule are encountered (Fig. 27). Grimes (21) found "marked epithelial hyperplasia" in one third of benign cystosarcomas, including four (13%)

Text continues on page 78

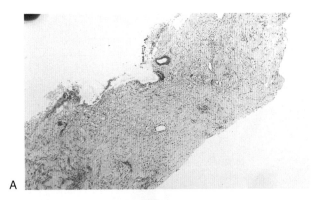

FIGURE 19. Cystosarcoma, benign. A,B: A needle core biopsy specimen. The border of the lesion is not included in this sample, which exhibits stromal overgrowth. **C:** A needle core biopsy specimen from another lesion, with an invasive border.

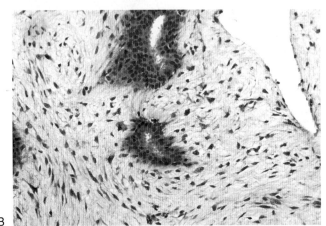

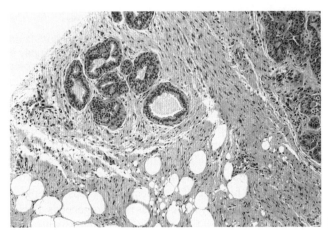

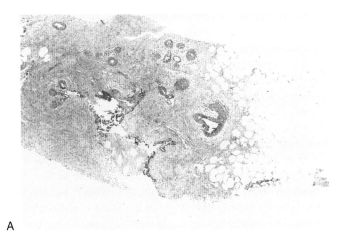

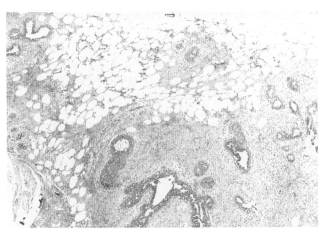

FIGURE 20. Cystosarcoma, benign. A: A needle core biopsy specimen showing an invasive border. **B:** The invasive growth pattern as seen in the excisional biopsy. Secondary nodules are present in the fat.

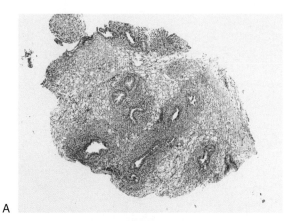

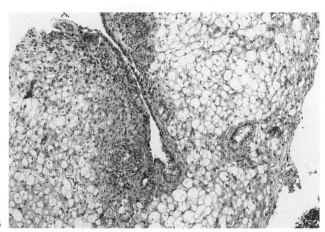

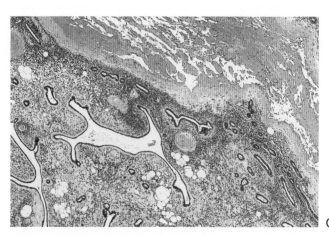

FIGURE 21. Cystosarcoma, benign with adipose differentiation. A,B: A needle core biopsy specimen in which the stroma consists of adipose tissue. Mitoses were absent. **C:** The excisional biopsy specimen of the tumor revealed diffuse adipose differentiation. There is angiomatous transformation adjacent to the tumor in the organizing hematoma resulting from the prior needle core biopsy.

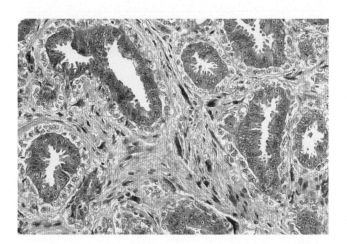

FIGURE 22. Cystosarcoma, benign with stromal giant cells. Multinucleated giant cells are present in the stroma.

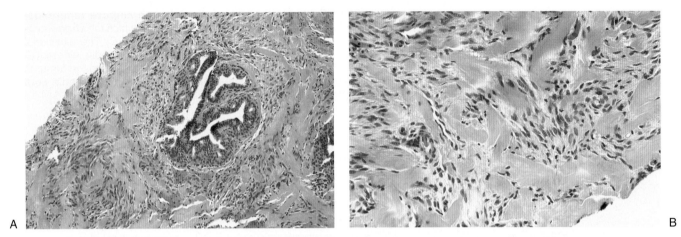

FIGURE 23. Cystosarcoma, benign with pseudoangiomatous stromal hyperplasia. A,B: This lesion has a prominent fascicular stromal pattern composed of bundles of myofibroblasts. The patient was a 75-year-old woman with a recently detected 1.5-cm tumor.

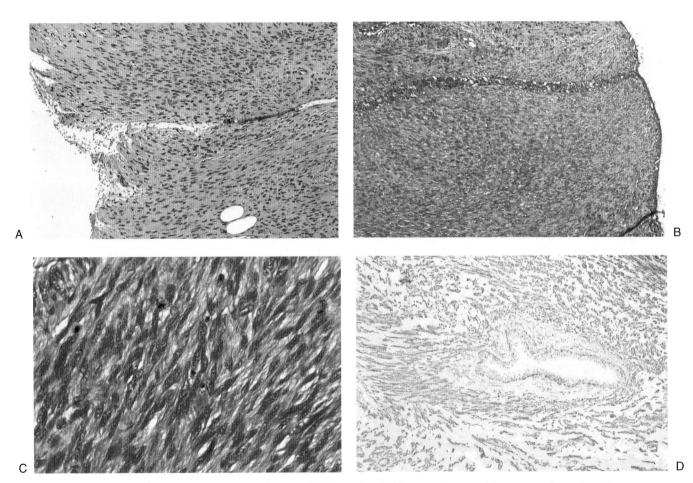

FIGURE 24. Cystosarcoma, malignant, high-grade. A: The needle core biopsy specimen is a fibrosarcomatous cystosarcoma. **B–D:** The epithelium-lined cleft in (B) is virtually obliterated in this needle core biopsy specimen from a tumor with leiomyosarcomatous differentiation. The tumor cells are immunoreactive for actin in (D) (immunoperoxidase: smooth-muscle actin).

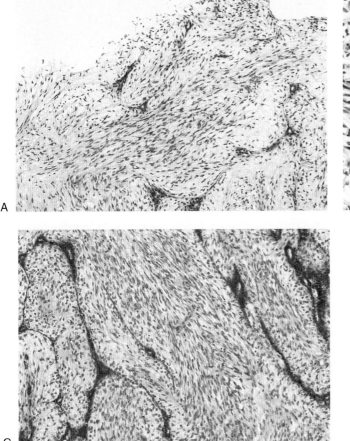

FIGURE 25. Cystosarcoma, malignant, low-grade. A,B: A needle core biopsy specimen showing moderately cellular stroma and tightly compressed epithelial slits. **C:** Excisional biopsy specimen of the tumor showing low-grade fibrosarcomatous stroma with rare mitotic figures.

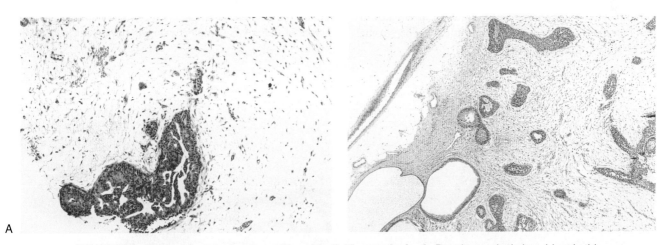

FIGURE 26. Cystosarcoma, benign with epithelial hyperplasia. A: Duct hyperplasia is evident in this needle core biopsy specimen. **B:** The excisional biopsy specimen shows cysts and duct hyperplasia.

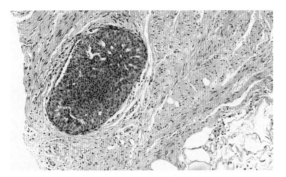

FIGURE 27. Cystosarcoma, benign with florid epithelial hyperplasia. The stromal component in this needle biopsy specimen is not notably cellular in the region of the hyperplastic epithelium.

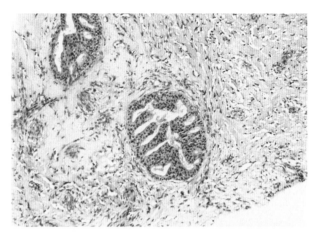

FIGURE 29. Cystosarcoma, benign with intraductal carcinoma. The intraductal carcinoma in this needle core biopsy specimen has micropapillary and cribriform features.

with atypia, and in 26% of malignant cystosarcomas. Atypical epithelial hyperplasia is sometimes extreme, leading to consideration of the diagnosis of intraductal carcinoma (Fig. 28). The cystosarcomatous character of the tumor may be overlooked if the stromal component is interpreted as reactive rather than as an intrinsic part of the neoplasm. However, the epithelial proliferation rarely reaches a level acceptable as intraductal carcinoma, and the diagnosis of intraductal carcinoma in a cystosarcoma is very infrequent (29) (Fig. 29). Lobular carcinoma *in situ* can also develop in a cystosarcoma. Squamous metaplasia of ductal epithelium, which occurs in benign and malignant tumors, is found in about 10% of cystosarcomas (21). Apocrine metaplasia has also been reported in the epithelium of cystosarcomas (21). The stroma of cystosarcomas is vimentin-positive. Actin and desmin reactivity are present in a variable proportion of tumors that exhibit myoid differentiation (30). The stromal cells rarely show S-100 reactivity.

The classification of a cystosarcoma as benign or low- or high-grade malignant reflects an estimate of the probable clinical course as determined by the histologic appearance of the tumor. A benign cystosarcoma will not metastasize, and the probability of local recurrence is low (approximately 20%) after local excision (31). With a low-grade malignant cystosarcoma, there is a slight probability (<5%) of metastasis, but such a tumor is more likely than a benign cystosarcoma to recur locally unless it is widely excised. Metastases occur in about 25% of high-grade malignant cystosarcomas, and these lesions are also very prone to local recurrence. Fewer than 1% of high-grade cystosarcomas give rise to axillary lymph node metastases (21,32). The fundamental principle of therapy is complete excision to prevent local recurrence (32–35).

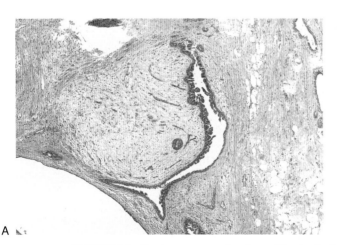

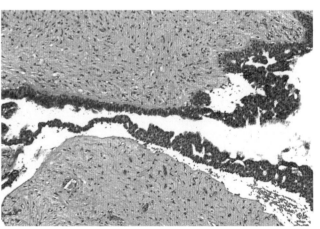

A   B

FIGURE 28. Cystosarcoma, benign with atypical epithelial hyperplasia. A,B: A needle core biopsy specimen showing atypical micropapillary epithelium.

REFERENCES

1. Kovi J, Chu HB, Leffall L Jr. Sclerosing lobular hyperplasia manifesting as a palpable mass of the breast in young black women. *Hum Pathol* 1984;15:336–340.
2. Poulton TB, Shaw de Pardeds E, Baldwin M. Sclerosing lobular hyperplasia of the breast: imaging features in 15 cases. *AJR Am J Roentgenol* 1995;165:291–294.
3. Dupont WD, Page DL, Parl FF, et al. Long-term risk of breast cancer in women with fibroadenoma. *N Engl J Med* 1994;331:10–15.
4. Foster ME, Garrahan N, Williams S. Fibroadenoma of the breast: a clinical and pathological study. *J R Coll Surg Edinb* 1988; 33:16–19.
5. Oberman HA. Breast lesions in the adolescent female. *Pathol Annu* 1979;14:175–201.
6. Moross T, Lang AP, Mahoney L. Tubular adenoma of breast. *Arch Pathol Lab Med* 1983;107:84–86.
7. Tesluk H, Amott T, Goodnight JE. Apocrine adenoma of the breast. *Arch Pathol Lab Med* 1986;110:351–352.
8. Gusterson BA, Sloane JP, Middwood C, et al. Ductal adenoma of the breast—a lesion exhibiting a myoepithelial/epithelial phenotype. *Histopathology* 1987;11:103–110.
9. Chen KTK. Pleomorphic adenoma of the breast. *Am J Clin Pathol* 1990;93:792–794.
10. Goodman ZD, Taxy JB. Fibroadenomas of the breast with prominent smooth muscle. *Am J Surg Pathol* 1981;5:99–101.
11. Powell CM, Rosen PP. Adipose differentiation in cystosarcoma phyllodes. *Am J Surg Pathol* 1994;18:720–727.
12. Powell CM, Cranor ML, Rosen PP. Multinucleated stromal giant cells in mammary fibroepithelial neoplasms. A study of 11 patients. *Arch Pathol Lab Med* 1994;118:912–916.
13. Meyer JE, Lester SC, DiPiro PJ, Ferraro FA, Frenna TH, Denison CM. Occult calcified fibroadenomas. *Breast Dis* 1995;8:29–38.
14. Fechner RE. Fibroadenomas in patients receiving oral contraceptives: a clinical and pathologic study. *Am J Clin Pathol* 1970;53:857–864.
15. Mechtersheimer G, Kruger KH, Born IA, Moller P. Antigenic profile of mammary fibroadenoma and cystosarcoma phyllodes. A study using antibodies to estrogen and progesterone receptors and to a panel of cell surface molecules. *Pathol Res Pract* 1990;186:427–438.
16. Rao BR, Meyer JS, Fry CG. Most cystosarcoma phyllodes and fibroadenomas have progesterone receptor but lack estrogen receptor: a stromal localization of progesterone receptor. *Cancer* 1981;47:2016–2021.
17. Tobin CE, Hendrix TM, Geyer SJ, Mendelson EB, Resnikoff LB. Breast imaging case of the day. *Radiographics* 1996;16:1225–1226.
18. Pike A, Oberman HA. Juvenile (cellular) adenofibromas. A clincopatholgic study. *Am J Surg Pathol* 1985;9:730–736.
19. Mies C, Rosen PP. Juvenile fibroadenoma with atypical epithelial hyperplasia. *Am J Surg Pathol* 1987;11:184–190.
20. Cohn-Cedermark G, Rutqvist LE, Rosendahl I, Silverswärd C. Prognostic factors in cystosarcoma phyllodes. A clinicopathologic study of 77 patients. *Cancer* 1991;68:2017–2022.
21. Grimes MM. Cystosarcoma phyllodes of the breast: histologic features, flow cytometry analysis, and clinical correlations. *Mod Pathol* 1992;5:232–239.
22. Rajan PB, Cranor ML, Rosen PP. Cystosarcoma phyllodes in adolescent girls and young women: a study of 45 patients. *Am J Surg Pathol* 1998;22:64–69.
23. Reinfuss M, Mitus J, Smolak K, Stelmach A. Malignant phyllodes tumours of the breast. A clinical and pathological analysis of 55 cases. *Eur J Cancer* 1993;29A:1252–1256.
24. Buchberger W, Strasser K, Heim K, Müller E, Schröcksnadel P. Phyllodes tumor: findings on mammography, sonography, and aspiration cytology in 10 cases. *AJR Am J Roentgenol* 1991;157:715–719.
25. Liberman L, Bonaccio E, Hamele-Bena D, Abramson AF, Cohen MA, Dershaw DD. Benign and malignant phyllodes tumors: mammographic and sonographic findings. *Radiology* 1996;198:121–124.
26. Cosmacini P, Zurrida S, Veronesi P, Bartoli C, Coopmans de Yoldi GF. Phyllode tumor of the breast: mammographic experience in 99 cases. *Eur J Radiol* 1992;15:11–14.
27. Barnes L, Pietruszka M. Rhabdomyosarcoma arising within a breast cystosarcoma phyllodes and its mimic: An immunohistochemical study. *Am J Surg Pathol* 1978;2:423–429.
28. Powell CM, Rosen PP. Adipose differentiation in cystosarcoma phyllodes. *Am J Surg Pathol* 1994;18:720–727.
29. Knudsen PJ, Ostergaard J. Cystosarcoma phyllodes with lobular and ductal carcinoma *in situ. Arch Pathol Lab Med* 1987;111:873–875.
30. Aranda FI, Laforga JB, Lopez JI. Phyllodes tumor of the breast. An immunohistochemical study of 28 cases with special attention to the role of myofibroblasts. *Path Res Pract* 1994;190:474–481.
31. Reinfuss M, Mitus J, Duda K, Stelmach A, Rys J, Smolak K. The treatment and prognosis of patients with phyllodes tumor of the breast. An analysis of 170 cases. *Cancer* 1996;77:910–916.
32. Treves N, Sunderland DA. Cystosarcoma phyllodes of the breast: a malignant and a benign tumor. A clinicopathological study of seventy-seven cases. *Cancer* 1951;4:1286–1332.
33. Bartoli C, Zurrida S, Veronesi P, et al. Small-sized phyllodes tumor of the breast. *Eur J Surg Oncol* 1990;16:215–219.
34. McGregor GI, Knowling MA, Este FA. Sarcoma and cystosarcoma phyllodes tumors of the breast—a retrospective review of 58 cases. *Am J Surg* 1994;167:477–480.
35. Salvadori B, Cusumano F, Del Bo R, et al. Surgical treatment of phyllodes tumors of the breast. *Cancer* 1989;63:2532–2536.

CHAPTER 8

Ductal Hyperplasia and Intraductal Carcinoma

DUCTAL HYPERPLASIA—ORDINARY AND ATYPICAL

The distinction between intraductal hyperplasia and intraductal carcinoma is important for patient management (1). In most instances, intraductal proliferations are readily classified by pathologists on the basis of generally accepted histopathologic features as either hyperplasia or *in situ* carcinoma (2). There exists a small subset for which assignment to either of these categories is less certain. The existence of these "borderline" lesions, which may be diagnosed as atypical hyperplasia or *in situ* carcinoma depending on which criteria are employed, is not a compelling reason for abandoning the existing practice of distinguishing pathologically and clinically between ductal hyperplasia and *in situ* carcinoma. Studies of interobserver differences in the diagnosis of highly selected examples of these lesions have focused attention on this troublesome diagnostic problem that applies to a small percentage of proliferative breast changes (3–5).

No clinical features are specifically associated with ductal hyperplasia. The alterations caused by epithelial proliferation in individual ducts or in groups of ducts are microscopic in dimension and consequently often not palpable. Ductal hyperplasia in various forms is a frequent constituent of "fibrocystic changes" that may be detected by mammography or as a palpable tumor. The lesion complex can also include sclerosing adenosis, cystic and papillary apocrine metaplasia, duct stasis, fibrosis or pseudoangiomatous stromal hyperplasia, and lobular hyperplasia. An important corollary to the lack of clinical indicators of ductal hyperplasia is an inability to determine the duration of these lesions. The date on which a patient with ductal hyperplasia has undergone biopsy is customarily used as if it were the date of "onset." This practice, which is the consequence of an inability to determine the preclinical duration of hyperplastic ductal lesions, can be a source of bias when the precancerous significance of proliferative lesions in an individual patient is assessed.

The mammographic manifestations of duct hyperplasia include altered duct patterns, parenchymal distortion, nonpalpable mass lesions, calcification, and asymmetry when both breasts are compared. Calcifications are the most frequent mammographic indication of atypical ductal hyperplasia in the absence of a palpable abnormality (6–8). Lesions described on mammography as radial scars often have a component of ductal hyperplasia. Some but not all radial scar lesions contain microcalcifications. In the era that preceded the widespread use of mammography, when the indication for biopsy was a palpable abnormality, ductal hyperplasia was found in 25% or fewer of specimens obtained (9,10). Not more than 5% of these biopsy specimens had atypical ductal hyperplasia. The frequency of these atypical abnormalities is higher in patients who undergo mammographically directed biopsies, including surgical excisions and stereotaxic core biopsies (11,12).

Ductal hyperplasia can be found in female patients at virtually any age. After age 60, ductal hyperplasia becomes less frequent, and when present, the growth pattern is usually less florid than in younger women. However, an occasional woman older than 60 years may be found to have extensive proliferative changes with florid ductal hyperplasia. The use of exogenous estrogens can be documented in some but not all of these cases.

Ductal hyperplasia describes a proliferative condition that is manifested histologically as an increase in the cellularity of epithelium in ducts. Because the normal resting epithelium consists of a continuous monolayer of cuboidal-to-columnar epithelial cells supported by a discontinuous layer of myoepithelial cells, an increase in the cellularity of this two-layer configuration constitutes hyperplasia. The increased thickness of the epithelial layer results in partial or complete obstruction of the duct lumen at the site of the proliferative abnormality. If intraductal hyperplasia is traced in serial sections, it is often possible to observe the discontinuous and multifocal nature of the condition. Various distortions of the basic ductal architecture occur when hyperplastic ducts become more sinuous or are incorporated into complex proliferative lesions, such as papillomas or "radial scars."

Ordinary (Usual) Ductal Hyperplasia

When individual cell borders are inconspicuous, the cellular proliferation in ductal hyperplasia has a syncytial appearance. Cytoplasmic vacuolization may occur. True intracytoplasmic microlumina containing secretion that stains positively with the mucicarmine or alcian blue-PAS (periodic acid–Schiff) stains are extremely uncommon in hyper-

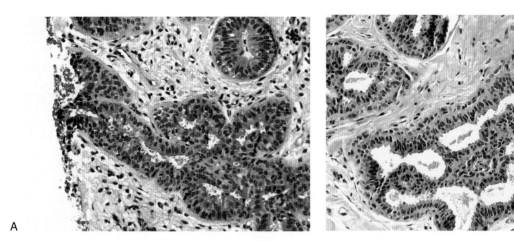

FIGURE 1. Ductal hyperplasia, mild. A: The small ducts in this needle core biopsy specimen are lined by epithelium that is one or two cells in thickness. **B:** Minimal papillary hyperplasia in another needle core biopsy specimen. Hyperplasia of myoepithelial cells is also evident.

plastic ductal epithelium (13). The presence of intracytoplasmic mucin-containing microlumina is an atypical feature that should occasion careful consideration of a diagnosis of intraductal carcinoma. In duct hyperplasia, nuclear spacing is uneven, so that in some areas the cells appear crowded and the nuclei seem to overlap. Nucleoli are inapparent or inconspicuous unless there is a prominent element of apocrine metaplasia. Mitotic figures are very infrequent and when present have a regular configuration.

Mild hyperplasia may affect the entire epithelium circumferentially in a duct cross section or only a segment of the duct. It occurs as an increase in the amount of epithelium, which rarely exceeds three cells in thickness. The epithelium may be focally papillary (Fig. 1).

In moderate hyperplasia, the epithelium tends to be more than three cells in thickness. Intraluminal proliferation is more pronounced than in mild hyperplasia, resulting in the formation of secondary glandular lumina (Fig. 2). Part of the

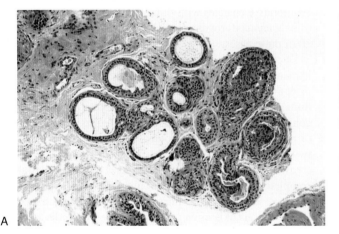

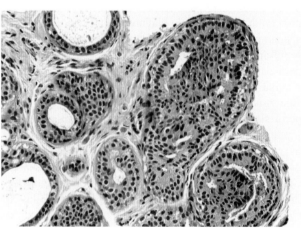

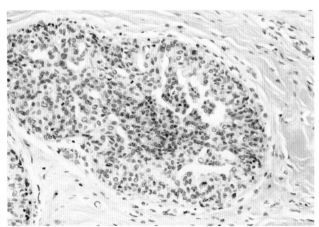

FIGURE 2. Ductal hyperplasia, moderate. A,B: This hyperplastic focus in a needle core biopsy specimen has a radial scar pattern. Note the persistent columnar duct epithelium at the periphery of hyperplastic ducts. **C:** This duct from another specimen is nearly filled with hyperplastic epithelium. Note condensation of the cells with diminished cytoplasm in the center of the duct, and a single epithelial mitosis near the lower right corner.

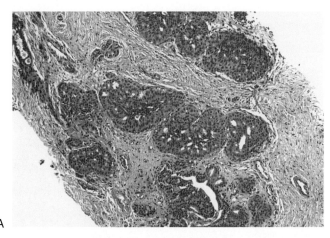 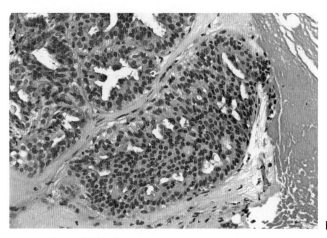

FIGURE 3. Ductal hyperplasia, moderate. A,B: Hyperplastic epithelium fills the ducts in this needle core biopsy specimen, forming a fenestrated pattern. Cells in the center have small, condensed nuclei and scant cytoplasm. Columnar epithelium is present at the periphery.

duct lumen may remain as a crescentic space or spaces at the edge of the duct in this cribriform-like hyperplasia (Fig. 3). Micropapillary hyperplasia is part of the spectrum of mild and moderate ductal hyperplasia (Fig. 4). The papillae are blunt or slender, irregularly shaped fronds of epithelium in which cells are smaller and have more condensed nuclei than do those in the adjacent basal epithelium. See Chapter 13 for a discussion of columnar cell hyperplasia and tubular carcinoma.

The nuclei in moderate hyperplasia are often overlapping and irregularly shaped, and they may be distributed in a "streaming" fashion (Fig. 5). Streaming refers to a growth pattern in which the nuclei of hyperplastic epithelial cells are oriented parallel to the long axes of the cells (Fig. 6). Because the cytoplasmic borders of these cells are often indistinct, streaming is usually detected as a parallel orientation of oval or spindle-shaped nuclei. Streaming occurs in most structural patterns of moderate, severe, and atypical intra-

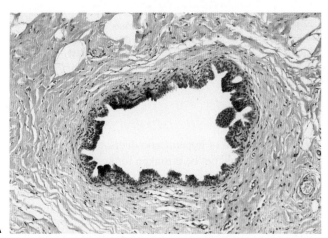 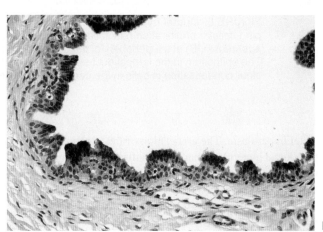

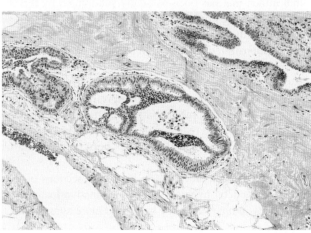

FIGURE 4. Ductal hyperplasia, micropapillary. A,B: The blunt micropapillary epithelium consists of columnar cells with dark, condensed nuclei and scant cytoplasm. **C:** Well-preserved columnar ductal epithelium is present at the periphery of this duct, with a complex micropapillary proliferation in the lumen.

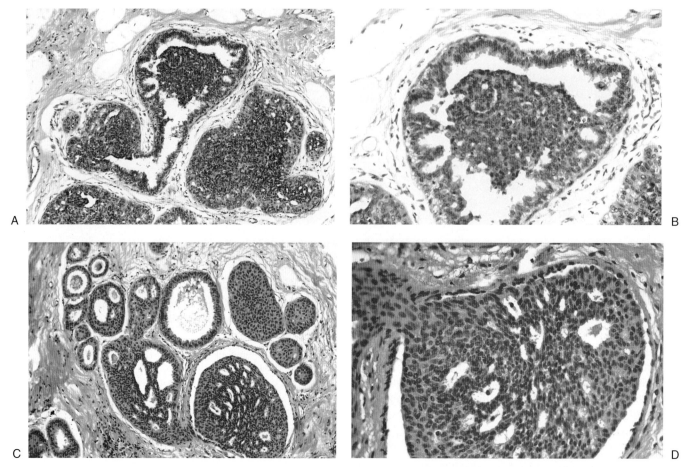

FIGURE 5. Ductal hyperplasia, florid. A,B: In this needle core biopsy specimen, the dense, overlapping cellular proliferation has solid and papillary patterns. Columnar and micropapillary hyperplasia are apparent in (B) at the periphery of the duct. **C,D:** Solid and fenestrated hyperplasia is seen in this lesion. The epithelium in the largest duct structure has a streaming pattern. Note the loss of cytoplasm and nuclear condensation in cells in the center of the ducts.

ductal hyperplasia. The association of the streaming pattern with ductal hyperplasia has been confirmed by computerized morphometric analysis of the orientation of nuclei in proliferative duct lesions (14).

The distinction between moderate and florid hyperplasia is not sharp, but lesions are generally placed in the latter category when the affected ducts are appreciably enlarged in comparison with nonhyperplastic counterparts. Florid hyperplasia has the papillary and bridging growth patterns that are encountered in moderate hyperplasia, but the overall proliferation tends to be more cellular and complex than in moderate hyperplasia (Fig. 7). Foci of florid hyperplasia are more likely to fill the entire duct lumen in a solid or fenestrated fashion.

Necrotic cellular debris is rarely present in hyperplastic ducts, and when found, it is usually associated with florid sclerosing papillary hyperplasia (Fig. 8). Hyperplastic ducts with necrosis are indistinguishable cytologically and structurally from adjacent ducts with non-necrotic hyperplastic epithelium. Histiocytes or foam cells are found relatively of-

ten in the lumina of hyperplastic ducts, and the presence of these cells should not be mistaken for necrosis (Fig. 9).

The fenestrated growth pattern that occurs in moderate and severe ductal hyperplasia results from the formation of epithelial bridges that become joined as they traverse the duct lumen. The fenestrations represent portions of the original lumen that has been passively subdivided by the complex arborizing epithelial proliferation. Using a serial-section, three-dimensional reconstruction method, Ohuchi et al. (15) demonstrated that the lumina that appear to be separated from each other in a two-dimensional histologic section of papillary intraductal hyperplasia are actually part of a network of channels surrounded by the proliferating epithelium. By contrast, three-dimensional reconstruction of intraductal carcinoma revealed that the fenestrations in these lesions are newly formed disconnected spaces bordered by polarized neoplastic cells.

The spaces that are found in histologic sections of fenestrated intraductal hyperplasia have distinctive features. The secondary lumina tend to be larger and more numerous at the

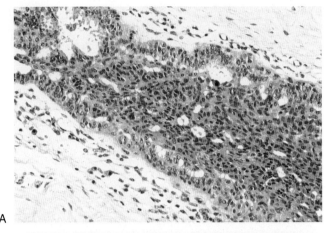

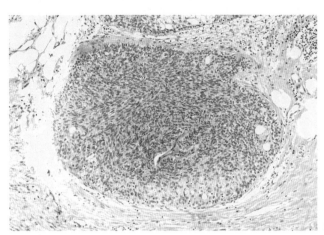

A

B

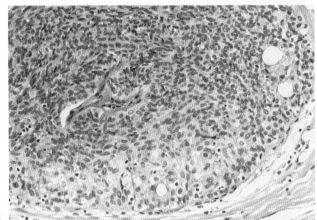

C

FIGURE 6. Ductal hyperplasia, florid with streaming. A: The hyperplastic epithelium in the lumen of this duct is composed of cells with a streaming pattern. Note the persistent columnar ductal epithelium and microlumina at the border of the duct. **B,C:** This solid ductal hyperplasia is composed of spindle cells with a streaming pattern. Cuboidal cells and microlumina are present at the perimeter of the duct.

periphery of the duct than centrally, but the reverse distribution may be encountered. Cells outlining these spaces are arranged in a haphazard fashion except at the edge of the duct, where residual columnar or cuboidal duct epithelium composed of cells with more regularly oriented nuclei may persist. The shapes of the spaces in a given duct are usually varied (ovoid, crescentic, irregular, or serpiginous) rather than rounded as

they tend to be in cribriform carcinoma (Figs. 3,5–7,10). The spaces formed in intraductal hyperplasia may be empty or may contain secretion and histiocytes. Fine calcifications can develop in the glandular lumina of intraductal hyperplasia.

A layer of myoepithelial cells is often evident at the edge of the hyperplastic duct (Fig. 11). These cells may accompany the proliferation into the duct lumen when the fibrovascular

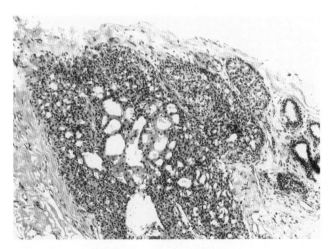

FIGURE 7. Ductal hyperplasia, florid. The hyperplastic duct in this needle core biopsy specimen is enlarged and filled by epithelium with solid and fenestrated areas. Apocrine metaplasia is present in the center.

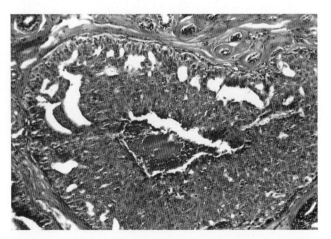

FIGURE 8. Ductal hyperplasia, florid with necrosis. Necrosis is present in the center of this hyperplastic duct, which was part of sclerosing papillary duct hyperplasia. Columnar epithelium can be seen at the periphery of the duct, where there are microlumina of various sizes and shapes.

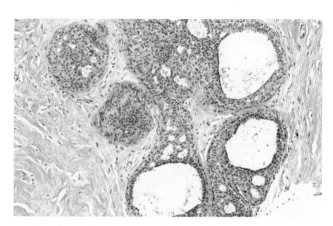

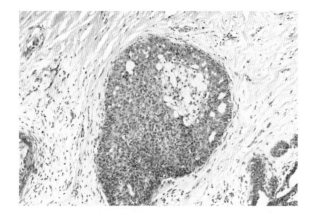

FIGURE 9. Ductal hyperplasia, florid with histiocytes. The epithelial proliferation in this enlarged duct is solid with peripheral fenestrations.

FIGURE 10. Ductal hyperplasia, florid. Microlumina and the main duct lumina are apparent in these ducts obtained by needle core biopsy.

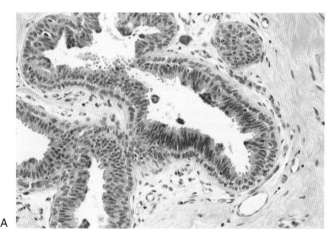

A

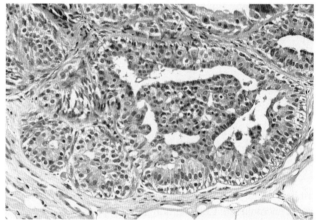

B

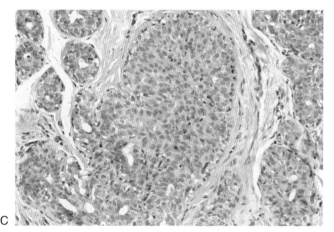

C

FIGURE 11. Ductal hyperplasia with myoepithelial cells. Three different samples show progressively more florid epithelial hyperplasia and diminishing myoepithelial cell hyperplasia. **A:** Columnar cell hyperplasia. **B:** Papillary hyperplasia. **C:** Solid hyperplasia.

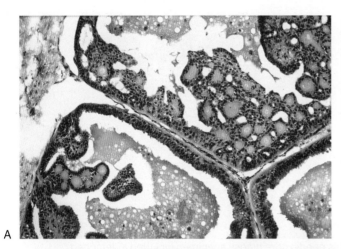

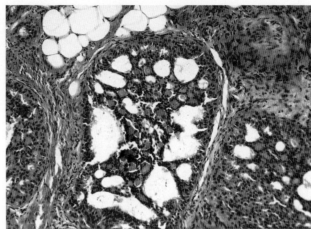

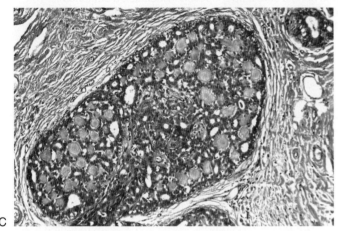

FIGURE 12. Ductal hyperplasia with collagenous spherulosis. Three patterns of hyperplasia with collagenous spherulosis. **A:** Papillary growth with prominent eosinophilic spherules. **B:** Cribriform hyperplasia with small spherules amidst the microlumina. **C:** Solid hyperplasia with prominent laminated spherules.

stromal framework of papillary hyperplasia is present. Because myoepithelial cells can persist at the periphery of ducts with intraductal carcinoma or with intraductal hyperplasia, their presence or absence is not a reliable criterion for distinguishing between these lesions. Collagenous spherulosis is a special form of duct hyperplasia wherein persistent myoepithelial cells contribute to the formation of nodular subepithelial deposits of basement membrane material (Fig. 12).

Atypical Ductal Hyperplasia

There is broad agreement on the general description of atypical ductal hyperplasia as a proliferative lesion that fulfills some but not all criteria for a diagnosis of intraductal carcinoma. By extension, it can be stated that atypical ductal hyperplasia has features of ordinary hyperplasia and of intraductal carcinoma. The difficulty in arriving at a more precise definition lies in the specifics. In general, these can be considered under two headings: quantitative and qualitative. The former refers to the extent of a proliferative abnormality, whereas the latter is concerned with microscopic structural and cytologic details.

Quantitative criteria for distinguishing between ductal hyperplasia and intraductal carcinoma have been based on the number of duct cross sections that exhibit the abnormality or

the dimension of the affected area. Some investigators have classified proliferative lesions limited to a single duct as atypical ductal hyperplasia, even if the abnormality is qualitatively consistent with intraductal carcinoma (10). Based on the criterion requiring at least two fully involved duct cross sections for a diagnosis of intraductal carcinoma, cases with one qualitatively diagnostic duct are arbitrarily assigned to the category of atypical hyperplasia.

Another scheme emphasizes the microscopic dimensions of a lesion as one of the bases for a diagnosis of atypical ductal hyperplasia (16). According to these criteria, foci measuring less than 2 mm are diagnosed as atypical ductal hyperplasia, regardless of the number of duct cross sections, even if the individual ducts qualify as intraductal carcinoma. The 2-mm criterion was selected because ". . . it was at the level of one or more small ducts or ductules measuring around 2 mm in aggregate cross-sectional diameter that most pathologists felt hesitant in diagnosing a lesion as intraductal carcinoma" (17). Another explanation offered by the proponents of this criterion was that "questions about quantity are raised generally when dispersed lesions add up to from 1.6 to 2.7 mm in aggregate size. Therefore, we arbitrarily chose 2 mm as a cutoff point" (16).

No scientific studies have compared the clinical significance of different quantitative criteria. There is no *a priori* reason for choosing two duct cross sections or 2 mm as crit-

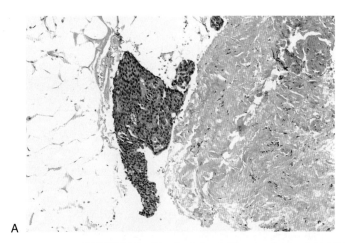
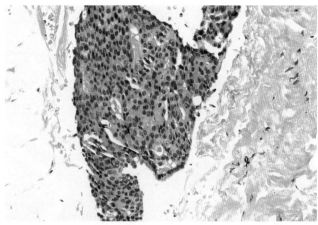

A   B

FIGURE 13. Atypical ductal hyperplasia. A,B: This needle core biopsy specimen included a detached fragment of nearly solid proliferative duct epithelium. There is a suggestion of streaming in the upper left corner, and a slender line of cuboidal ductal cells is seen along the border in the 6 o'clock axis.

ical decision points in relation to risk. For example, no data exist regarding the respective risks for subsequent development of carcinoma in patients with biopsy specimens containing proliferative lesions qualitatively consistent with intraductal carcinoma limited to one, two, or three duct cross sections. Regarding the dimensions of these lesions, no analysis comparing foci measuring 1.5 mm, 2.0 mm, 2.5 mm, or larger has been reported.

There are a number of technical issues that hamper the application of quantitative criteria, especially in the analysis of needle core biopsy findings. What appear to be two contiguous cross sections may prove in serial sections to be part of a single duct, or deeper sections of what appears to be a single-duct lesion may uncover additional involved duct cross sections. How close must two duct cross sections be to be considered contiguous? Is stroma between duct cross sec-

tions included in the measurement? Quantitative criteria assume that the ducts in question have been sectioned transversely. How to assess ducts cut longitudinally has not been adequately addressed. If the longitudinal dimension of a duct in a section exceeds 2 mm but the transverse diameter is 1 mm, should this focus be considered intraductal carcinoma when the 2-mm criterion is employed?

Others have rejected quantitative factors in the diagnosis of atypical ductal hyperplasia. This position was elaborated by Fisher et al. (18), who stated that "our definition of atypical ductal hyperplasia consists of a ductal epithelial alteration approximating but not unequivocally satisfying the criteria for a diagnosis of DCIS. It does not include arbitrarily established quantities of unequivocal DCIS (less than 2.0 mm or 2 'spaces')." In their study of the prognostic significance of proliferative breast disease, Bodian et al. (9) re-

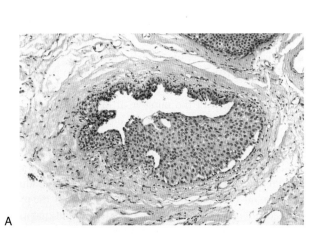
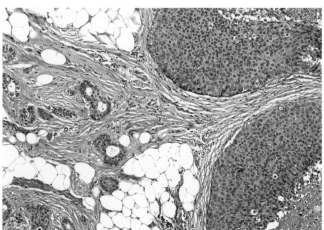

A   B

FIGURE 14. Atypical ductal hyperplasia. A: The needle core biopsy specimen from this patient contained this duct, part of which is occupied by a solid epithelial proliferation of monomorphic cells. Myoepithelial cells are apparent around most of the perimeter of the duct. This partially involved duct is an indication for excisional biopsy. **B:** The excisional biopsy specimen revealed intraductal and infiltrating duct carcinoma. The area of intraductal carcinoma has a more dense and cytologically more atypical cellular population than does the duct in (A).

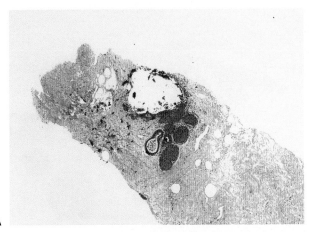 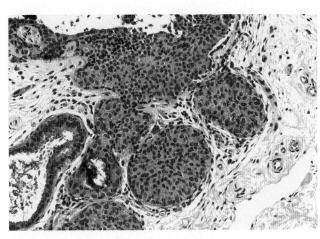

A B

FIGURE 15. Atypical ductal hyperplasia. A: This needle core biopsy specimen of mammographically detected calcifications shows a ductular proliferation that arose from a duct with calcification. The large intraductal calcification was fractured during preparation of the slide, causing blue-stained fragments to be deposited on the adjacent breast stroma. **B:** One ductule is uninvolved by the proliferative process, and another contains a small calcification. The site of the needle core biopsy in the subsequent excisional biopsy specimen contained no additional proliferative lesions.

ported that ". . . during the course of many years, intraductal carcinoma has been diagnosed if the characteristic features are present in only one ductal space."

The role of quantitative factors in the diagnosis of proliferative ductal lesions seems to lie between these extremes. The use of rigid criteria, such as two duct cross sections or 2 mm, can be justified in a research setting to ensure a homogeneous study group or to assess a particular criterion, but the strict application of these arbitrary rules in a clinical setting is difficult for the technical reasons stated above and poorly substantiated by existing data. Given the limitations of current methods for diagnosing intraductal lesions, quantitative factors sometimes play a role in the assessment of a particular lesion in material obtained by needle core biopsy. This situation arises when the specimen contains detached fragments of cytologically atypical epithelium (Fig. 13), or

when only part of one duct with changes suggestive of intraductal carcinoma is represented (Figs. 14–17). The same issue arises when a process that suggests lobular extension of ductal carcinoma is present (Fig. 18).

In many instances, the diagnosis of atypical hyperplasia depends on the presence of structural elements of intraductal carcinoma mingling with hyperplasia. Architecturally, this may be manifested by a cribriform pattern partially involving a duct (Figs. 19,20). Columnar cell, micropapillary and true papillary foci involving hyperplastic ducts constitute other architectural manifestations of atypical ductal hyperplasia (Fig. 21). Atypical hyperplasia can be encountered in ducts exhibiting apocrine metaplasia (Figs. 21,22). Cytologic atypia may involve individual cells, focal groups of cells, or the entire population of a proliferative lesion. Atypical features include nuclear enlargement with an increased

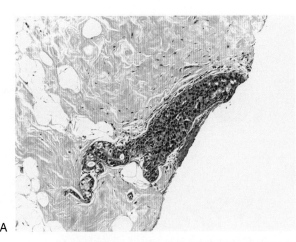 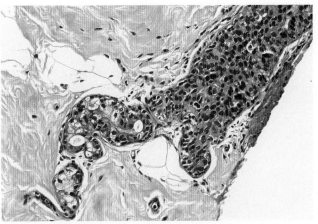

A B

FIGURE 16. Atypical ductal hyperplasia, solid. A,B: The duct at the edge of this specimen contained the only significant abnormality in this needle core biopsy specimen. Note the overlapping pattern of hyperchromatic, pleomorphic nuclei and the transition to clear-cell apocrine change in the narrowest part of the duct. Excisional biopsy yielded a 3-mm focus of atypical ductal hyperplasia similar to what is seen in this duct.

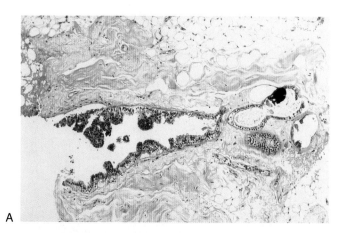

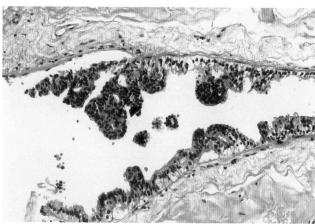

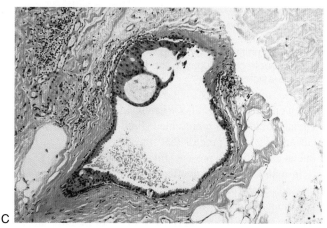

FIGURE 17. Atypical ductal hyperplasia, micropapillary. A: Mammographically detected calcifications led to this needle core biopsy. Calcifications are apparent in the duct lumina on the right. **B:** The left portion of the duct has an atypical micropapillary proliferation in which the micropapillae are composed of cells with small, overlapping, hyperchromatic nuclei. **C:** This focus of atypical micropapillary hyperplasia with apocrine change was found next to the core biopsy site in the excisional biopsy specimen.

nuclear-to-cytoplasmic ratio, nuclear hyperchromasia, an irregular chromatin pattern, or the presence of nucleoli (Fig. 23).

The most challenging atypical ductal proliferations, sometimes referred to as "borderline" lesions, feature marked cytologic and architectural atypia. Most of these foci retain a minor characteristic of hyperplasia, such as persistent columnar ductal epithelium or nuclear overlap, with a structure otherwise typical of intraductal carcinoma (Figs. 23–25). These slight variations will be disregarded by observers who classify the lesions as intraductal carcinoma, whereas others may diagnose atypical hyperplasia. Similarly, those who place credence in quantitative criteria will

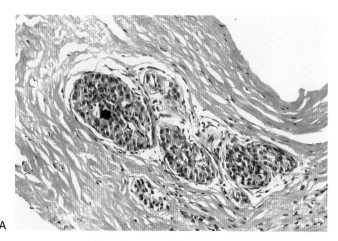

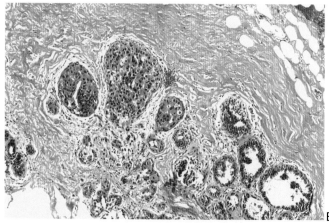

FIGURE 18. Atypical ductal hyperplasia, lobular extension. Two foci of intralobular proliferation raise concern about lobular extension of intraductal carcinoma. **A:** A thin layer of persistent glandular epithelium outlines a narrow, slit-shaped lumen next to a calcification in the largest lobular gland. Solid intraductal carcinoma was found in the excisional biopsy specimen. **B:** An irregular proliferation of cells with apocrine differentiation fills three lobular glands in this needle core biopsy specimen. Excisional biopsy revealed foci of atypical apocrine ductal hyperplasia.

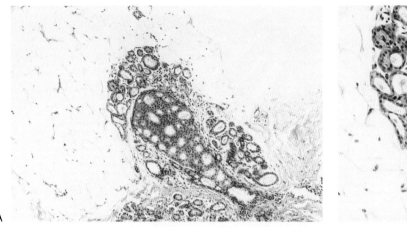
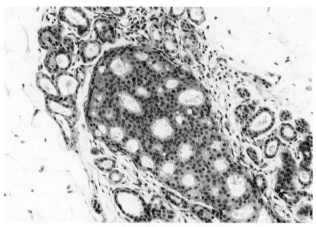

FIGURE 19. Atypical ductal hyperplasia, cribriform. A,B: The only proliferative abnormality in the needle core biopsy specimen in this case was one focus of cribriform proliferation in an intralobular duct. Part of the duct in the lower right corner of (A) is not involved by the proliferation, and it does not extend into lobular glands. Sclerosing adenosis with calcifications was found at the needle biopsy site in the excisional biopsy specimen.

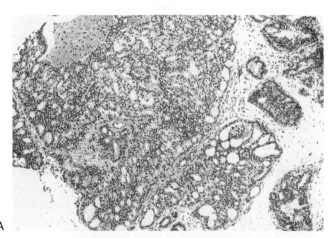
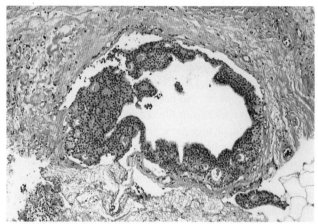

FIGURE 20. Atypical ductal hyperplasia, cribriform. A: The florid hyperplasia in this needle core biopsy specimen of a papillary lesion has areas of cribriform microlumen formation. **B:** This was one of several ducts with cribriform intraductal carcinoma in the excisional biopsy specimen next to the site from which the needle core biopsy specimen in (A) was obtained. Disrupted epithelium and the displaced epithelial fragment (*lower right*) can be present in the vicinity of a prior needle core biopsy.

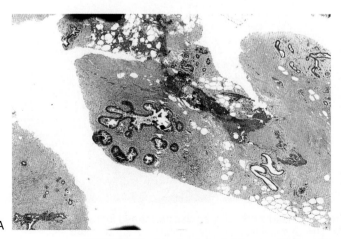
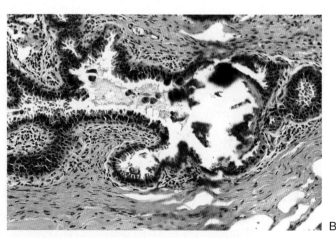

FIGURE 21. Atypical ductal hyperplasia, columnar cell and micropapillary. Three different needle core biopsy specimens. **A,B:** Hyperplasia composed of columnar cells with hyperchromatic nuclei is a precursor to atypical micropapillary hyperplasia. A fractured calcification is present in the duct lumen. *Figure continues.*

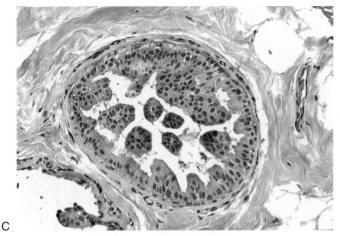

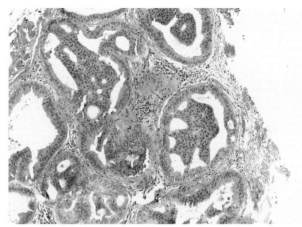

C

D

FIGURE 21. Atypical ductal hyperplasia, columnar cell and micropapillary. *Continued* **C:** Crowding and hyperchromasia of shrunken nuclei in some micropapillae are apparent in this duct. The cells have apocrine cytoplasm, there is a ring of evenly spaced nuclei at the periphery of the duct, and some myoepithelial cells are present. **D:** A monomorphic population of cells forms bridges across these ducts, creating cribriform microlumina. Epithelium at the perimeter of each duct consists of nonproliferative cuboidal or low columnar cells with evenly spaced, basally oriented nuclei. One weakly stained calcification is present near the center.

diagnose atypical hyperplasia because the extent of a lesion is not sufficient, while others, not adhering to these rules, will diagnose intraductal carcinoma.

Insufficient emphasis has been placed on diagnosing specific proliferative lesions in the context of the overall spectrum of histologic changes in a given biopsy specimen. In a research setting, a pathologist can be required to make a diagnosis that is based only on one or more selected foci on a single slide. This situation, duplicated to a large extent in assessing needle core biopsy specimens, is different from the circumstances under which the various diagnostic criteria were originally refined, in which multiple histologic samples were reviewed (10,16,18). When faced with a ductal proliferative lesion in a needle core biopsy specimen, the patholo-

gist should obtain serial sections of the specimen, and if they are available, slides from previous biopsies should be reviewed for comparison. The diagnosis of "borderline" intraductal proliferations is best made in the context of the spectrum of pathologic changes present in current and prior specimens. A focus of concern may be found to be substantially more atypical and different qualitatively from the overall proliferative level in a given case, or it may prove to be part of a spectrum of changes lacking distinct histologic boundaries. The former situation would tend to support a diagnosis of intraductal carcinoma in the lesional area, whereas the latter suggests atypical hyperplasia.

Atypical ductal hyperplasia has been diagnosed in fewer than 10% of patients subjected to stereotaxic needle core

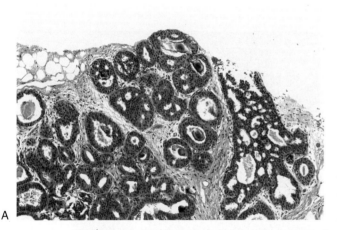

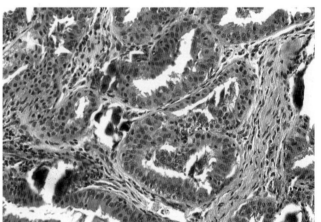

A

B

FIGURE 22. Atypical ductal hyperplasia, apocrine. This needle core biopsy was performed for mammographically detected clustered calcifications. **A:** The atypical ductal hyperplasia with a columnar cell–cribriform pattern and hyperplastic epithelium in lobular glands shows apocrine differentiation. There are numerous calcifications in the lobular glands. **B:** The excisional biopsy specimen contained residual atypical apocrine hyperplasia with calcifications.

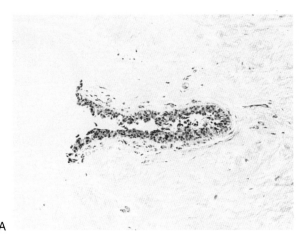

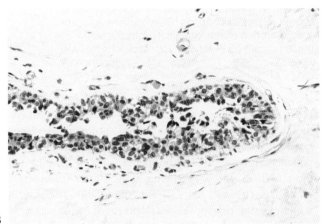

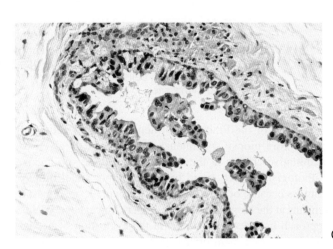

FIGURE 23. Atypical ductal hyperplasia with severe cytologic atypia. A,B: The only proliferative abnormality in this needle core biopsy specimen was this duct at the edge of one tissue sample. The epithelial layer is thickened and composed of cells distributed in a disordered pattern. Many nuclei are hyperchromatic, especially at the luminal border, and there is some nuclear overlap. The proliferation has micropapillary traits. **C:** The subsequent surgical excision revealed micropapillary intraductal carcinoma with marked nuclear pleomorphism. Periductal reactive changes and vascularity are more pronounced than around the duct in (A), and there is a fully developed micropapillary structure.

biopsy (7,8,19). In these studies, approximately 50% of patients with atypical hyperplasia in the needle biopsy specimen were proved to have carcinoma, usually intraductal, in a subsequent surgical biopsy. At least 80% of subsequent biopsies reveal additional proliferative lesions, either because the needle biopsy sample was incomplete or the entire abnormality was included in the needle biopsy and the excisional specimen had other foci of hyperplasia. The approximately 50% frequency of carcinoma detected in excisional biopsy specimens after a diagnosis of atypical ductal hyperplasia in a needle core biopsy sample dictates that surgical excision should be performed promptly in this setting (7,8).

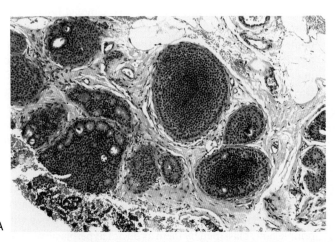

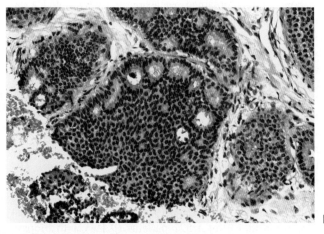

FIGURE 24. Atypical ductal hyperplasia, borderline. A,B: The ducts in this needle core biopsy specimen have a solid central population of small, monomorphic cells. Microlumina are formed at the periphery of some ducts, outlined by cells oriented around the rounded fenestrations, which form a continuous ring around the ducts.

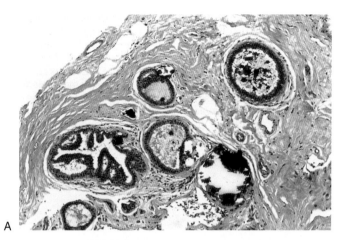
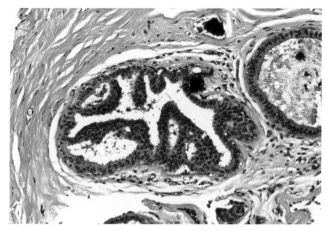

A

B

FIGURE 25. Atypical ductal hyperplasia, borderline. A,B: The needle core biopsy that yielded the specimen containing this lesion was performed for clustered microcalcifications. Calcifications are present in cysts and the stroma. The proliferation has the appearance of micropapillary intraductal carcinoma, but some of the nonpapillary peripheral epithelium is composed of regular cuboidal cells that are indistinguishable from cells lining the adjacent nonproliferative cysts. The micropapillary abnormality was limited to this site.

Because of the limited and often fragmented nature of needle core biopsy specimens, added weight is given to quantitative criteria in the assessment of these specimens. Pathologists should avoid overinterpreting small biopsy samples because of the expectation that more lesional tissue remains at the biopsy site. In the proper clinical context, this approach has merit. However, in the evaluation of needle core biopsy specimens of breast lesions, especially those evident only by mammography, it must be anticipated that the material seen in the needle biopsy sample may be the most extreme and potentially the only abnormality present. Atypical ductal hyperplasia may be diagnosed if detached fragments of abnormal epithelium are present that suggest carcinoma, or if only part of a duct with features of carcinoma is contained in the sample. The importance of quantitative criteria and adequate sampling was documented by Jackman et al. (7) who ". . . progressively increased the average number of core samples obtained per lesion and have found a decrease in both the number of ADH (atypical duct hyperplasia) lesions and the discordance of ADH lesion." The greater success in diagnosis was attributable to more lesions being diagnosed as intraductal carcinoma rather than as atypical ductal hyperplasia, a result of more complete sampling (7).

The major clinical concern attributable to ordinary and atypical intraductal hyperplasia is the risk for subsequent development of carcinoma. In a minority of women with biopsy findings classified as nonproliferative or proliferative, carcinoma subsequently develops in either breast. The overall proportion of women in whom breast carcinoma later develops rarely exceeds 10%, even with follow-up of two decades or more. Bodian et al. (9) detected subsequent breast carcinoma in 139 of 1,521 patients (9.1%) with biopsy-proven proliferative changes, and in 18 of 278 (6.5%) with nonproliferative biopsy findings within a follow-up period of 21 years. Overall, breast carcinoma developed in 8.7% of

the patients. In other reports involving at least 1,000 patients, the proportions of women in whom carcinoma developed were 2.2% (20), 4.1% (21), and 4.9% (22). The proportion of patients with subsequent carcinoma tends to increase with the length of follow-up, being highest after follow-up of more than a decade (21,22). This observation is consistent with the rising risk for the development of breast carcinoma with advancing age.

The risk for the development of carcinoma subsequent to unilateral biopsy-proven proliferative changes affects both breasts. The bilaterality of risk was noted by Davis et al. (23) in a review of 297 patients with "cystic disease." These authors also tabulated data from 11 articles with at least 100 patients to show that carcinoma subsequently developed in 0.7% to 4.9% of patients, with 50% of cases arising in the contralateral breast.

Krieger and Hiatt (22) found that only 56% of subsequent carcinomas occurred in the previously sampled breast with benign proliferative changes. Laterality of subsequent carcinoma was not significantly influenced by the type of antecedent proliferative change or the age at biopsy. The mean interval to subsequent ipsilateral carcinomas (11.2 years) was less than that for contralateral carcinomas (14 years). Page et al. (24) reported that 8 of 18 (44%) carcinomas subsequent to atypical ductal hyperplasia occurred in the contralateral breast. Involvement of the contralateral breast in similar proportions of patients was also described by Connolly et al. (25).

An exception to the foregoing reports of bilateral risk was described by Tavassoli and Norris (26), who found carcinoma in the ipsilateral breast of 10 of 14 (71%) women with prior lesions classified by them as ductal hyperplasia or atypical ductal hyperplasia. Although this unusual distribution of laterality could have been a chance event in a relatively small series of cases, it is more likely reflective of the authors' criteria for defining atypical hyperplasia, which probably include a substantial proportion of small intraductal carcinomas, lesions associated with increased ipsilateral risk.

The chances for development of breast carcinoma are influenced by factors that can modify the level of risk associated with benign proliferative changes. Age at diagnosis is inversely related to subsequent risk. Carter et al. (27) found that the rate of subsequent breast carcinoma, when compared with that of normal women, was increased 3.7-fold in women with atypical hyperplasia who were 46 to 55 years of age and 2.3-fold in women older than 55. London et al. (28) also observed an inverse relationship of age and risk, in which the relative risk increased 2.6-fold among premenopausal women who had biopsy-proven atypia in comparison with postmenopausal subjects.

A history of breast carcinoma among first-degree female relatives is a particularly strong additive factor in women who have atypical hyperplasia. Page et al. (24) and Dupont and Page (29) found that the risk associated with atypical duct hyperplasia in women with a positive family history was more than double that of women without this factor. London et al. (28) also reported that the increased risk associated with family history was strongest in patients with atypical hyperplasia. The relative risk was not increased by a positive family history in women with nonproliferative biopsy findings.

Among women who have had a benign result on breast biopsy, the risk for subsequent development of carcinoma is related to the histologic components of the antecedent biopsy. When assessed independently, sclerosing adenosis has been associated with an increased risk in several studies (20,26,29,30). Some of these investigators reported a greater increase in risk for relatively small groups of women who had atypical hyperplasia and sclerosing adenosis (26,29,31).

The proportion of patients in whom carcinoma develops is highest in the group of women with atypical ductal hyperplasia, intermediate in those with proliferative ductal changes without atypia, and least in those without proliferative changes. Proliferative changes were identified in 152 (85%) of 1,799 biopsy specimens studied by Bodian et al. (9). Moderate-to-severe atypia was present in 70 specimens, representing 3.8% of all cases and 4.6% of specimens with proliferative changes. Follow-up revealed that the relative risk (RR) for development of carcinoma (in comparison with the general population, represented by the Connecticut Tumor Registry) was higher in women with any proliferative changes (RR of 2.2) than in those with nonproliferative findings on biopsy (RR of 1.6). The relative risk associated with severe ductal atypia was 3.9. Page et al. (24) found the relative risk to be 4.7 for women with atypical ductal hyperplasia in comparison with women who had nonproliferative biopsy results. The relative risk for women with atypical duct hyperplasia and a family history of breast carcinoma was increased further in comparison with women who had nonproliferative biopsy results and a positive family history (24). Ma and Boyd (30) undertook a metaanalysis of studies that investigated the association between atypical hyperplasia and breast cancer risk. Fifteen reports between 1960 and 1992 fulfilled the authors' requirements for inclusion in the study, resulting in a total sample size of 182,980 women. The overall odds ratio in comparison with controls for the development of carcinoma in women with atypical hyperplasia was 3.67 (95% CI, 3.16 to 4.26).

INTRADUCTAL CARCINOMA

A 1996 review of data included in the National Cancer Institute's Surveillance, Epidemiology and End Results (SEER) Program demonstrated a striking increase in the incidence of intraductal carcinoma after 1983 (32). Among women 30 to 39 years of age, the average annual increase in the incidence rate changed from 0.3% between 1973 and 1983 to 12.0% between 1983 and 1992. Similar increases were found for women 40 to 49 years old (0.4% to 17.4%) and for women 50 years and older (5.2% to 18.1%). The estimated total number of cases of intraductal carcinoma in 1992 was 200% higher than expected based on 1983 rates. Review of the records of the Connecticut Tumor Registry revealed a yearly increase in the number of cases of intraductal carcinoma reported (33). In 1979, the 33 diagnoses of intraductal carcinoma represented 1.8% of breast carcinomas, and in 1988, the 200 cases constituted 7.4% of breast carcinomas (33). The beneficial effects of mammography as a diagnostic and screening modality are reflected in these trends (34).

Mammography is the most sensitive diagnostic procedure for detecting intraductal carcinoma because a substantial proportion of the lesions are not palpable. Of nonpalpable carcinomas detected by mammography, 25% to 30% are intraductal lesions (35–37). Mammographically detected calcifications are found in at least 70% of intraductal carcinomas (36,37). Other radiologic findings that lead to the detection of a small proportion of intraductal carcinomas are densities and asymmetric soft-tissue changes, sometimes with microcalcifications. Calcifications alone are more likely to be the mammographic indicator of intraductal carcinoma in women younger than 50 years, whereas coexistent soft-tissue abnormalities are evident more often in women older than 50, a distinction that probably results from differences in breast density between these age groups rather than from intrinsic tumor differences (37).

Calcifications associated with intraductal carcinoma are generally described as linear "casts" or as granular in mammograms. Round or oval, well-circumscribed calcifications are less common in intraductal carcinoma. The mammographic distribution of calcifications has been used as a guide to the extent of intraductal carcinoma or the dimensions of the involved area. However, these measurements may underestimate the size of the lesion in comparison with careful histologic sampling (38). When the extent of lesions is measured both mammographically and pathologically, discrepancies are found more often between the interpretations for cases that are predominantly cribriform or micropapillary than for intraductal comedocarcinomas. A discrepancy of more than 20 mm was found in 44% of pure cribriform-micropapillary lesions, in 12% of pure comedocarcinomas, and in 50% of cases with both patterns (38). The likelihood of detecting multifocal intraductal carcinoma radiologically and pathologically is related to the size of the lesion as determined by either procedure. Multifocality is appreciably more frequent in lesions larger than 2.0 to 2.5 cm than in smaller foci of intraductal carcinoma (39).

The mammographic appearance of microcalcifications bears some relationship to the histologic type of the lesion, but as noted by Stomper and Connolly (40), "there is considerable overlap, and the predominant histologic subtype cannot be predicted on the basis of the microcalcification type with a high degree of accuracy." Predominantly linear calcifications are found significantly more often in comedocarcinomas than in cribriform, papillary, or solid types, which typically contain granular calcifications (38,40). Nonetheless, 22% of linear calcifications were associated with non-comedocarcinomas, and 47% of granular calcifications occurred in comedocarcinomas in one series (40). Abnormal mammogram findings without calcifications are more likely to call attention to intraductal carcinoma of the small-cell type than the large-cell type, regardless of the growth pattern (solid, cribriform, or mixed) of the lesion (41). Linear calcifications are a marker of necrosis, and

small, punctate, or granular calcifications are associated with intraductal carcinoma without necrosis (41). Intraductal carcinomas that express the HER2/neu oncogene are more likely to have calcifications detected by mammography than are HER2/neu-negative carcinomas (42).

Intraductal carcinoma in women occurs throughout the age range of breast carcinoma generally. The mean age at diagnosis of patients in multiple studies is between 50 and 59 years. There are no significant differences in the age distribution of structural subtypes of intraductal carcinoma (43).

Intraductal carcinoma can be recognized in frozen sections, but if any difficulty is encountered, the decision should be immediately deferred to permanent sections because there is a significant risk of trimming away the lesional area as more sections are made (Fig. 26). Needle core biopsy samples are not suitable for frozen-section examination unless there are exceptional circumstances. In one study of intraductal carcinomas, 50% of the lesions were diagnosed at the time of frozen section: 36% were reported to be benign, 8% were deferred, 5% were diagnosed as atypical hyperplasia, and one case was diagnosed as invasive (44). Approximately 3% of lesions reported to be benign at frozen section prove to contain carcinoma when paraffin sections are examined (45). Because the amount of tissue that can be examined by frozen section during surgery is limited, approximately 20% of patients with a frozen-section diagnosis of intraductal carcinoma in a surgical biopsy prove to have invasion when it is

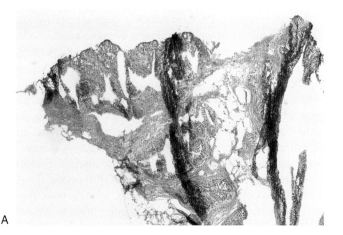

A

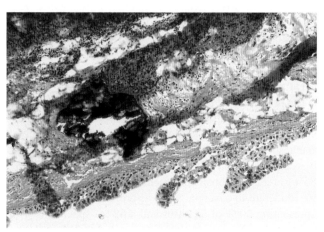

B

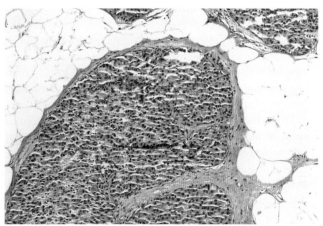

C

FIGURE 26. Intraductal carcinoma, frozen section. The patient had a needle core biopsy for nonpalpable calcifications, and this sample was submitted for frozen section. **A:** The frozen section slide has folds and tears. **B:** A displaced calcification is present near the center, and a band of atypical cells is present at the lower border of the tissue. The diagnosis was deferred. **C:** Solid intraductal carcinoma with frozen-section artifact in a section of the paraffin-embedded tissue after examination by frozen section.

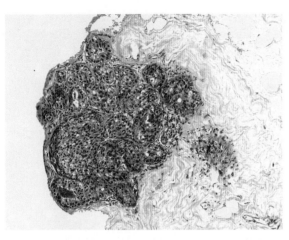
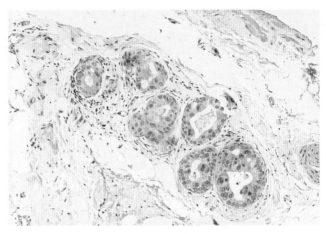

A

B

FIGURE 27. Intraductal carcinoma, lobular extension (lobular cancerization). A: This enlarged lobular complex at the border of a needle core biopsy specimen is involved by intraductal carcinoma, solid type with poorly differentiated nuclear grade. **B:** Lobular involvement by apocrine intraductal carcinoma in another needle core biopsy specimen.

possible to examine multiple paraffin sections of the same biopsy specimen (46). Frozen section is not recommended for the diagnosis of needle core or surgical biopsy specimens of mammographically detected nonpalpable lesions unless there are exceptional clinical circumstances.

The microanatomic site of origin of many intraductal carcinomas appears to be in the terminal duct-lobular unit. The most convincing evidence for this conclusion comes from the subgross microdissection studies of Wellings et al. (47). A histologic correlate of this is the presence of the neoplastic process in the epithelium of lobular glands, termed lobular cancerization (Fig. 27). Greatly expanded terminal duct-lobular units sometimes resemble primary or secondary segmental ducts, but their lobular origin is suggested by the excessive number of duct structures within a low-power microscopic field. The relative frequencies of origin from the terminal duct-lobular unit and from larger duct structures and the clinical significance of this distinction remains to be determined.

In standard histologic sections, intraductal carcinoma appears to be confined within the lumina of ducts and lobules involved in the process. When studied by immunohistochemistry, basement membranes in intraductal carcinomas are intact or focally discontinuous (48). The diagnosis of intraductal carcinoma alone does not apply to lesions in which commingling with invasive foci is present, even if the latter comprise a minimal portion of the lesion.

The presence or absence of mitotic figures is not a definitive feature in the diagnosis of intraductal carcinoma because very infrequent mitoses may also be found in normal lobules and in duct hyperplasia. The finding of numerous mitoses, such as one or more per high-power field, suggests intraductal carcinoma. Myoepithelial cells do not accompany the neoplastic proliferation within the duct lumen in intraductal carcinoma, but these cells are variably retained and occasionally hyperplastic at the periphery of the duct (Fig. 28). Carcinoma cells at the periphery of the duct exhibit loss of basal polarity as a manifestation of cellular crowding. Rarely, remnants of non-neoplastic normal or hyperplastic duct epithelium persist in ducts involved by intraductal carcinoma (Fig. 29).

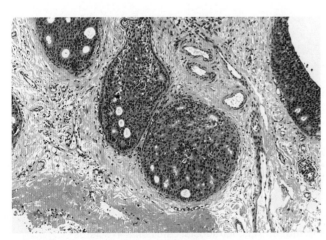

FIGURE 28. Intraductal carcinoma. Myoepithelial cells are evident at the perimeter of one of these duct cross sections involved by cribriform intraductal carcinoma.

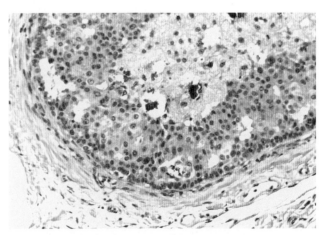

FIGURE 29. Intraductal carcinoma. Microlumina are present at the perimeter of the duct between intraductal carcinoma and an incomplete ring of evenly spaced cuboidal ductal epithelial cells.

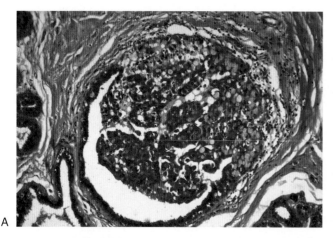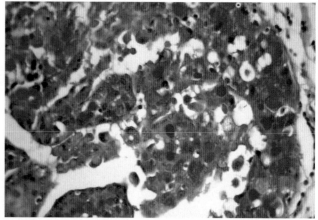

FIGURE 30. Intraductal carcinoma, signet-ring cells. A: Papillary intraductal carcinoma with signet-ring cells. **B:** The intracytoplasmic mucin is stained magenta with the mucicarmine stain.

A broad range of cell types is found in intraductal carcinomas. Certain distinct variants have been identified and described by specific names. *Signet-ring cells*, usually associated with lobular carcinoma, also occur in intraductal carcinomas, most often in the papillary and cribriform types (Fig. 30). Signet-ring cells have eccentric nuclei that are often indented by a cytoplasmic mucin vacuole. A minute droplet of secretion may be apparent in the vacuole. Intracytoplasmic mucin sometimes imparts a pale blue color to the cytoplasm without forming distinct vacuoles (Fig. 31). Clear holes in the cytoplasm can be mistaken for signet-ring vacuoles. These cytoplasmic defects, sometimes the site of glycogen accumulation, are not reactive with the mucicarmine stain, they do not indent the nucleus, and there is ordinarily no secretion evident in the lumen. *Clear-cell* intraductal carcinoma is a poorly defined variant typically encountered with solid and comedo patterns. Some clear-cell intraductal carcinomas are composed of cells with an arrangement described as "mosaic" because of the appearance

created by sharply defined cell borders (Fig. 32). A subset of lesions classified under this heading are a form of apocrine carcinoma. Occasionally, clear-cell intraductal carcinomas have strongly mucicarmine-positive cytoplasm. Other clear-cell lesions are the *in situ* forms of lipid-rich or glycogen-rich carcinomas, discussed in Chapter 20. *Apocrine* cytology is encountered in all the structural types of intraductal carcinoma (Figs. 27,33). These cells have abundant cytoplasm that ranges from granular and eosinophilic to vacuolated or clear. There is variable nuclear pleomorphism, sometimes manifested by prominent nucleoli. *Spindle-cell* intraductal carcinomas may express neuroendocrine markers such as synaptophysin and neuron-specific enolase (Fig. 34). Small-cell intraductal carcinoma is extremely uncommon (Fig. 35).

The cellular composition of intraductal carcinomas is usually described as *monomorphic*, a term applied especially to cribriform, solid, and micropapillary carcinomas. In this context, monomorphic means that there is overall homogeneity in the cytologic appearance of the lesion, although all cells

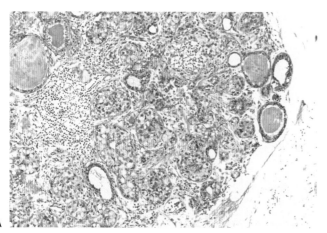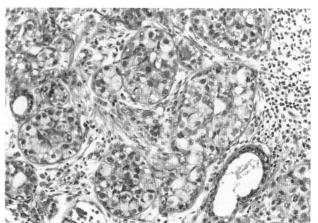

FIGURE 31. Intraductal carcinoma, intracytoplasmic mucin. A,B: Intraductal carcinoma in sclerosing adenosis in a needle core biopsy specimen. The cells have pale blue cytoplasm that was reactive with the mucicarmine stain.

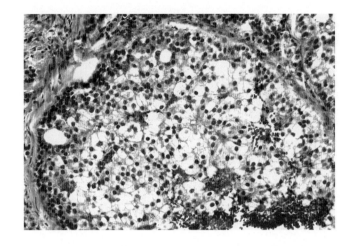

FIGURE 32. Intraductal carcinoma, clear-cell type. The cells have sharply defined cell borders and low-grade nuclei.

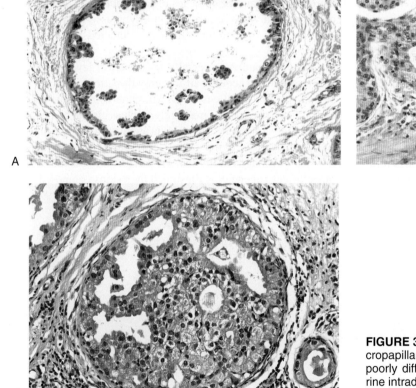

FIGURE 33. Intraductal carcinoma, apocrine type. A: Micropapillary intraductal carcinoma with apocrine cytology and poorly differentiated nuclear grade. **B:** Micropapillary apocrine intraductal carcinoma. **C:** Cribriform apocrine intraductal carcinoma with cytoplasmic granularity and slight clearing.

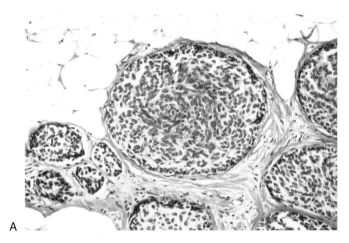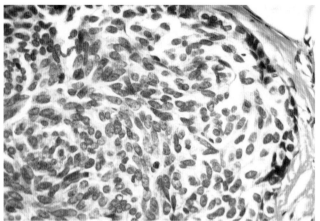

A B

FIGURE 34. Intraductal carcinoma, spindle-cell type. A,B: The swirling spindle-cell proliferation mimics the streaming pattern of ductal hyperplasia. The monomorphic spindle cells extend to the perimeter of the duct in this needle core biopsy specimen.

are not identical in regard to such features as amount of cytoplasm or nuclear size. Cell and nuclear shape may be altered by the presence or absence of crowding in one or another part of the duct. The presence of a myoepithelial cell layer is not a consideration in judging whether a ductal proliferation is monomorphic, as long as these cells are confined to the periphery of the duct. Dimorphic variants of intraductal carcinoma, consisting of two distinctly different populations of epithelial cells, are unusual (see Fig. 35). The majority of dimorphic intraductal carcinomas are papillary carcinomas.

Intraductal carcinoma in a given patient can have more than a single microscopic structural, cytologic, or immunocytochemical phenotype (43). Mixed histologic patterns are found in 30% to 40% of cases. Whereas some structural combinations, such as papillary- or micropapillary-cribri-

form and solid-comedo, occur relatively more often than others, there is considerable heterogeneity with respect to growth patterns (49). The probability of structural variability increases with the size of the lesion, a phenomenon that must be considered when needle core biopsy is used for the subclassification of mammographically detected intraductal carcinoma.

Cytologic features, especially at the nuclear level, tend to be more homogeneous than the growth pattern in a given case. Some combinations of growth patterns and cytologic appearances occur more frequently, such as classic comedocarcinoma, composed of poorly differentiated pleomorphic cells with necrosis, or the low nuclear grade typically present in micropapillary carcinoma. However, the considerable range of heterogeneity is illustrated by lesions composed of

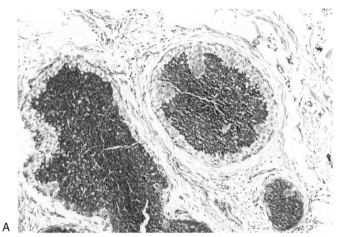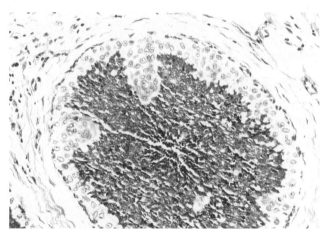

A B

FIGURE 35. Intraductal carcinoma, small-cell type. A,B: This extraordinary lesion consists of a central, nearly syncytial mass of small undifferentiated carcinoma cells and an outer zone of larger polygonal cells. Two papillary mounds of large cells show apical traces of squamous differentiation, a feature that was more pronounced in other ducts. Persistent myoepithelial cells that were immunoreactive for actin are indicated by the small, dark, elongated nuclei at the outer border of the duct.

small, cytologically low-grade nuclei growing in a solid pattern with central comedo necrosis, and others having a papillary pattern composed of cells with high-grade nuclei, found in some examples of clinging carcinoma. When multiple architectural patterns are encountered in a single case, they should be listed separately with the most abundant type cited first.

Micropapillary intraductal carcinoma consists of ducts lined by a layer of neoplastic cells that give rise intermittently to slender papillary fronds or arcuate formations, which protrude into the lumen (Figs. 28,33,36). The papillae are variable in appearance, ranging from bumps or mounds to pronounced slender processes. They almost all lack a fibrovascular core and are composed of cytologically homogeneous carcinoma cells. Arcuate structures, commonly referred to as Roman bridge arches, develop when microlumina are formed beneath adjacent coalescent fronds or within a mound of neoplastic cells. These fenestrations resemble the lumina formed in cribriform intraductal carcinoma. In conjunction with micropapillae, they are a feature of micropapillary intraductal carcinoma.

The appearance of the micropapillary fronds varies somewhat with the plane of individual histologic sections. Whereas some micropapillae are cut in a plane perpendicular to their long axis, others are seen sectioned tangentially or transversely, resulting in irregular nests of seemingly detached cell clusters in the duct lumen (see Fig. 36). Aside from the epithelial proliferation, ducts with low nuclear grade micropapillary intraductal carcinoma are usually relatively free of cellular debris or inflammatory cells, but they may contain calcifications.

Micropapillary intraductal carcinoma is usually composed of cytologically low-grade, small, homogeneous cells with a high nuclear-to-cytoplasmic ratio and dense, hyperchromatic nuclei (see Fig. 36). The nuclei typically vary very little in size and chromatin density between cells at the base

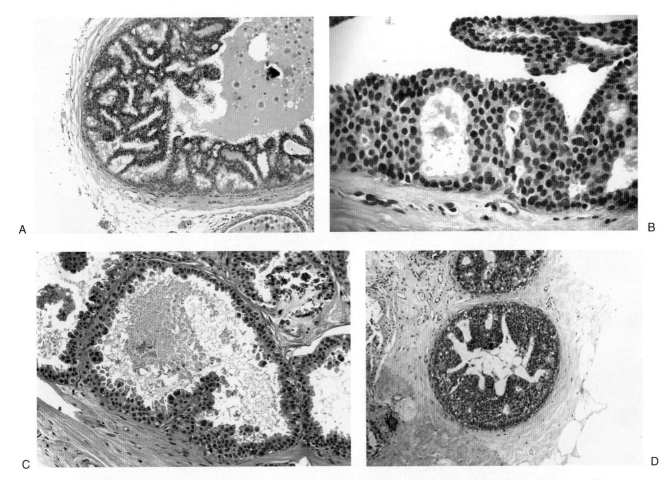

FIGURE 36. Intraductal carcinoma, micropapillary type. A: Slender fronds of micropapillary carcinoma with low nuclear grade form a network of arches at the periphery of this duct in a needle core biopsy specimen. **B:** Thick bands of monomorphic cells with low nuclear grade outline microlumina in this duct. **C:** Micropapillary intraductal carcinoma in a needle core biopsy specimen with apocrine cytology and high nuclear grade. Calcifications are present. Part of this lesion is in the form referred to as "flat" micropapillary carcinoma. **D:** Micropapillary intraductal carcinoma with intermediate and high nuclear grade in these duct sections was the only evidence of carcinoma in this needle core biopsy specimen.

and tip of micropapillae. They may be slightly smaller and darker at the surface, but marked disparity in these characteristics is a feature of micropapillary hyperplasia. At the margin of the duct, between papillary and arcuate structures, the neoplastic cells typically form a thin layer between one to not more than three or four cells deep. Persistent non-neoplastic epithelium between micropapillae is a feature of micropapillary hyperplasia rather than micropapillary carcinoma. Mitoses are rarely evident. In most instances, the cells are so crowded that their individual borders and cytoplasm cannot be identified. Occasionally, the cells have slightly more abundant cytoplasm, with apocrine-type protrusions at the luminal border. In one variant of this cell type, the nuclei of the tumor cells are contained in cytoplasmic blebs that are extruded into the duct lumen.

A minority of carcinomas with a micropapillary structural phenotype are composed of cells with intermediate- or high-grade (poorly differentiated) cytologic characteristics (see Figs. 33,36). This type of micropapillary carcinoma tends to occur in women 35 to 50 years of age. It is multifocal and sometimes bilateral. The microscopic foci are mainly localized in terminal duct lobular units. Cells forming this type of carcinoma differ from those in the conventional micropapillary lesions in that they are larger, with more abundant cytoplasm. Nuclei are also correspondingly larger, and nucleoli may be apparent. Mitoses can be seen in this epithelium, and

the cells often have a distinctly apocrine appearance. The cytologically high-grade form of micropapillary intraductal carcinoma is more likely to have calcifications than the low-grade variant, and necrotic cellular debris may be found in the duct lumen. Florid micropapillary proliferation tends to result in fusion of the epithelial fronds and the formation of cribriform microlumina. Consequently, it is not unusual to find intraductal carcinomas with a combination of micropapillary and cribriform features. *Cystic hypersecretory intraductal carcinoma* is a special subtype of micropapillary carcinoma that is discussed in Chapter 19.

Cribriform intraductal carcinoma is a fenestrated epithelial proliferation in which microlumina are formed in the neoplastic epithelium bridging most or all of the duct lumen (Fig. 37). Extension into lobular epithelium (so-called lobular cancerization) or into the main lactiferous ducts of the nipple is uncommon. Dilated ducts with cribriform intraductal carcinoma can be mistaken for adenoid cystic carcinoma or a complex papilloma. In rare instances, intraductal carcinoma that has in a cribriform pattern can develop in collagenous spherulosis, which is usually associated with hyperplastic duct lesions.

The secondary lumina tend to be round or oval, with smooth edges bordered by cuboidal cells. The distribution of microlumina is variable. In some instances, the spaces are spread across the entire duct, but in others, they are concen-

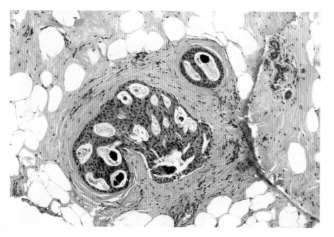

A

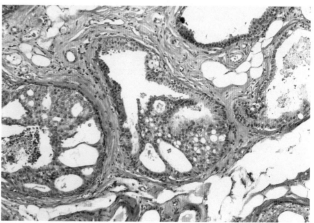

B

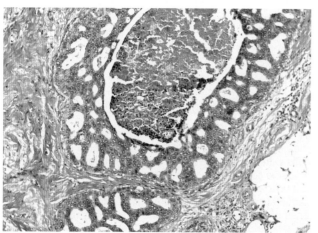

C

FIGURE 37. Intraductal carcinoma, cribriform type.
A: A small duct with cribriform intraductal carcinoma of low nuclear grade and apocrine cytology in a needle core biopsy specimen. Punctate calcifications are present. **B:** Necrosis is present in a duct on the left in this lesion with low nuclear grade. **C:** A florid example of cribriform intraductal carcinoma with a central area of necrosis.

trated toward the center or in a zone largely at the periphery of the duct. Microlumina surrounded by a homogeneous cell population that is uniformly distributed throughout the duct are a hallmark of cribriform intraductal carcinoma. The microlumina may contain secretion, small numbers of degenerated or necrotic cells, and punctate calcification.

Bands of neoplastic cells between and around the microlumina are described as "rigid," a term that refers to the uniform, not overlapping distribution of polygonal cells, which is in contrast to the streaming pattern of overlapping, frequently oval cells in duct hyperplasia. Polarization of the cells in a radial fashion around the microlumina contributes to the "rigid" appearance. The most orderly type of cribriform intraductal carcinoma is composed of cytologically low-grade cuboidal-to-low columnar monomorphic cells. Nucleoli are inconspicuous or absent, and mitoses are rarely encountered. The cells usually have sparse cytoplasm. Other lesions are composed of cells with nuclei of intermediate to high grade. Necrosis may be present in such foci.

Solid intraductal carcinoma is formed by neoplastic cells that fill most or all of the duct space (Fig. 38). Microlumina and papillary structures are absent, but calcifications may be present. Patients with comedocarcinoma often have coexistent foci of solid intraductal carcinoma. The polygonal cells are typically of a single type with a low to moderate nuclear grade. The cytoplasm exhibits a spectrum of appearances, including clear, granular, amphophilic, and apocrine.

Intraductal comedocarcinoma is composed of carcinoma cells with poorly differentiated nuclei, central necrosis with calcification, and in many cases a high mitotic rate (Fig. 39). The myoepithelial cell layer is sometimes completely eliminated by the carcinomatous proliferation, but in other instances it may be hyperplastic and produce a distinct ring (see Fig. 28). The latter configuration is usually accompanied by accentuation of the basement membrane itself, as well as a circumferential periductal collar of desmoplastic stroma. Neovascularization in many instances is represented by a partial or complete ring of capillaries immediately external to the basement membrane (50). A variable inflammatory infiltrate is present in the periductal stroma, with a granulomatous reaction in foci where the duct wall is partially disrupted, and it appears that necrotic contents of the duct have been discharged into the stroma. Calcification can also be displaced from the duct into the stroma (Fig. 40).

It is important to distinguish between comedo necrosis and the accumulation of secretion accompanied by an inflammatory reaction, which occurs in duct stasis. Both conditions are prone to the formation of microcalcifications that are difficult to distinguish on mammography. Cellular necrosis is rarely seen in duct stasis, and when present, the degenerated cells are usually histiocytes. The duct contents in comedocarcinoma consist of necrotic carcinoma cells represented by ghost cells and karyorrhectic debris with little or

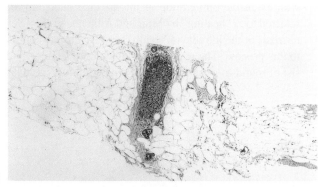

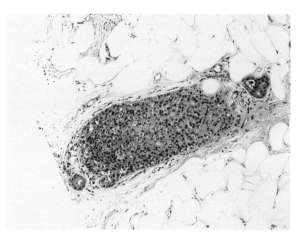

A

B

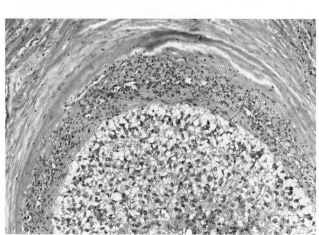

C

FIGURE 38. Intraductal carcinoma, solid type. A,B: The only evidence of carcinoma in this needle core biopsy specimen was this single duct with a solid growth pattern. The excisional biopsy contained additional foci of intraductal carcinoma. **C:** An unusual example of solid, clear-cell intraductal carcinoma with very marked periductal angiogenesis.

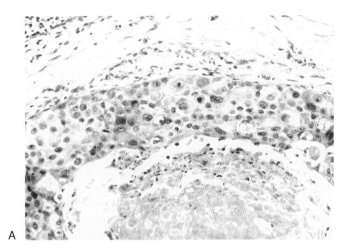 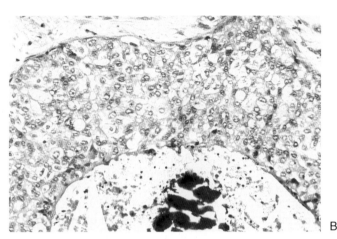

A / B

FIGURE 39. Intraductal carcinoma, comedo type. A: Solid growth with a high nuclear grade is present at the perimeter of a duct with comedo-type central necrosis. Slight angiogenesis is evident in the periductal tissue. **B:** Calcification and comedo necrosis are apparent in this duct.

no intraductal inflammation. There is typically a sharp demarcation between viable carcinoma cells and the necrotic core. A space may be formed between the surviving and dead elements. Dying cells at the inner edge of the viable zone have pyknotic nuclei and frayed cytoplasmic borders. The outlines of necrotic cells may be visible in the center of the duct (ghost cells) (Fig. 41).

Dystrophic calcification develops in the necrotic core. The calcification tends to be finely granular and mixed with cellular debris in some instances, whereas in others, it forms more solid, irregular fragments. Calcifications in comedocarcinoma almost always consist of calcium salts, mainly calcium phosphate, rather than crystalline calcium oxalate, which is typically found in benign lesions. In routine hematoxylin and eosin-stained sections, calcium phosphate calcifications are magenta to purple, whether in comedocarcinoma or other va-

rieties of intraductal carcinoma. Calcifications and necrotic debris may become dislodged in a needle core biopsy, and rarely this material is the only component of the lesion found in a needle core biopsy specimen. When this occurs, serial sections of the biopsy specimen should be prepared. An excisional biopsy is indicated even if no epithelial elements are found in the needle core biopsy sample (Fig. 42). If a dislodged fragment of carcinoma becomes embedded in stroma or fat in a needle core biopsy specimen, the resulting appearance can be mistaken for invasive carcinoma (Fig. 43).

Marked periductal fibrosis can on occasion be associated with extensive obliteration of the affected ducts, a process referred to as "healing" by Muir and Aitkenhead (51). Severe necrosis of the intraductal lesion (see Fig. 41) can contribute to this process. The residual ductal structures typically consist of round-to-oval scars comprising circumferential layers

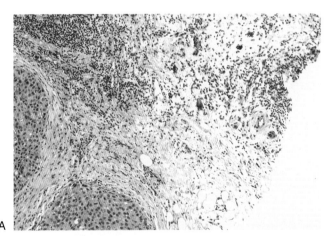 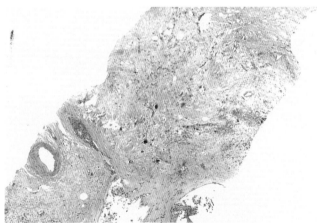

A / B

FIGURE 40. Intraductal carcinoma, comedo type with stromal calcification. A: Fine granular calcifications are present in the stroma in an area of lymphocytic reaction in this needle core biopsy specimen with intraductal comedocarcinoma. **B:** Another needle core biopsy specimen, with more conspicuous stromal calcification and minimal evidence of intraductal carcinoma. No carcinoma cells are seen in the areas of stromal calcification in either specimen. The finding of stromal calcifications such as these alone in a needle core biopsy specimen should raise concern about associated intraductal carcinoma.

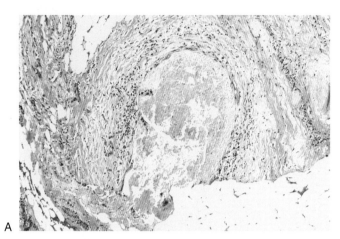 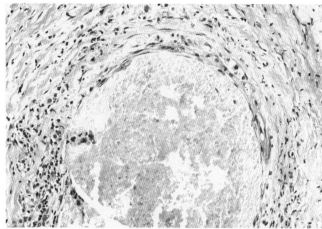

A   B

FIGURE 41. Intraductal carcinoma, comedo type with severe central necrosis. A,B: The intraductal carcinoma is almost totally necrotic in this needle core biopsy specimen. A few degenerating tumor cells are visible in (B).

of collagen and elastic tissue (Fig. 44). The core of the scar, representing the center of the duct, is often less dense, and it may contain a few residual carcinoma cells, histiocytes, fragments of calcification, and granulation tissue. End-stage scars of periductal mastitis are not distinguishable from those of obliterated comedocarcinoma (52). When this type of scar is found in a needle core biopsy specimen, multiple serial sections should be obtained because small foci of carcinoma cells may be present. The very limited histologic evidence for carcinoma found in some of these cases may result in a diagnosis of atypical ductal hyperplasia.

Papillary intraductal carcinoma is distinguished by the presence of a fibrovascular stromal architecture supporting one or more of the structural patterns described above (see Chapter 11).

Intraductal carcinoma arising in sclerosing adenosis assumes the structural configuration of the underlying adeno-

sis and may be mistaken for invasive carcinoma (53–55). Because sclerosing adenosis is fundamentally a lesion formed by altered lobules, this presentation can be viewed as a form of intralobular extension of the ductal lesion (Fig. 45). The condition usually occurs focally rather than diffusely and is diagnosed when the proliferative epithelium has the structural and cytologic appearance of intraductal carcinoma. The growth patterns are usually solid and cribriform. An organoid appearance can result from the alveolar expansion of lobular structures in the adenosis. Microcalcifications may be present in the underlying adenosis or as part of the intraductal carcinoma. Intraductal carcinoma can be limited to the sclerosing adenosis, or there may be additional intraductal foci in the surrounding breast (54). The underlying architecture of sclerosing adenosis can be appreciated with stains for basement membranes, such as PAS, reticulin, or laminin, and immunostains for actin to identify myoepithe-

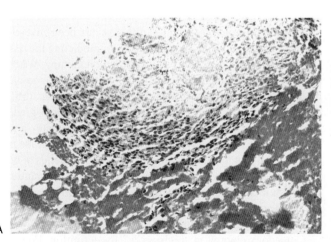 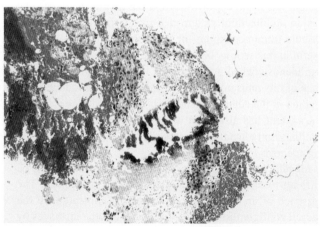

A   B

FIGURE 42. Probable intraductal carcinoma, comedo type. A,B: The needle core biopsy specimen contained these fragments of calcification, comedo-type necrosis, and atypical cells. A needle core biopsy specimen such as this is an indication for prompt excisional biopsy to determine if comedocarcinoma is present.

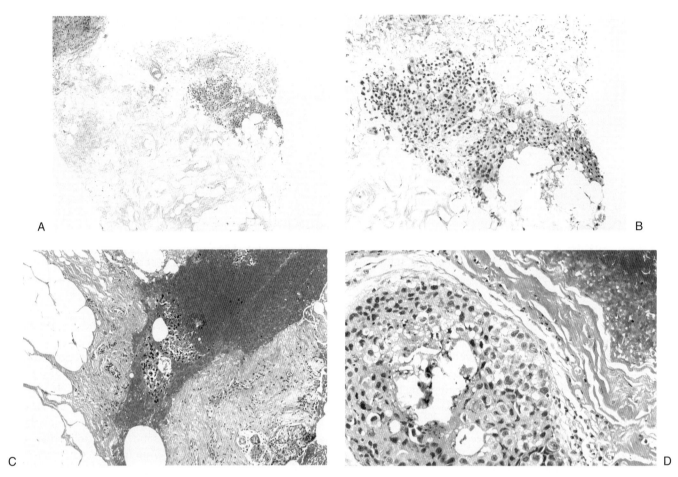

FIGURE 43. Displaced epithelium mistaken for invasive carcinoma in a needle core biopsy specimen. A,B: This fragment of carcinoma displaced in fibrofatty tissue was interpreted as invasive carcinoma in a needle core biopsy specimen. **C:** The subsequent excisional biopsy specimen contained similar detached fragments of carcinoma, such as the one here in an area of hemorrhage caused by the needle biopsy procedure. **D:** The excisional biopsy specimen contained intraductal comedocarcinoma with no intrinsic invasion.

lial cells (54). Invasive carcinoma arising in sclerosing adenosis is very difficult to detect unless the invasive component has clearly grown beyond the area of adenosis and has an architectural pattern that differs from the adenosis. Double immunostaining for cytokeratin and actin may be useful in this setting. Nerves can be incorporated in sclerosing adenosis when no carcinoma is present (56). The presence of this unusual finding coexisting with intraductal carcinoma in the adenosis is not indicative of invasion. Neural entrapment has also been observed in areas of sclerosing papillary intraductal carcinoma not associated with sclerosing adenosis (57).

Intraductal carcinoma in radial sclerosing lesions may be difficult to distinguish from atypical duct hyperplasia. The presence of an underlying radial scar is indicated by the overall configuration of the lesion, and in some instances by the presence of benign proliferative elements, such as cysts, sclerosing adenosis, and apocrine metaplasia (Fig. 46). Incomplete samples of radial scar lesions obtained in a needle core biopsy are difficult to assess for the presence of intraductal carcinoma or for invasion, and they may be reported as atypical hyperplasia.

The grading of intraductal carcinoma has been investigated to determine if it would be useful for predicting the risk for local recurrence after breast conservation therapy. When an invasive element is associated with intraductal carcinoma, both components tend to have similar nuclear grades (58). Grading schemes consisting of two categories (high-grade and all others) and three categories (high-, intermediate-, and low-grade) have been devised. The determination of grade is based mainly on nuclear cytology. Nuclear grade tends to be relatively constant in a given patient, even when substantial variation in architectural pattern is noted (58). The presence or absence of necrosis and the architecture of the intraductal carcinoma may also be considered.

Comedocarcinoma is "high-grade" by definition. Poorly differentiated nuclei, sometimes accompanied by necrosis, are infrequently encountered in papillary, micropapillary,

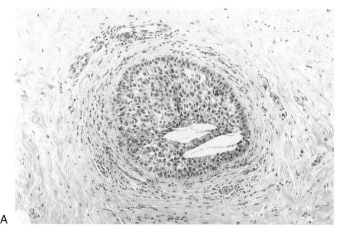

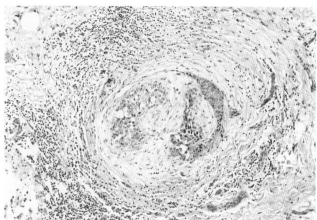

A

B

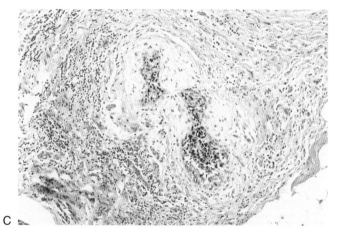

C

FIGURE 44. Intraductal carcinoma with obliterative sclerosis. A–C: Different areas in a needle core biopsy specimen arranged in a sequence that suggests the progressive replacement of degenerating intraductal carcinoma by circumferential sclerosis of the ducts.

and cribriform intraductal carcinomas (58). Intraductal carcinoma is considered to be in the intermediate-grade category when it has a cribriform, solid, or papillary pattern with necrosis but lacks the nuclear anaplasia of comedocarcinoma, or if one of these growth patterns is comprised of

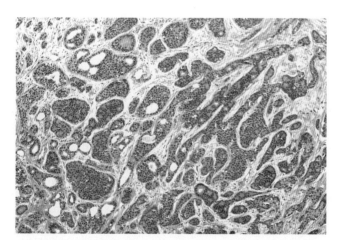

FIGURE 45. Intraductal carcinoma in sclerosing adenosis. The carcinoma has solid and cribriform growth patterns with low nuclear grade. Some of the underlying architecture is tubular adenosis.

high-grade carcinoma cells in the absence of necrosis. Any pattern of intraductal carcinoma composed of uniform cells without atypia or necrosis is classified as low-grade. A case is usually classified on the basis of the highest grade present.

Silverstein et al. (59) proposed a classification of intraductal carcinoma based on nuclear grade (high or not high) and the presence or absence of necrosis. Three prognostic categories resulted from consideration of these variables. Group 1 is a not-high nuclear grade without necrosis; group 2 is a not-high nuclear grade with necrosis; group 3 is a high nuclear grade with or without necrosis. Follow-up revealed a significant correlation between this classification of intraductal carcinoma and the risk for local recurrence after breast conservation therapy. The 8-year actuarial disease-free survivals for the three groups of patients were 93%, 84%, and 61%, respectively. Long-term follow-up will be necessary to determine if this classification simply reflects differences in the time to recurrence related to these histologic features or if they indicate other biologic differences. This classification scheme was later incorporated into the Van Nuys Prognostic Index, a scoring system that also includes margin status and tumor size (60).

Grading has been a component of most attempts to develop classification schemes to assess the effectiveness of

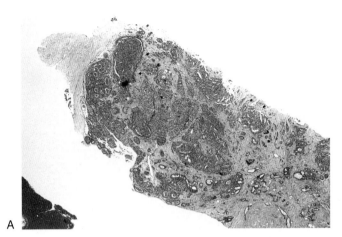

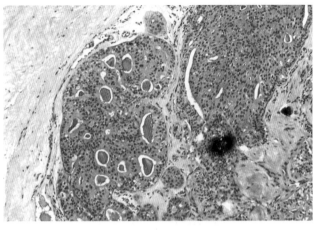

FIGURE 46. Intraductal carcinoma in a radial sclerosing lesion. A: Cribriform intraductal carcinoma is present in the upper left portion of this needle core biopsy specimen, atypical duct hyperplasia occupies the midportion, and sclerosing adenosis with calcification is present at the lower right. **B:** The area of cribriform intraductal carcinoma.

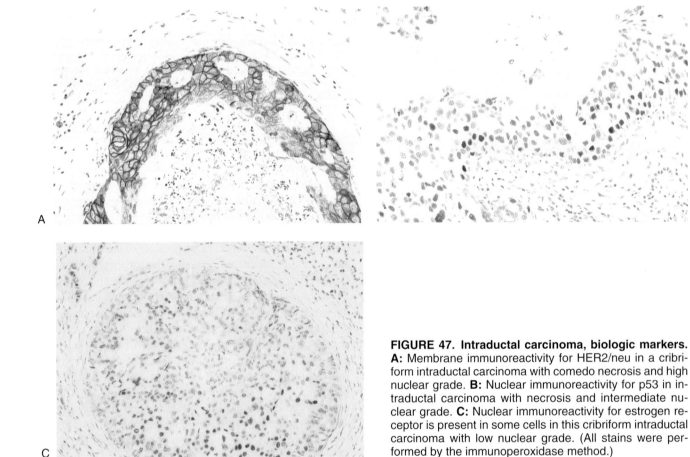

FIGURE 47. Intraductal carcinoma, biologic markers. A: Membrane immunoreactivity for HER2/neu in a cribriform intraductal carcinoma with comedo necrosis and high nuclear grade. **B:** Nuclear immunoreactivity for p53 in intraductal carcinoma with necrosis and intermediate nuclear grade. **C:** Nuclear immunoreactivity for estrogen receptor is present in some cells in this cribriform intraductal carcinoma with low nuclear grade. (All stains were performed by the immunoperoxidase method.)

breast conservation therapy in the treatment of intraductal carcinoma. Including those cited above, at least six classifications have been proposed (61). These have been based on some or all of the following features: architecture, nuclear grade, presence or absence of necrosis, lesion size, and cell polarity. Most classifications have emphasized nuclear grade, necrosis, and architecture. Generally, three grades have been proposed: high, intermediate, and low. There is a significant correlation between the grade of intraductal carcinoma and a corresponding invasive component, if present, regardless of grading system (61). The grading categories also have significant associations with biologic characteristics of intraductal carcinoma, especially lesions classified as high-grade and low-grade. High-grade lesions exhibit the following features: absence of estrogen and progesterone receptor expression, aneuploidy, high proliferative rate, periductal angiogenesis, membrane reactivity for HER2/neu, nuclear reactivity for p53, and abnormal bcl-2 expression (Fig. 47). Conversely, low-grade intraductal carcinomas have been characterized by the following: presence of estrogen and progesterone receptors, absence of aneuploidy, low proliferative rate, little periductal angiogenesis, absence of HER2/neu and p53 expression, and normal bcl-2 expression. Intermediate-grade intraductal carcinomas tend to have mixed patterns of biologic marker expression.

Currently, the classification of intraductal carcinoma is frequently expressed in terms of grade as well as architectural subtype. No single grading system has been adopted universally, but there is a consensus that the histomorphologic features most important in clinical practice as predictors of risk for local recurrence after breast conservation therapy are nuclear grade, necrosis, and microscopic structure (62). Margin status and size are also critical features relating to overall lesional characteristics. Presently, there is no single widely accepted method for combining these data into a grading system, and the recommended practice is to provide documentation for each of the individual features separately (62).

There is no reliable method for measuring the actual size of intraductal carcinoma in most cases. Many intraductal carcinomas currently detected by mammography do not form a clinically or pathologically palpable lesion. It is sometimes possible to determine the size of a lesion microscopically if it is limited to a single group of contiguous ducts (unifocal), especially when the area is confined to the histologic section from a single paraffin block containing tissue from a surgical excisional biopsy. A needle core biopsy cannot be relied on to measure the size of an intraductal carcinoma because the specimen rarely provides a single intact sample of the lesion. Many patients have more then one procedure performed (e.g., needle core biopsy, excision, repeated excision), with intraductal carcinoma in more than one specimen. It is not possible to reassemble the intraductal foci from multiple samples to obtain a single measurement. For these reasons, a consensus report on the classification of intraductal carcinoma left the issue of size largely unanswered (62). A classification system for intraductal carcinoma that includes measured lesion size is currently impractical.

The diagnosis of intraductal carcinoma by needle core biopsy cannot be relied on in all cases to exclude invasive carcinoma in the affected breast. Several studies have reported the frequency of invasive carcinoma detected by excisional biopsy after a needle core biopsy diagnosis of intraductal carcinoma to be in the range of 15% to 20% (7,63,64). The diagnosis of intraductal carcinoma was reported to be more reliable with a directional vacuum-assisted biopsy procedure than with an automated needle biopsy system in one study (64).

Ultrastructural studies have detected foci of discontinuity in the basement membranes of ducts with intraductal carcinoma (65), and similar observations have been reported in tissues studied by immunohistochemistry (66). Breaks in the basement membrane are more common when intraductal carcinoma is of the comedo type or has a high nuclear grade. In such regions, the neoplastic epithelium appears to protrude from the duct, coming in contact with the stroma while it remains connected to the intraductal neoplasm (67). This finding often elicits diagnostic uncertainty, reflected in such caveats as "microinvasion suspected" or "microinvasion cannot be ruled out." When *microinvasion* is present, carcinoma cells are distributed singly or as small groups that have irregular shapes in the periductal stroma with no particular orientation relative to the intraductal carcinoma (Fig. 48). The stroma sometimes appears less dense at sites of microinvasion than in other areas around ducts and lobules containing intraductal carcinoma. Detecting carcinoma cells in the stroma can be difficult when a marked periductal reaction is present. Microinvasion should be suspected at sites of pronounced lymphocytic reaction around ducts with intraductal carcinoma. A granulomatous reaction may be elicited at foci of microinvasion (68). In this setting, tumor cells can resemble histiocytes, and immunostains for cytokeratin may be required to confirm their presence outside the ducts (see Fig. 48). Microinvasion is more often associated with comedocarcinoma but may occur in other types (43). Carcinomatous epithelium displaced by needling procedures should not be misinterpreted as intrinsic invasive carcinoma (see Fig. 43).

There is no consensus as to the amount or extent of invasive carcinoma described by the term microinvasion. It is preferable to use the term *microinvasion* for lesions with no single focus of invasive carcinoma that is 1.0 mm or larger in diameter. This definition provides a descriptive identity for these unusually small invasive lesions that are otherwise not separately categorized. When multiple foci of such microinvasion are present, there is no precise method for estimating their aggregate diameter, and these cases still qualify as intraductal carcinoma with microinvasion. Foci larger than 1 mm are diagnosed as invasive duct carcinoma and measured (Fig. 49).

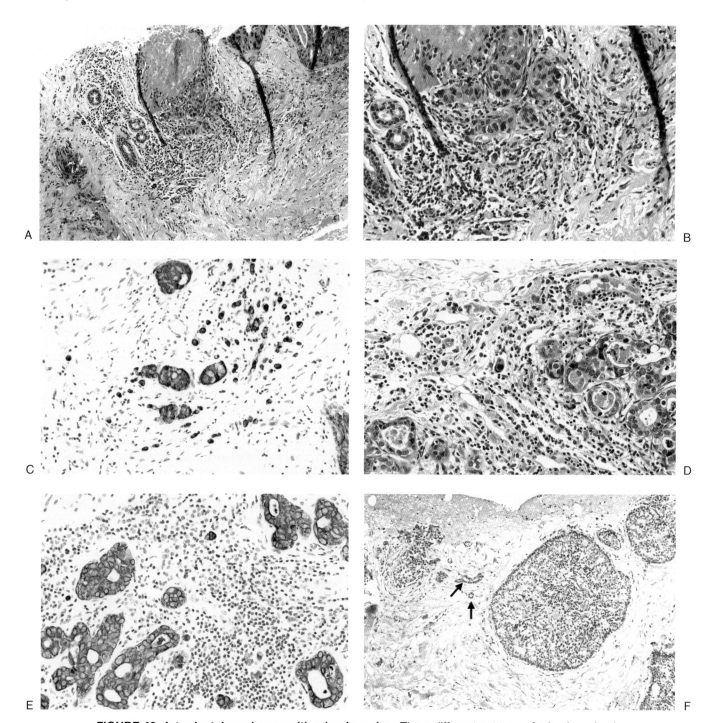

FIGURE 48. Intraductal carcinoma with microinvasion. Three different patterns of microinvasion in needle core biopsy specimens. **A–C:** Microinvasion here consists of a linear strand of tumor cells extending into the stroma surrounded by a lymphocytic reaction. Carcinoma cells in the stroma are highlighted here by cytokeratin immunohistochemistry (immunoperoxidase: CAM5.2). **D,E:** Another needle core biopsy specimen, with isolated carcinoma cells in the perilobular stroma. The invasive carcinoma cells are highlighted by an immunostain for cytokeratin (immunoperoxidase: CAM5.2). **F:** Well-differentiated infiltrating carcinoma is represented by two glands in the stroma to the left of the large duct (*arrows*). A small duct on the extreme left has been disrupted by the procedure and does not constitute invasive carcinoma.

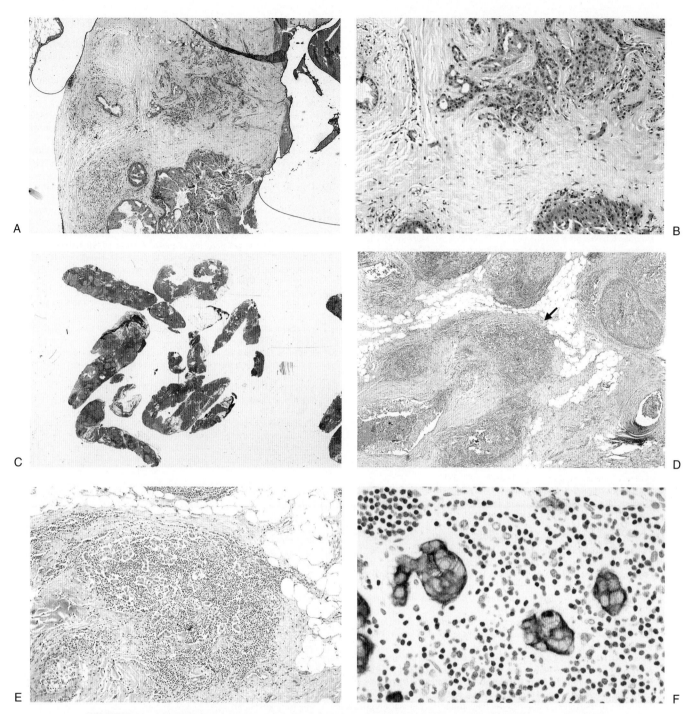

FIGURE 49. Intraductal carcinoma with invasion. A,B: A 1-mm focus of orderly invasive apocrine duct carcinoma is present in the upper half of this needle core biopsy specimen. Apocrine intraductal carcinoma is apparent below in the invasive area. **C:** This specimen consisted of multiple needle core biopsy samples with extensive intraductal carcinoma. **D:** The specimen in (C) contained these areas of solid, high-grade intraductal carcinoma and a 2-mm focus of invasive ductal carcinoma with a marked lymphocytic reaction, shown here in the center (*arrow*). **E:** A magnified view of the invasive ductal carcinoma. **F:** Groups of carcinoma cells in the invasive focus are highlighted with a keratin immunostain (immunoperoxidase: CAM5.2).

REFERENCES

1. Connolly JL, Schnitt SJ. Benign breast disease. Resolved and unresolved issues. *Cancer* 1993;71:1187–1189.
2. Bodian CA, Perzin KH, Lattes R, Hoffman P. Reproducibility and validity of pathologic classifications of benign breast disease and implications for clinical applications. *Cancer* 1993;71:3908–3913.
3. Rosai J. Borderline epithelial lesions of the breast. *Am J Surg Pathol* 1991;15:209–221.
4. Schnitt SJ, Connolly JL, Tavassoli FA, et al. Interobserver reproducibility in the diagnosis of ductal proliferative breast lesions using standardized criteria. *Am J Surg Pathol* 1992;16:1133–1143.
5. Palli D, Galli M, Bianchi S, et al. Reproducibility of histological diagnosis of breast lesions: results of a panel in Italy. *Eur J Cancer* 1996; 32A:603–607.
6. Helvie MA, Hessler C, Frank TS, Ikeda DM. Atypical hyperplasia of the breast: mammographic appearance and histologic correlation. *Radiology* 1991;179:759–764.
7. Jackman RJ, Nowels KW, Shepard MJ, Finkelstein SI, Marzoni MA Jr. Stereotaxic large-core needle biopsy of 450 nonpalpable breast lesions with surgical correlation in lesions with cancer or atypical hyperplasia. *Radiology* 1994;193:91–95.
8. Liberman L, Cohen MA, Abramson AF, Hann LE, Rosen PP. Atypical ductal hyperplasia diagnosed at stereotaxic core biopsy of breast lesions: an indication for surgical biopsy. *AJR Am J Roentgenol* 1995; 164:1111–1113.
9. Bodian CA, Perzin KH, Lattes R, Huffman P, Abernathy TG. Prognostic significance of benign proliferative breast disease. *Cancer* 1993;71: 3896–3907.
10. Page DL, Rogers LW. Combined histologic and cytologic criteria for the diagnosis of mammary atypical ductal hyperplasia. *Hum Pathol* 1992;23:1095–1097.
11. Rubin E, Visscher DW, Alexander RW, Urist MM, Maddox WA. Proliferative disease and atypia in biopsies performed for nonpalpable lesions detected mammographically. *Cancer* 1988;61:2077–2082.
12. Stomper PC, Cholewinski SP, Penetrante RB, Harlos JP, Tsangaris TM. Atypical hyperplasia: frequency and mammographic and pathologic relationships in excisional biopsies guided by mammography and clinical examination. *Radiology* 1993;189:667–671.
13. Arapantoni-Dadioti P, Panayiotides J, Georgakila H, Lekka J. Significance of intracytoplasmic lumina in the differential diagnosis between epithelial hyperplasia and carcinoma *in situ* of the breast. *Breast Dis* 1996;9:277–282.
14. Ozaki D, Kondo Y. Comparative morphometric studies of benign and malignant intraductal proliferative lesions of the breast by computerized image analysis. *Hum Pathol* 1995;26:1109–1113.
15. Ohuchi N, Abe R, Takahashi T, Tezuka F, Kyogoku M. Three-dimensional atypical structure in intraductal carcinoma differentiating from papilloma and papillomatosis of the breast. *Breast Cancer Res Treat* 1985;5:57–65.
16. Tavassoli FA, Norris HJ. A comparison of the results of long-term follow-up for atypical intraductal carcinoma of the breast. *Cancer* 1990; 65:518–529.
17. Tavassoli FA. Intraductal hyperplasias, ordinary and atypical. In: *Pathology of the breast*. New York: Elsevier Science, 1992:155–191.
18. Fisher ER, Costantino J, Fisher B, Palekar AS, Redmond C, Mamounas E, for the National Surgical Adjuvant Breast and Bowel Project Collaborating Investigators. Pathologic findings from the National Surgical Adjuvant Breast Project (NSABP) Protocol B-17. Intraductal carcinoma (ductal carcinoma *in situ*). *Cancer* 1995;75:1310–1319.
19. Tocino I, Garcia BM, Carter D. Surgical biopsy findings in patients with atypical hyperplasia diagnosed by stereotaxic core needle biopsy. *Ann Surg Oncol* 1996;3:483–488.
20. Kodlin D, Winger EE, Morgenstern NL, Chen V. Chronic mastopathy and breast cancer: a follow-up study. *Cancer* 1977;39:2603–2607.
21. Dupont WD, Page DL. Breast cancer risk associated with proliferative disease, age at first birth, and family history of breast cancer. *Am J Epidemiol* 1987;1225:769–779.
22. Krieger N, Hiatt RA. Risk of breast cancer after benign breast diseases. Variation by histologic type, degree of atypia, age at biopsy, and length of follow-up. *Am J Epidemiol* 1992;135:619–631.
23. Davis HH, Simons M, Davis JB. Cystic disease of the breast: relationship to carcinoma. *Cancer* 1964;17:957–978.
24. Page DL, DuPont WD, Rogers LW, Rados MS. Atypical hyperplastic lesions of the female breast. A long-term follow-up study. *Cancer* 1985;55:2698–2708.
25. Connolly J, Schnitt S, London S, Dupont W, Colditz G, Page D. Both atypical lobular hyperplasia (ALH) and atypical ductal hyperplasia (ADH) predict for bilateral breast cancer risk. *Lab Invest* 1992;66:13A.
26. Tavassoli FA, Norris HJ. A comparison of the results of long-term follow-up for atypical intraductal hyperplasia and intraductal hyperplasia of the breast. *Cancer* 1990;65:518–529.
27. Carter CL, Corle DK, Micozzi MS, Schatzkin A, Taylor PR. A prospective study of the development of breast cancer in 16,692 women with benign breast disease. *Am J Epidemiol* 1988;128:467–477.
28. London SJ, Connolly JL, Schnitt SJ, Colditz GA. A prospective study of benign breast disease and the risk of breast cancer. *JAMA* 1992;267: 941–944.
29. Dupont WD, Page DL. Risk factors for breast cancer in women with proliferative breast disease. *N Engl J Med* 1985;312:146–151.
30. Ma L, Boyd NF. Atypical hyperplasia and breast cancer risk: a critique. *Cancer Causes Control* 1992;3:517–525.
31. Jensen RA, Page DL, Dupont WD, Rogers LW. Invasive breast cancer risk in women with sclerosing adenosis. *Cancer* 1989;64:1977–1983.
32. Ernster VL, Barclay J, Kerlikowske K, Grady D, Henderson IC. Incidence of and treatment for ductal carcinoma *in situ* of the breast. *JAMA* 1996;275:913–918.
33. Ward BA, McKhann CF, Ravikumar TS. Ten-year follow-up of breast carcinoma *in situ* in Connecticut. *Arch Surg* 1992;127:1392–1395.
34. Chu KC, Tarone RE, Kessler LG, et al. Recent trends in U.S. breast cancer incidence, survival, and mortality rates. *J Natl Cancer Inst* 1996; 88:1571–1579.
35. Ciatto S, Cataliotti L, Distante V. Nonpalpable lesions detected with mammography: review of 512 consecutive cases. *Radiology* 1987;165: 99–102.
36. Dershaw DD, Abramson A, Kinne DW. Ductal carcinoma *in situ*: mammographic findings and clinical implications. *Radiology* 1989; 170:411–415.
37. Stomper PC, Connolly JL, Meyer JE, Harris JR. Clinically occult ductal carcinoma *in situ* detected with mammography: analysis of 100 cases with radiologic-pathologic correlation. *Radiology* 1989;172: 235–241.
38. Holland R, Hendriks JHCL, Verbeek ALM, Mravunac M, Schuurmans-Stekhoven JH. Extent, distribution, and mammographic/histological correlations of breast ductal carcinoma *in situ*. *Lancet* 1990;335: 519–522.
39. Lagios MD. Multicentricity of breast carcinoma demonstrated by routine correlated subgross and radiographic examination. *Cancer* 1977; 40:1726–1734.
40. Stomper PC, Connolly JL. Ductal carcinoma *in situ* of the breast: correlation between mammographic calcification and tumor subtype. *AJR Am J Roentgenol* 1992;159:483–485.
41. Evans A, Pinder S, Wilson R, et al. Ductal carcinoma *in situ* of the breast: correlation between mammographic and pathologic findings. *AJR Am J Roentgenol* 1994;162:1307–1311.
42. Evans AJ, Pinder SE, Ellis IO, et al. Correlations between the mammographic features of ductal carcinoma *in situ* (DCIS) and c-erb-s oncogene expression. *Clin Radiol* 1994;49:559–562.
43. Patchefsky AS, Schwartz GF, Finkelstein SD, et al. Heterogeneity of intraductal carcinoma of the breast. *Cancer* 1989;63:731–741.
44. Cheng L, Al-Kaisi NK, Liu AY, Gordon NH. The results of intraoperative consultations in 181 ductal carcinomas *in situ* of the breast. *Cancer* 1997;80:75–79.
45. Rosen PP. Frozen section diagnosis of breast lesions. Recent experience with 556 consecutive biopsies. *Ann Surg* 1978;187:17–19.
46. Rosen PP, Senie R, Schottenfeld D, Ashikari R. Noninvasive breast carcinoma: frequency of unsuspected invasion and implication for treatment. *Ann Surg* 1979;189:98–103.
47. Wellings SR, Jensen HM, Marcum RG. An atlas of subgross pathology of the human breast with special reference to possible precancerous lesions. *J Natl Cancer Inst* 1975;55:231–273.
48. Barsky SH, Siegal GP, Jannotta F, Liotta LA. Loss of basement membrane components by invasive tumors but not by their benign counterparts. *Lab Invest* 1983;49:140–147.
49. Lennington WJ, Jensen RA, Dalton LW, Page DL. Ductal carcinoma *in situ* of the breast. Heterogeneity of individual lesions. *Cancer* 1994;73: 118–124.
50. Bose S, Lesser ML, Norton L, Rosen PP. Immunophenotype of intraductal carcinoma. *Arch Pathol Lab Med* 1996;100:81–85.

51. Muir R, Aitkenhead AC. The healing of intraduct carcinoma of the mamma. *J Pathol Bacteriol* 1934;38:117–127.
52. Davies JD. Hyperelastosis, obliteration and fibrous plaques in major ducts of the human breast. *J Pathol* 1973;110:13–26.
53. Chan JKC, Ng WF. Sclerosing adenosis cancerized by intraductal carcinoma. *Pathology* 1987;19:425–428.
54. Eusebi V, Collina G, Bussolati G. Carcinoma *in situ* in sclerosing adenosis of the breast: an immunocytochemical study. *Semin Diagn Pathol* 1989;6:146–152.
55. Oberman HA, Markey BA. Non-invasive carcinoma of the breast presenting in adenosis. *Mod Pathol* 1991;4:31–35.
56. Taylor HB, Norris HJ. Epithelial invasion of nerves in benign diseases of the breast. *Cancer* 1967;20:2245–2249.
57. Tsang WYW, Chan JKC. Neural invasion in intraductal carcinoma of the breast. *Hum Pathol* 1992;23:202–204.
58. Goldstein NS, Murphy T. Intraductal carcinoma associated with invasive carcinoma of the breast. A comparison of the two lesions with implications for intraductal carcinoma classification systems. *Am J Clin Pathol* 1996;106:312–318.
59. Silverstein MJ, Poller DN, Waisman JR, et al. Prognostic classification of breast ductal carcinoma-in-situ. *Lancet* 1995;345:1154–1157.
60. Silverstein MJ, Lagios MD, Craig PH, et al. A prognostic index for ductal carcinoma *in situ* of the breast. *Cancer* 1996;77:2267–2274.
61. Douglas-Jones AG, Gupta SK, Attanoos RL, Morgan JM, Mansel RE. A critical appraisal of six modern classifications of ductal carcinoma *in situ* of the breast (DCIS): correlation with grade of associated invasive carcinoma. *Histopathology* 1996;29:397–409.
62. Consensus Conference on the Classification of Ductal Carcinoma *In Situ*. The Consensus Conference Committee. *Cancer* 1997;80: 1798–1802.
63. Liberman L, Dershaw DD, Rosen PP, et al. Stereotaxic core biopsy of breast carcinoma: accuracy at predicting invasion. *Radiology* 1995; 194:379–381.
64. Burbank F. Stereotactic breast biopsy of atypical ductal hyperplasia and ductal carcinoma *in situ* lesions: improved accuracy with directional, vacuum-assisted biopsy. *Radiology* 1997;202:843–847.
65. Ozzello L. Ultrastructure of intra-epithelial carcinomas of the breast. *Cancer* 1971;28:1508–1515.
66. Rajan PB, Perry RH. A quantitative study of patterns of basement membrane in ductal carcinoma *in situ* (DCIS) of the breast. *Breast J* 1995;1: 315–321.
67. Ozzello L. The behavior of basement membranes in intraductal carcinoma of the breast. *Am J Pathol* 1959;35:887–899.
68. Coyne J, Haboubi NY. Micro-invasive breast carcinoma with granulomatous stromal response. *Histopathology* 1992;20:184–185.

CHAPTER 9

Invasive Duct Carcinoma

This largest group of malignant mammary tumors constitutes 65% to 80% of mammary carcinomas. A generic term sometimes employed is invasive duct carcinoma, not otherwise specified (NOS), which is a useful designation that recognizes the distinction between these tumors and other, specific forms of duct carcinoma, such as tubular, medullary, metaplastic, colloid, and adenoid cystic carcinomas.

Invasive duct carcinoma includes a subset of tumors that express in part characteristics of one of the specific types of breast carcinoma but do not constitute pure examples of the individual tumors. One example of this phenomenon is invasive duct carcinoma with an infiltrating lobular carcinoma component (Fig. 1). Foci of tubular, mucinous, or papillary differentiation can be found in invasive duct carcinomas. When evidence of a mixed growth pattern is present in a needle core biopsy specimen, the findings should be reported descriptively, with final classification reserved for the excisional biopsy specimen. The relatively favorable prognosis associated with some specific histologic types has been found to apply only to those tumors that exhibit entirely or in very large part the designated pattern.

The tissue obtained in a needle core biopsy procedure often includes multiple samples of tumor tissue (Fig. 2). On occasion, only a small fragment of the lesion may be present (Fig. 3). All tissue on a slide must be carefully examined to ensure that this very limited material is not overlooked. In the most extreme circumstance, the evidence is so scant that a diagnosis of carcinoma cannot be made with confidence, and an excisional biopsy is necessary to determine if carcinoma is present. Although it is technically possible to examine needle core biopsy specimens by frozen section, this is not a standard practice and should be done only rarely, in exceptional situations (Fig. 4).

There are no specific clinical features that distinguish invasive duct carcinoma from other types of invasive carcinoma and some benign tumors. The lesions occur throughout the age range of breast carcinoma, being most common in patients in their middle to late fifties. Invasive duct carcinoma invariably forms a solid tumor. Cystic change in this group of lesions is extremely uncommon but may be a manifestation of necrosis, usually accompanied by hemorrhage in the degenerated area.

The measured gross *size* of a mammary carcinoma is one of the most significant prognostic variables. Survival decreases with increasing tumor size of invasive duct carcinoma and most of the subtypes of breast carcinoma, and there is a coincidental rise in the frequency of axillary nodal metastases (1,2). This phenomenon applies not only to the overall spectrum of primary tumor size, but also within subsets, such as those defined by TNM (tumor-node-metastasis) staging. For example, among T_1 breast carcinomas (≤ 2 cm in diameter), there is a significant relationship between size, frequency of nodal metastases, and prognosis when the tumors are stratified in 5-mm groups (3,4). The interaction of the number of involved lymph nodes and tumor size is important prognostically in stage II patients. Quiet et al. (5) found that long-term disease-free survival after mastectomy was 81% in patients with one lymph node metastasis and a tumor 2 cm or smaller, compared with 59% if the tumor was larger than 2 cm.

Because most carcinomas have asymmetric shapes, the measurement of size is generally reported in terms of the greatest diameter. The gross measurement of the size of a carcinoma is only an approximation of the actual amount of invasive tumor present (6,7). Measurement of the invasive component exclusive of peripheral extensions of intraductal carcinoma is recommended when it is practical. It is rarely possible to measure the size of an invasive carcinoma in a needle core biopsy specimen because it is difficult to ensure that the sample represents a complete diameter in the largest dimension. Correlation with the dimensions of a small lesion seen on a mammogram can be useful in some circumstances to confirm the size of a carcinoma and to assess the contour of the tumor.

Histologic grading of infiltrating carcinomas is an estimate of structural differentiation, limited to the invasive portion of the tumor (Fig. 5). The most widely used histologic grading system is based on criteria established by Bloom and Richardson (8) and Elston and Ellis (9). The parameters measured are the extent of tubule formation, degree of nuclear hyperchromasia or size, and mitotic rate. Histologic grade is usually expressed in three categories: well-differentiated (grade 1), intermediate (grade 2), and poorly differentiated (grade 3). A modified Scarff-Bloom-Richardson system presented by Robbins et al. (10) is outlined in Table 1.

Text continues on page 119

115

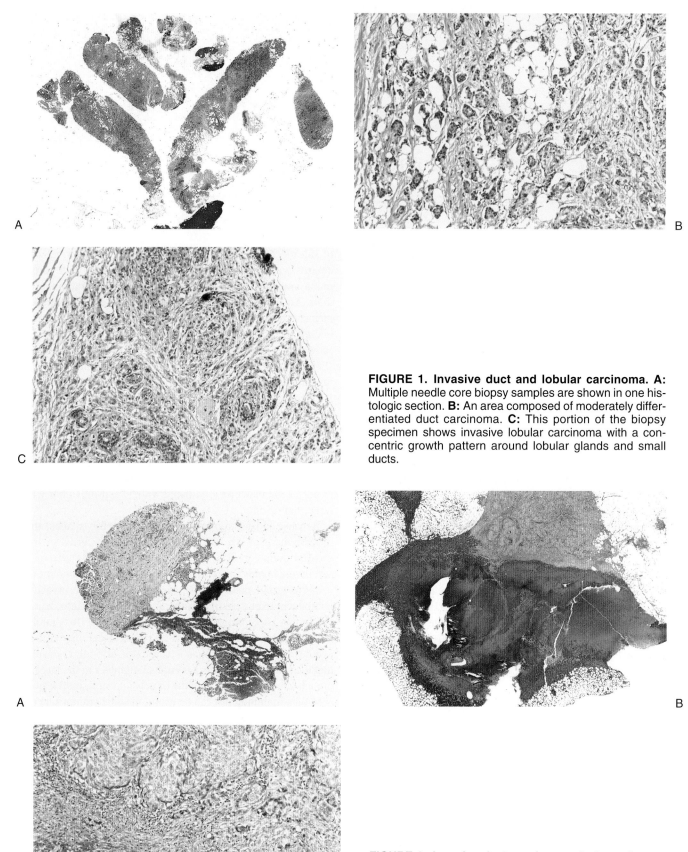

FIGURE 1. Invasive duct and lobular carcinoma. A: Multiple needle core biopsy samples are shown in one histologic section. **B:** An area composed of moderately differentiated duct carcinoma. **C:** This portion of the biopsy specimen shows invasive lobular carcinoma with a concentric growth pattern around lobular glands and small ducts.

FIGURE 2. Invasive duct carcinoma. A: A needle core biopsy sample of carcinoma with hemorrhage and a displaced fragment of carcinoma in the fat in the lower right corner. **B:** A low-magnification view of the excised tumor showing hemorrhage at the needle biopsy site. **C:** Granulation tissue is present between the poorly differentiated invasive duct carcinoma above and the blood clot.

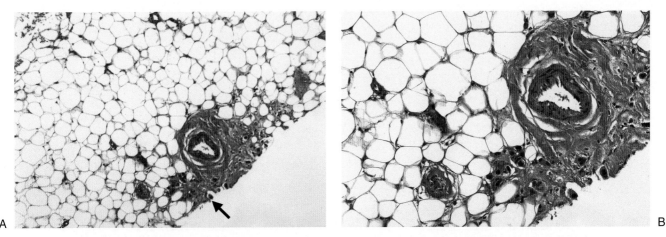

FIGURE 3. Invasive duct carcinoma. A,B: A small group of atypical cells in fat (*arrow*) around a blood vessel in this needle core biopsy specimen was the only evidence of carcinoma in this case. The material was not considered diagnostic, and excisional biopsy of an 8-mm circumscribed tumor revealed invasive, poorly differentiated duct carcinoma.

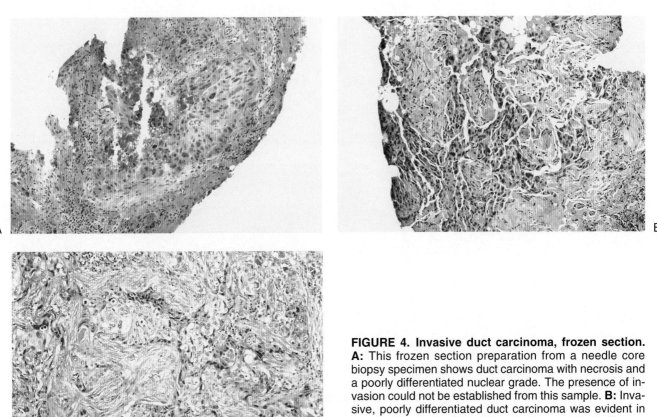

FIGURE 4. Invasive duct carcinoma, frozen section. A: This frozen section preparation from a needle core biopsy specimen shows duct carcinoma with necrosis and a poorly differentiated nuclear grade. The presence of invasion could not be established from this sample. **B:** Invasive, poorly differentiated duct carcinoma was evident in the paraffin section from the same tissue sample. The tissue is distorted by frozen-section artifact. **C:** The appearance of the tumor without frozen-section artifact is shown here in the excisional biopsy specimen.

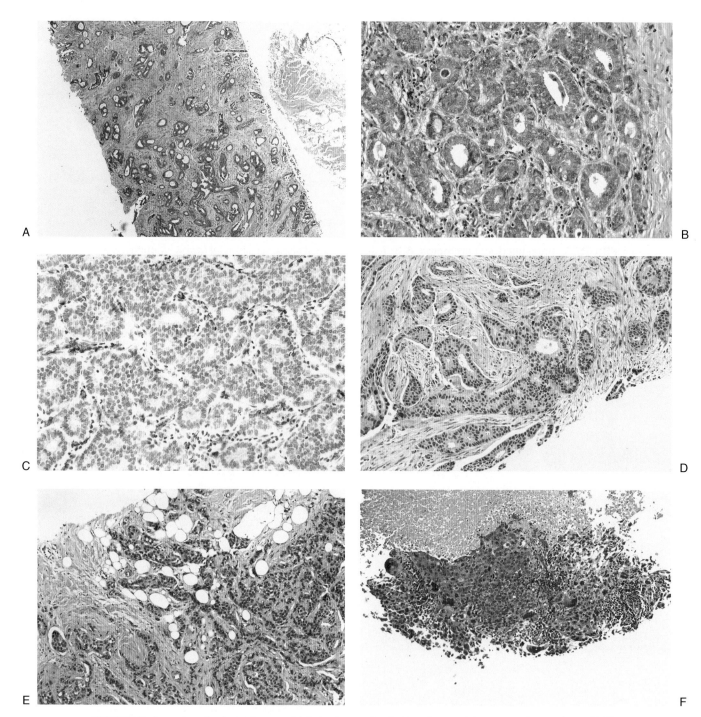

FIGURE 5. Invasive duct carcinoma, histologic grade. A: Needle core biopsy specimen of a well-differentiated carcinoma is characterized by distinct glands with lumina, partly with a cribriform pattern. The complexity of the glandular arrangement exceeds the appearance of tubular carcinoma. **B:** This unusual form of invasive duct carcinoma with well-differentiated histologic grade resembles florid adenosis. The nuclear grade is intermediate. **C:** The immunostain for actin shown here failed to detect myoepithelial cells around the neoplastic glands (immunoperoxidase: smooth-muscle actin). **D,E:** Two needle core biopsy specimens of invasive duct carcinoma with moderate histologic grade. In (D), the carcinoma cells are arranged in distinct glands, whereas in (E), the tumor is composed of irregular bands with ill-defined lumina. **F:** Poorly differentiated invasive duct carcinoma consists of solid nests of tumor cells without gland formation. The tumor cell nuclei are intermediate and poorly differentiated. This poorly differentiated invasive duct carcinoma has anaplastic giant cells and focal necrosis.

TABLE 1. *Modified Scarff-Bloom-Richardson grading system*

Extent of tubule formation
Score 1: >75% of tumor
Score 2: 10%–75% of tumor
Score 3: <10% of tumor
Nuclear size
Score 1: tumor cell nuclei similar to normal duct cell nuclei (2–3 × RBC)
Score 2: intermediate-size nuclei
Score 3: very large nuclei, usually vesicular with prominent nucleoli
Mitotic count
Based on 10 fields from edge of tumor (40× objective, 400× magnification, field area 0.196 mm²)
Score 1: 0–7 mitoses
Score 2: 8–14 mitoses
Score 3: ≥15 mitoses

RBC, red blood cell.
From ref. 10, with permission.

Nuclear grading is the cytologic evaluation of tumor nuclei in comparison with the nuclei of normal mammary epithelial cells (Fig. 6). Because nuclear grading does not involve an assessment of the growth pattern of the tumor, this procedure is applicable not only to invasive duct carcinoma but also to other subtypes of mammary carcinoma. The most widely employed system for nuclear grading, introduced by Black et al. (11) and Cutler et al. (12), is usually reported in terms of three categories: well-differentiated, intermediate, and poorly differentiated. By convention, the sequence of numerical designations originally used for nuclear grading was the reverse of that for histologic grading, but more recently there has been a trend to employ a numbering system that conforms to histologic grading (grade 1, well-differentiated; grade 2, moderate; grade 3, poorly differentiated). Because of the potential for confusion on this issue, it is preferable to employ descriptive terms for nuclear grading rather than numerals.

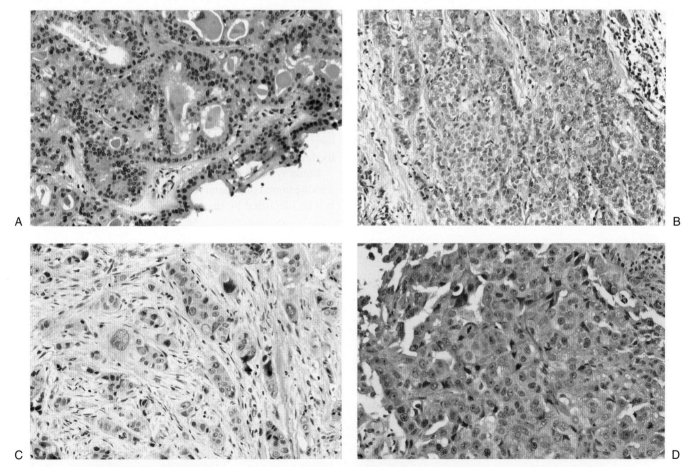

FIGURE 6. Invasive duct carcinoma, nuclear grade. A: A well-differentiated nuclear grade is characterized by cells having small, regular, round nuclei with even chromatin lacking nucleoli and mitoses. **B:** A moderately differentiated nuclear grade is characterized by modest nuclear pleomorphism and enlargement with nucleoli in some nuclei. The nuclei are only slightly hyperchromatic. **C,D:** A poorly differentiated nuclear grade features marked nuclear pleomorphism and enlargement with hyperchromasia.

The histologic and nuclear grades of a given tumor coincide in many but not all invasive duct carcinomas (13). Nuclear and histologic grade have been shown to be useful indicators of prognosis for patients stratified by stage of disease, especially those without axillary lymph node metastases (14,15). Increasing tumor grade has been associated with several factors related to an increased risk for local recurrence after breast conservation therapy, including greater tumor size, diagnosis at a relatively young age, and absence of estrogen receptor expression. Although some investigators found a significant relationship between grade and local recurrence (16), others concluded that grade was not significant (17). In patients with relatively favorable stage I carcinomas treated by lumpectomy without radiotherapy, tumors recurred sooner and with greater frequency after a median follow-up of 58 months in patients with high-grade carcinomas (18).

Women with BRCA1 mutations have a significantly higher frequency of poorly differentiated carcinomas in comparison with women not carrying this mutation. BRCA1 mutations occurring in sporadic and familial breast carcinomas have been associated with similar patterns of poorly differentiated growth (19). This is manifested by a nuclear grade denoting poor differentiation (19), low frequency of estrogen receptor positivity (19), and a high histologic grade (20). Mammography did not detect a significant difference in the radiographic appearance of carcinomas in BRCA1 carriers (21).

The *stromal lymphoplasmacytic infiltration* within and around invasive duct carcinomas usually consists of mature lymphocytes with a variable admixture of plasma cells and macrophages (Fig. 7). Nonmedullary duct carcinomas with a prominent lymphocytic reaction tend to be poorly differentiated and also are almost always negative for estrogen and progesterone receptors. Studies of the lymphocyte subgroups infiltrating mammary carcinomas indicate that they

are largely T lymphocytes (22) consisting mainly of T4 (CD4+) helper and T8 (CD8+) cytotoxic suppressor cells (23).

The presence of *lymphatic tumor emboli* (Fig. 8) in the breast is an unfavorable prognostic finding. For this purpose, lymphatics are defined as vascular channels lined by endothelium without supporting smooth muscle. Most do not contain red blood cells, but undoubtedly some blood capillaries are included in this definition. Artifactual spaces can be formed around nests of tumor cells within an invasive carcinoma as a result of tissue shrinkage during processing (Fig. 9). Because it may be difficult to distinguish shrinkage artifacts from true lymphatic spaces, assessment for lymphatic invasion is more reliably accomplished in breast parenchyma adjacent to or well beyond the invasive tumor margin, where these artifacts are less often present (24,25). An unusual pattern of necrosis in carcinoma that involves pseudoangiomatous stromal hyperplasia can simulate lymphatic invasion by carcinoma (Fig. 10).

Extratumoral lymphatic tumor emboli in the breast are found associated with approximately 15% of invasive duct carcinomas that have been examined in excisional biopsy specimens. The majority of these patients also have axillary lymph node metastases, but lymphatic tumor emboli are found in the breast surrounding invasive duct carcinomas in 5% to 10% of patients who have pathologically negative lymph nodes. Several studies have shown that lymphatic emboli are prognostically unfavorable in node-negative patients treated by mastectomy (5,26–28) and by breast conservation therapy (29). Lymphatic tumor emboli do not predispose to local recurrence in patients treated by mastectomy (27), but they are associated with an increased risk for recurrence in the breast after breast conservation therapy (29).

Blood vessel invasion is defined as penetration by tumor into the lumen of an artery or vein. These vascular structures can be identified by the presence of a smooth-muscle wall

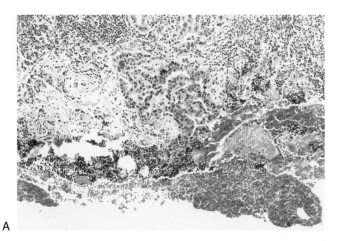
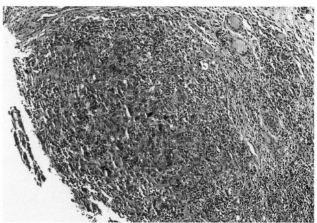

A   B

FIGURE 7. Invasive duct carcinoma, lymphoplasmacytic infiltration. A: A needle core biopsy specimen showing slight lymphocytic reaction associated with invasive duct carcinoma. **B:** Extreme lymphoplasmacytic infiltration in a needle core biopsy sample from a poorly differentiated duct carcinoma. Medullary carcinoma was ruled out when invasive areas were found in the excisional biopsy specimen.

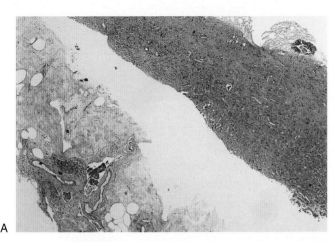

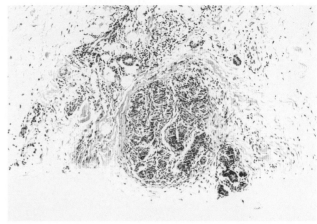

FIGURE 8. Invasive duct carcinoma with lymphatic tumor emboli. A: This needle core biopsy specimen shows clusters of carcinoma cells in dilated lymphatic spaces among small blood vessels adjacent to a sample of invasive, poorly differentiated duct carcinoma. **B:** Lymphatic tumor emboli are located in the stroma around a lobule in a needle core biopsy specimen.

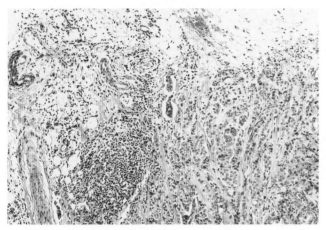

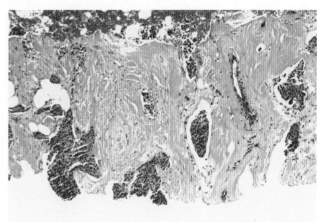

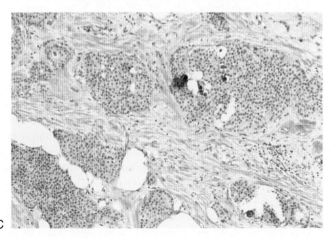

FIGURE 9. Invasive duct carcinoma with shrinkage artifact. A: Two clusters of carcinoma cells are present in a bilobed space in the midst of this needle core biopsy specimen. The contour of the space closely duplicates the shape of the carcinoma that it contains. This is a hallmark of shrinkage artifact. **B:** Shrinkage artifact in a needle core biopsy specimen from an invasive duct carcinoma. **C:** No shrinkage artifact was present in this excisional biopsy specimen of the tumor in (B).

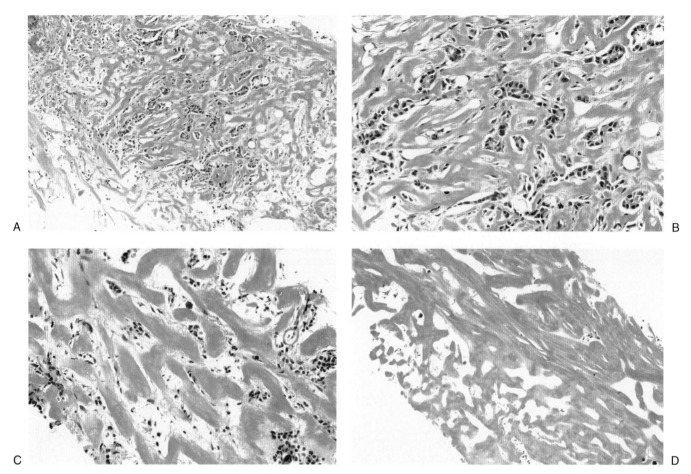

FIGURE 10. Invasive duct carcinoma with necrosis. A,B: The invasive duct carcinoma in this needle core biopsy specimen is growing in stroma that has a pseudoangiomatous architecture. **C,D:** The pseudoangiomatous pattern is accentuated in areas of necrosis.

supported by elastic fibers. It is usually necessary to employ special histochemical procedures (e.g., orcein or Verhoeff-van Gieson stains) that selectively stain elastic tissue to detect this component of the vascular wall. Elastic fibers are often deposited around ducts that contain intraductal carcinoma within an invasive tumor, and the resulting appearance in an elastic tissue stain may be difficult to distinguish from vascular invasion. Because larger vascular components in the breast usually consist of a paired artery and vein, vascular invasion should be diagnosed with confidence only when tumor is demonstrated within one or both of a pair of vessels by an elastic tissue stain.

The *angiogenesis* associated with breast carcinomas reflects the capacity of neoplastic tissue to induce vascular proliferation (30). Tumor growth is enhanced not only by increased perfusion associated with neovascularization, but also by the paracrine mitogenic effects of growth factors produced by endothelial cells (30). Pathologic studies of angiogenesis in breast carcinoma have examined the relevance of tumor vascularity to known prognostic markers and prognosis. To perform such studies, histologic sections or paraffin-

embedded tissue are stained with an immunohistochemical marker for endothelial cells (31) (Fig. 11). Vessel counts are recorded in foci of greatest vascular density, so-called hot spots, by counting the number of immunostained structures in a predetermined number of fields at a fixed magnification (32). A significant problem in the method of assessment based on detecting hot spots is the heterogeneity of vascularity with breast carcinomas. A study of angiogenesis in multiple blocks from individual carcinomas revealed an average coefficient of variation (CV) of 11.1% for vessel counts in hot spots in different sections from a single paraffin block and a CV of 24.4% when hot spots in sections from different blocks from the same tumor were compared (33). The authors concluded that "one must carefully scan all the available tumor material in each case for the best spot." Counts based on limited samples, such as needle core biopsy specimens or one section of a tumor, could be highly misleading. Consequently, conventional needle core biopsy specimens are not suitable for estimating angiogenesis by current methods.

Perineural invasion can be found in approximately 10% of invasive carcinomas (Fig. 12). It tends to occur in high-

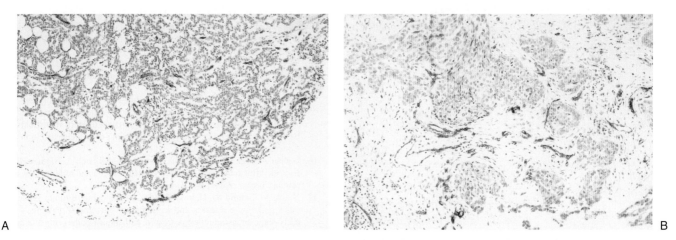

FIGURE 11. Invasive duct carcinoma with angiogenesis. A,B: Vascularity is demonstrated in the needle core biopsy specimens of two invasive duct carcinomas with the immunostain for CD34. The tumor invades fat in (A) and fibrous stroma in (B).

grade tumors, frequently associated with lymphatic tumor emboli, but it has not been proved to have independent prognostic significance.

Abundant *elastosis* in the stroma of an invasive duct carcinoma is significantly associated with estrogen receptor positivity (Fig. 13). The importance of elastosis as an independent prognostic variable remains controversial (34,35).

Attention has been directed to the pattern and distribution of *intraductal carcinoma* as a prognostic variable in patients with invasive duct carcinoma. The presence of intraductal carcinoma in a needle core biopsy specimen from an invasive duct carcinoma should be noted. Included in the diagnostic report should be a description of the structural pattern, nuclear grade, and the presence or absence of necrosis and calcifications.

Invasive duct carcinomas vary in the relative proportions of intraductal and invasive components. As the proportion of intraductal carcinoma increases for any gross tumor size,

there is a trend to decreased nodal metastases and a more favorable prognosis. Lesions with a prominent intratumoral intraductal component tend to be associated with intraductal carcinoma outside the main tumor and to have multicentric foci of carcinoma in other quadrants of the breast. The distribution of intraductal carcinoma in and around the primary tumor appears to correlate with the risk for recurrence in the breast after lumpectomy and radiation therapy (36) but has no bearing on the risk for systemic recurrence in women treated by mastectomy (37). Recurrence is more frequent in the breast after lumpectomy and radiation therapy in women who have intraductal comedocarcinoma or extensive intraductal carcinoma, defined as intraductal carcinoma within and around an invasive tumor that comprises at least 25% of the neoplasm. The increased risk for local recurrence attributable to an extensive intraductal component is probably a manifestation of a greater probability of the presence of carcinoma at the margin of excision, so that it remains in the

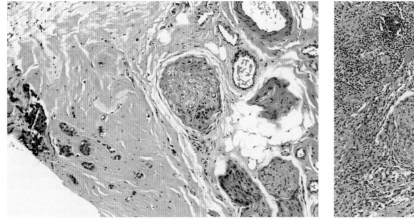

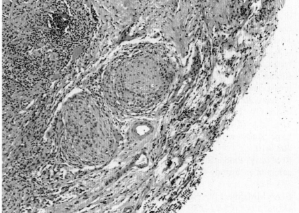

FIGURE 12. Invasive duct carcinoma with perineural infiltration. A,B: Carcinoma cells are shown invading nerves in needle core biopsy specimens from two patients.

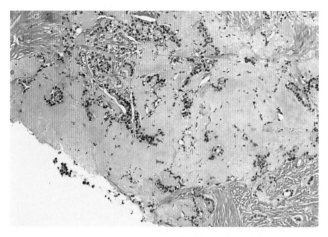

FIGURE 13. Invasive duct carcinoma with stromal elastosis. The stroma in this needle core biopsy specimen contains homogeneous masses of amphophilic elastin in invasive duct carcinoma.

breast. In patients with negative margins, the presence of extensive intraductal carcinoma does not increase the risk for local recurrence in the breast after breast conservation therapy (38,39). A reliable estimate of the proportion of intraductal carcinoma in the lesion and its extent beyond the invasive area cannot be determined from conventional needle core biopsy samples.

REFERENCES

1. Say CC, Donegan WL. Invasive carcinoma of the breast: prognostic significance of tumor size and involved axillary lymph nodes. *Cancer* 1974;34:468–471.
2. Smart CR, Myers MH, Gloecker LA. Implications for SEER data on breast cancer management. *Cancer* 1978;41:787–789.
3. Rosen PP, Saigo PE, Braun DW Jr, Weathers E, DePalo A. Predictors of recurrence in stage I ($T_1N_0M_0$) breast carcinoma. *Ann Surg* 1981; 193:15–25.
4. Rosen PP, Saigo PE, Braun DW Jr, Weathers E, Kinne DW. Prognosis in stage II ($T_1N_1M_0$) breast cancer. *Ann Surg* 1981;194:576–584.
5. Quiet CA, Ferguson DJ, Weichselbaum RR, Hellman S. Natural history of node-positive breast cancer: the curability of small cancers with a limited number of positive nodes. *J Clin Oncol* 1996;14:3105–3111.
6. Seidman JD, Schnaper LA, Aisner SC. Relationship of the size of the invasive component of the primary breast carcinoma to axillary lymph node metastasis. *Cancer* 1995;75:65–71.
7. Silverberg SG, Chitale AR. Assessment of significance of proportions of intraductal and infiltrating tumor growth in ductal carcinoma of the breast. *Cancer* 1978;32:830–837.
8. Bloom HJG, Richardson WW. Histological grading and prognosis in breast cancer. A study of 1049 cases, of which 359 have been followed 15 years. *Br J Cancer* 1957;11:359–377.
9. Elston CW, Ellis IO. Pathological prognostic factors in breast cancer. I. The value of histological grade in breast cancer: experience from a large study with long-term follow-up. *Histopathology* 1991;19: 403–410.
10. Robbins P, Pinder S, de Klerk N, et al. Histological grading of breast carcinomas: a study of interobserver agreement. *Hum Pathol* 1995;26: 873–879.
11. Black MM, Speer FD. Nuclear structure in cancer tissues. *Surg Gynecol Obstet* 1957;105:97–105.
12. Cutler SJ, Black MM, Mork T, Harvei S, Freeman C. Further observations on prognostic factors in cancer of the female breast. *Cancer* 1969; 24:653–667.
13. Goldstein NS, Murphy T. Intraductal carcinoma associated with invasive carcinoma of the breast. A comparison of the two lesions with implications for intraductal carcinoma classification systems. *Am J Clin Pathol* 1996;106:312–318.
14. Dawson PJ, Ferguson DJ, Karrison T. The pathologic findings of breast cancer in patients surviving 25 years after radical mastectomy. *Cancer* 1982;50:2131–2138.
15. LeDoussal V, Tubiana-Hulin M, Friedman S, Hacene K, Spyratos F, Brunet M. Prognostic value of histologic grade/nuclear components of Scarff-Bloom-Richardson (SBR). An improved score modification based on a multivariate analysis of 1262 invasive ductal carcinomas. *Cancer* 1989;64:1914–1921.
16. Locker A, Ellis IO, Morgan DA, Elston CW, Mitchell A, Blamey RW. Factors influencing local recurrence after excision and radiotherapy for primary breast cancer. *Br J Surg* 1989;76:890–894.
17. Nixon AJ, Schnitt SJ, Gelman R, et al. Relationship of tumor grade to other pathologic features and to treatment outcome of patients with early-stage breast carcinoma treated with breast-conserving therapy. *Cancer* 1996;78:426–431.
18. Schnitt SJ, Hayman J, Gelman R, et al. A prospective study of conservative surgery alone in the treatment of selected patients with stage I breast cancer. *Cancer* 1996;77:1094–1100.
19. Karp SE, Tonin PN, Begin LR, et al. Influence of BRCA1 mutations on nuclear grade and estrogen receptor status of breast carcinoma in Ashkenazi Jewish women. *Cancer* 1997;80:435–441.
20. Breast Cancer Linkage Consortium. Pathology of familial breast cancer: differences between breast cancers in carriers of BRCA1 and BRCA2 mutations and sporadic cases. *Lancet* 1997;349:1505–1510.
21. Helvie MA, Roubidoux MA, Weber BL, Merajver SD. Mammography of breast carcinoma in women who have mutations of the breast cancer gene BRCA1: initial experience. *AJR Am J Roentgenol* 1997;168: 1599–1602.
22. Bilik R, Mor C, Haraz B, Moroz C. Characterization of T-lymphocyte subpopulations infiltrating breast cancer. *Cancer Immunol Immunother* 1989;28:143–147.
23. Whiteside TL, Miescher S, Hurlimann J, Moretta L, von Fliedner V. Clonal analysis and *in situ* characterization of lymphocytes infiltrating human breast carcinomas. *Cancer Immunol Immunother* 1986;23: 169–173.
24. Gilchrist KW, Gould VE, Hirschl S, et al. Interobserver variation in the identification of breast carcinoma in intramammary lymphatics. *Hum Pathol* 1982;13:170–172.
25. Rosen PP. Tumor emboli in intramammary lymphatics in breast carcinoma: pathologic criteria for diagnosis and clinical significance. *Pathol Annu* 1983;18(Pt 2):215–232.
26. Bettelheim R, Penman HG, Thornton-Jones H, Neville AM. Prognostic significance of peritumoral vascular invasion in breast cancer. *Br J Cancer* 1984;50:771–777.
27. Nime F, Rosen PP, Thaler H, Ashikari R, Urban JA. Prognostic significance of tumor emboli in intramammary lymphatics in patients with mammary carcinoma. *Am J Surg Pathol* 1977;1:25–30.
28. Lauria R, Perrone F, Carlomagno C, et al. The prognostic value of lymphatic and blood vessel invasion in operable breast cancer. *Cancer* 1995;76:1772–1778.
29. Clemente CG, Boracchi P, Andreola S, Del Vecchio M, Veronesi P, Rilke FO. Peritumoral lymphatic invasion in patients with node-negative mammary duct carcinoma. *Cancer* 1992;69:1396–1403.
30. Rak JW, St Croix BD, Kerbel RS. Consequences of angiogenesis for tumor progression, metastasis and cancer therapy. *Anticancer Drugs* 1995;6:3–18.
31. Horak ER, Leek R, Klenk N, et al. Angiogenesis, assessed by platelet/endothelial cell adhesion molecule antibodies, as indicator of node metastases and survival in breast cancer. *Lancet* 1992;340: 1120–1124.
32. Weidner N, Gasparini G. Determination of epidermal growth factor receptor provides additional prognostic information to measuring tumor angiogenesis in breast carcinoma patients. *Breast Cancer Res Treat* 1994;29:97–107.
33. de Jong JS, van Diest PJ, Baak JPA. Methods in laboratory investigation. Heterogeneity and reproducibility of microvessel counts in breast cancer. *Lab Invest* 1995;73:922–926.
34. Tamura S, Enjoji M. Elastosis in neoplastic and non-neoplastic tissues

from patients with mammary carcinoma. *Acta Pathol Jpn* 1988;38: 1537–1546.

35. Glaubitz LC, Bowen JH, Cox ED, McCarty KS. Elastosis in human breast cancer. Correlation with sex steroid receptors and comparison with clinical outcome. *Arch Pathol Lab Med* 1984;108:27–30.

36. Schnitt SJ, Connolly JL, Harris JR, Hellman S, Cohen RB. Pathologic predictors of early local recurrences in stage I and II breast cancer treated by primary radiation therapy. *Cancer* 1984;53:1049–1057.

37. Rosen PP, Kinne DW, Lesser ML, Hellman S. Are prognostic factors for local control of breast cancer treated by primary radiotherapy sig-

nificant for patients treated by mastectomy? *Cancer* 1986;57: 1415–1420.

38. Hurd TC, Sneige N, Allen PK, et al. Impact of extensive intraductal component on recurrence and survival in patients with stage I and II breast cancer treated with breast conservation therapy. *Ann Surg Oncol* 1997;4:119–124.

39. Schnitt SJ, Abner A, Gelman R, et al. The relationship between microscopic margins of resection and the risk of local recurrence in patients with breast cancer treated with breast-conserving surgery and radiation therapy. *Cancer* 1994;74:1746–1751.

CHAPTER 10

Tubular Carcinoma

Tubular carcinoma is "a highly differentiated invasive carcinoma whose cells are regular and arranged in well-defined tubules typically one cell-layer thick and surrounded by an abundant fibrous stroma" (1) (Fig. 1). The term tubular refers to the formation of neoplastic tubules that closely resemble breast ductules. This characteristic is the main source of difficulty in recognizing the lesion, especially in the limited sample obtained by needle core biopsy (Fig. 2).

The diagnosis of tubular carcinoma does not apply to carcinomas in which the tubular structures are formed by less well-differentiated cells or have a more complex growth pattern (Fig. 3). The pattern of glandular growth in nontubular well-differentiated duct carcinoma is partly tubular, but the proliferation is more florid in some areas and the epithelium of the glands may be more than one cell thick. Micropapillae, cribriform transluminal bridging, or microgland structures develop in some glands. An occasional mitotic figure may be encountered, but there is little cytologic pleomorphism. The intraductal component is more likely to be cribriform than micropapillary in well-differentiated nontubular duct carcinoma.

Pure tubular carcinomas constitute fewer than 2% of all female breast carcinomas. The incidence of this lesion is influenced by the nature of the population under investigation. Before the widespread use of mammography, 5% of 382 $T_1N_0M_0$ breast carcinomas in one series were classified as tubular (2). When stratified by size, 9% of lesions 1.0 cm or smaller were tubular, a substantially higher proportion than the 2% of tubular carcinomas among tumors that measured 1.1 to 2.0 cm. Tubular carcinoma was less frequent among women with $T_1N_1M_0$ disease (1.5% of 142 patients), reflecting the relatively low frequency of axillary metastases from these tumors (3). Tubular carcinomas have been encountered with increasing frequency as a result of the growing use of mammography. In the Breast Cancer Detection Demonstration Projects, 8% of invasive carcinomas 1.0 cm or less in diameter were of the tubular variety (4).

Tubular carcinomas have structural features that render the lesions detectable by mammography. Most tubular carcinomas are spiculated, and calcifications are variably present (5). Leibman et al. (6) reported that the average radiographic size of tubular carcinomas was 0.8 cm in patients with nonpalpable lesions and 1.2 cm when the lesions were palpable.

It may be difficult to distinguish tubular carcinoma from radial scar in mammograms, a problem compounded by the fact that tubular carcinoma can arise in a radial scar (7,8) (Fig. 4).

The median age at diagnosis is the middle to late forties (9,10). Tubular carcinoma usually occurs in peripheral portions of the breast. Superficial tumors are fixed to the skin, producing retraction in a small number of cases. When tubular carcinoma arises from the major lactiferous ducts in the nipple or slightly lower in the subareolar region, it is difficult to distinguish from florid papillomatosis of the nipple. The finding of Paget disease supports the diagnosis of tubular carcinoma in this setting. When studied by immunohistochemistry or biochemically, almost all tubular carcinomas have been positive for estrogen receptor (11) (Fig. 5).

The distribution of the small neoplastic glands or tubules is largely haphazard, but they tend to be relatively evenly spaced throughout the lesion. The glands may have virtually any shape, but the majority have irregular shapes and angular contours (see Fig. 2). In very well-differentiated tubular carcinomas, especially tumors smaller than 1 cm, it is possible to find round or oval glands of relatively uniform caliber that resemble microglandular adenosis (12) (see Fig. 2B). Cribriform or papillary growth may be focally present.

The glands of tubular carcinoma are composed only of neoplastic epithelial cells, typically distributed in a single layer (Fig. 6). The cells are cuboidal or columnar with round or oval hyperchromatic nuclei that tend to be basally oriented. Nucleoli are inapparent, and mitoses are very rarely present. Apocrine-type cytoplasmic "snouts" are often evident at the luminal cell border. The cytoplasm is usually amphophilic. Eosinophilic or nearly clear apocrine cytoplasm rarely occurs in a pure tubular carcinoma. An uncommon type of tubular carcinoma is composed of tumor cells with intracytoplasmic mucin and mucin in the neoplastic gland lumina (Fig. 7).

The primary consideration in the differential diagnosis of tubular carcinoma is sclerosing adenosis, a lesion composed in varying proportions of compact, whorled, elongated, and largely compressed glands with interlacing spindly myoepithelial cells. The lobulocentric distribution of sclerosing adenosis is absent in tubular carcinoma. Because prolifera-

Text continues on page 130

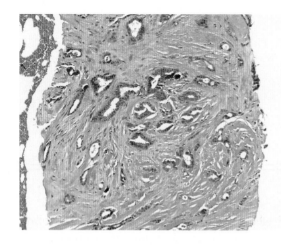

FIGURE 1. Tubular carcinoma. In this needle core biopsy small glands are evenly distributed throughout the specimen. Calcifications are present.

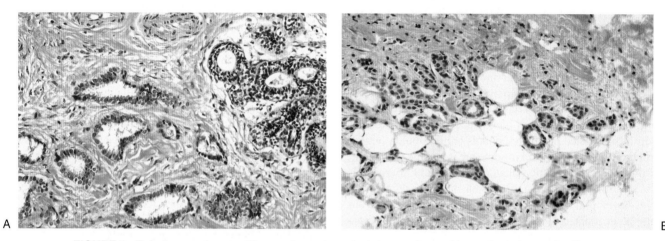

FIGURE 2. Tubular carcinoma. The carcinomatous ductules are formed by a single layer of uniform cuboidal cells. **A:** A normal terminal duct is shown on the right for contrast with the angular carcinomatous tubular structures. **B:** This carcinoma is composed mainly of ductular glands with rounded shapes.

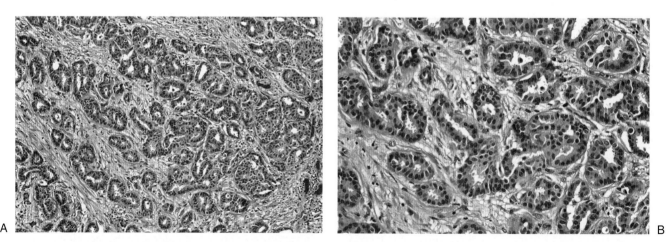

FIGURE 3. Well-differentiated invasive duct carcinoma. A,B: The glandular pattern is more complex than in tubular carcinoma. Intraglandular proliferation is evident.

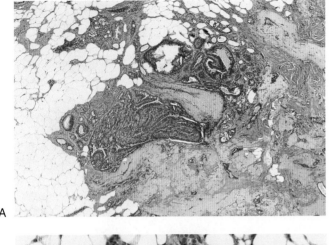
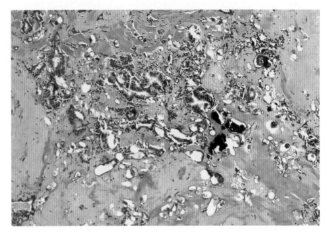
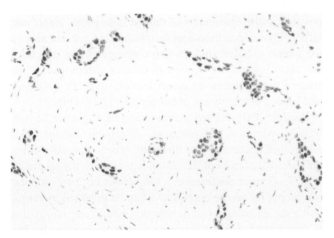

FIGURE 4. Tubular carcinoma arising in a radial scar. This nonpalpable lesion was detected as a mass with calcifications on mammography. **A:** This portion consists of sclerosing adenosis and papillary duct hyperplasia. The scleroelastotic core is seen on the right. **B:** A glandular proliferation in the sclerotic core with numerous calcifications. This area is not diagnostic of carcinoma. **C:** Tubular carcinoma invading fat at the periphery of the tumor.

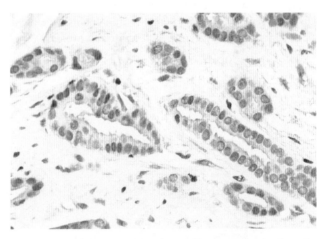

FIGURE 5. Tubular carcinoma. Nuclei in the carcinomatous glands are immunoreactive for estrogen receptor (immunoperoxidase).

FIGURE 6. Tubular carcinoma. The neoplastic ductular glands are formed by cuboidal or low columnar cells with basally oriented nuclei.

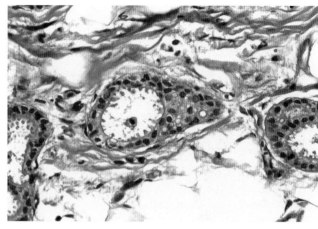

A

B

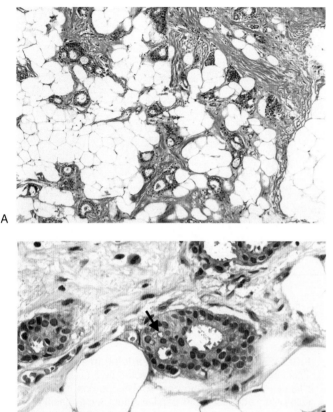

C

FIGURE 7. Tubular carcinoma with intracytoplasmic mucin. A,B: The carcinoma is composed mainly of rounded glands formed by cuboidal cells that have intracytoplasmic lumina. **C:** The lumina in some intracytoplasmic vacuoles are outlined in red (*arrow*) with the mucicarmine stain.

tion of myoepithelial cells is an integral part of sclerosing adenosis and these cells are not present in tubular carcinoma, it is occasionally helpful to employ immunohistochemical stains for actin when dealing with a difficult problem (13).

FIGURE 8. Tubular carcinoma. This immunostained preparation for type IV collagen highlights the basement membranes of a duct and small blood vessel. Immunoreactivity is faint or absent around tubular carcinoma glands in this needle core biopsy specimen (immunoperoxidase).

Immunostains for S-100 and 34BE12 are less reliable as markers for myoepithelial cells because they may also be positive in the epithelium of tubular carcinoma. Intact and largely continuous basement membranes are present around the glands of sclerosing adenosis, whereas these structures are absent or poorly formed in tubular carcinomas when studied with reagents to detect laminin, type IV collagen, and basement membrane proteoglycan (13,14) (Fig. 8).

Because of the limited sampling provided by a needle core biopsy specimen, the diagnosis of tubular carcinoma is sometimes uncertain. The difficulty arises especially when only a small portion of the lesion is present in the specimen (Fig. 9). Greater confidence in a diagnosis of "pure" tubular carcinoma by needle core biopsy can be obtained by correlating the pathologic and radiologic findings, especially if it is determined that the lesion seen mammographically has been completely or nearly completely removed by the biopsy procedure.

A tumor with areas of invasive lobular and tubular carcinoma is referred to as tubulolobular carcinoma (Fig. 10). The precise position of tubulolobular carcinoma in the classification of breast carcinomas is uncertain because it has been regarded as a variant of tubular carcinoma by some authors, and as a form of invasive lobular carcinoma by others. The majority of patients who have lobular carcinoma *in situ* co-

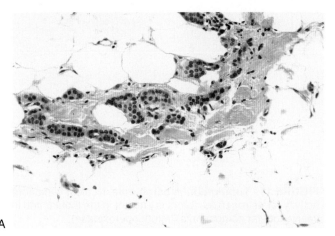 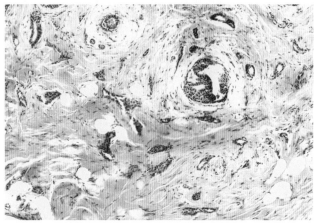

A B

FIGURE 9. Tubular carcinoma. A: This needle core biopsy specimen is from a nonpalpable focus of calcifications detected by mammography. These glands, the only abnormal finding in the specimen, were interpreted as adenosis. **B:** In retrospect, they proved to be a small peripheral sample from this tubular carcinoma diagnosed in a subsequent excisional biopsy shown here.

existing with tubular carcinoma have tubulolobular carcinoma, but patients with pure tubular carcinoma occasionally have separate, coexistent lobular carcinoma *in situ*. Patients with tubulolobular carcinoma are more likely to have axillary lymph node metastases than women with pure tubular carcinoma, and they have a prognosis between that of pure tubular and invasive lobular carcinoma (15). Almost all tubulolobular carcinomas are immunoreactive for estrogen and progesterone receptors (16) (Fig. 11). The prognosis of patients with tubulolobular carcinoma should be viewed as good, but not in the exceptionally favorable category of pure tubular carcinoma.

Tissue between the glands in tubular carcinomas often appears different from the stroma in the surrounding breast, sometimes as a result of the presence of abundant elastic tissue (17). However, elastosis can be a prominent feature of nontubular carcinomas and some benign lesions, particularly those with the "radial scar" pattern. Other stromal alterations

that may be seen include dense collagenization or loosening of the stroma caused by the accumulation of metachromatic ground substances. If present at all, there is at most a mild lymphocytic reaction. Blood vessel invasion and lymphatic tumor emboli are virtually never seen in tubular carcinoma. Calcifications are found in the majority of tubular carcinomas, distributed in the neoplastic glands, in the stroma, and often in the intraductal carcinoma component. Intraductal carcinoma can be found in at least two thirds of tubular carcinomas. It typically has a papillary or cribriform pattern or a mixture of the two (10) (Fig. 12). Micropapillary intraductal carcinoma is especially common, and the growth pattern is frequently so orderly that it is mistaken for hyperplasia.

Many patients with tubular and tubulolobular carcinoma have a distinctive type of associated proliferation in ducts and lobules that we have designated informally as "pretubular," or columnar cell, hyperplasia. Goldstein and O'Malley (18) have referred some of these lesions as "cancerization of

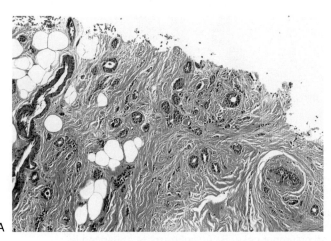 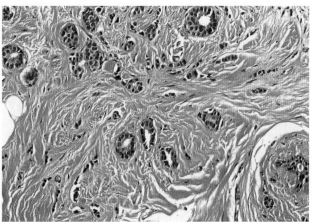

A B

FIGURE 10. Tubulolobular carcinoma. A,B: This needle core biopsy specimen has elements of invasive lobular and tubular carcinoma.

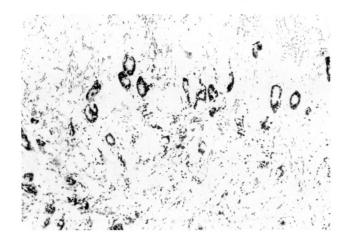

FIGURE 11. Tubulolobular carcinoma. Nuclear immunoreactivity for estrogen receptors is present in the tubular and invasive lobular components (immunoperoxidase).

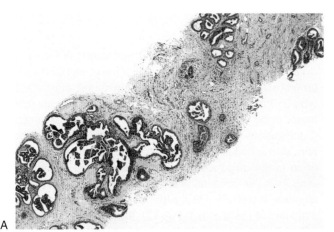

A

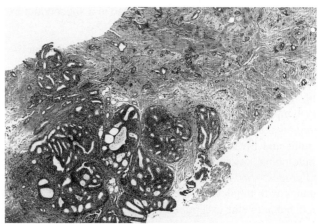

B

FIGURE 12. Tubular carcinoma with intraductal carcinoma. Two needle core biopsy specimens of tubular carcinoma. **A:** Papillary intraductal carcinoma. **B:** Cribriform intraductal carcinoma.

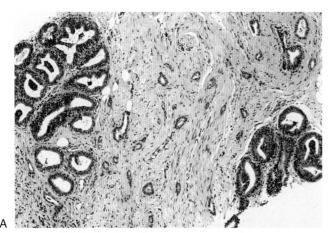

A

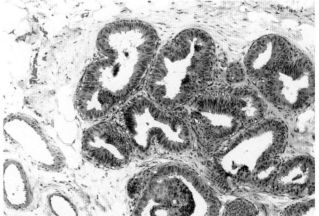

B

FIGURE 13. Columnar cell (pretubular) hyperplasia. A: Hyperplasia is present in ductules on the right and left borders of this needle core biopsy specimen showing tubular carcinoma in the center. The hyperplastic change consists of crowded cuboidal and columnar cells. **B:** A slightly more advanced lesion shows focal cell crowding resulting in the formation of small mounds of columnar cells. One papillary structure is present at the lower border. Myoepithelial cells with vacuolated cytoplasm are present at the outer border of the epithelium in many glands.

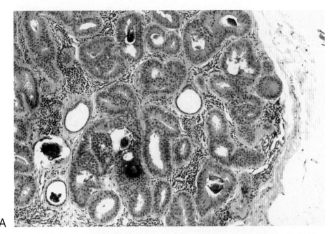

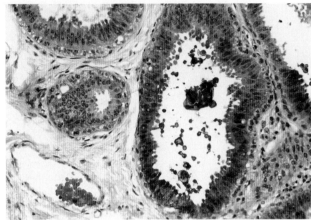

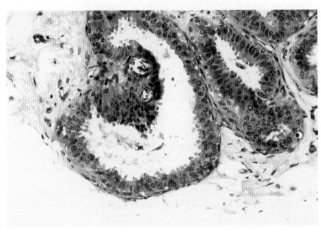

FIGURE 14. Columnar cell (pretubular) hyperplasia. A: Complex intraglandular proliferation with calcifications represents columnar cell hyperplasia with an adenosis pattern. **B:** The larger gland on the right shows severe cytologic atypia with a disorderly distribution of hyperchromatic nuclei. The two small glands on the left exhibit less atypia. Apical cytoplasmic blebs are prominent at the luminal borders, and the larger gland contains calcification. Hyperplastic myoepithelial cells are visible. **C:** A papillary frond with calcification.

small ectatic ducts of the breast by ductal carcinoma *in situ* cells with apocrine snouts." Features common to all phases of columnar cell hyperplasia are nuclear hyperchromasia, a high nuclear-to-cytoplasmic ratio, and apocrine snouts at the luminal borders of ducts and ductules that are usually dilated. This condition is most subtly expressed by cuboidal cells with the foregoing cytologic features distributed in a single layer (Fig. 13). Progressive hyperplasia is marked by crowding of cells that become increasingly compressed and columnar and have nuclei distributed in a haphazard pattern with respect to the basement membrane (Fig. 14). The appearance of papillary or micropapillary fronds composed of proliferative cells, sometimes with mitotic activity, is indicative of micropapillary intraductal carcinoma (Fig. 15). Excisional biopsy of the lesional area is recommended if columnar cell hyperplasia is found in a needle core biopsy specimen.

Lobular carcinoma *in situ* or atypical lobular hyperplasia often coexists close to the invasive tubular lesion, but it can also be more distant in the same breast or in the contralateral breast (Fig. 16). Lobular proliferative lesions are so commonly associated with tubular and tubulolobular carcinoma that their presence may be regarded as secondary evidence supporting a diagnosis of either lesion.

Most patients who prove to have tubular or tubulolobular carcinoma present with a single mass detected by palpation or mammography. However, sampling of surgical biopsy specimens reveals multifocal lesions of tubular carcinoma growing as seemingly separate foci in one or more quadrants in 20% of patients with tubular carcinoma and in nearly 30% of patients with tubulolobular carcinoma. Intraductal carci-

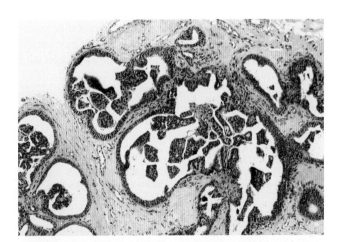

FIGURE 15. Tubular carcinoma with papillary intraductal carcinoma. Intraductal carcinoma in the same biopsy sample as Fig. 16. This proliferation might arise from pretubular hyperplasia.

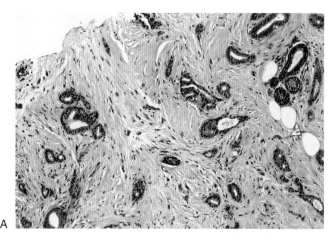 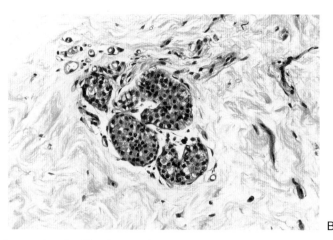

FIGURE 16. Tubular carcinoma and lobular carcinoma *in situ.* Needle core biopsy samples from a radiographically detected lesion. **A:** Pure tubular carcinoma. **B:** A separate focus of lobular carcinoma *in situ.*

noma indicative of independent lesions is often present in the individual carcinomatous areas. The frequency and prognostic significance of the multifocal variants have not been fully evaluated.

Tubular carcinoma has a relatively favorable prognosis when the diagnosis is restricted to "pure" tubular carcinoma (9,10). In a series of patients with $T_1N_0M_0$ breast carcinomas treated by modified or radical mastectomy and followed for a median of 18 years, there were no recurrences among patients with tubular carcinoma (19). The frequency of axillary lymph node metastases resulting from pure tubular carcinoma is about 10% (2,3,9–11). Axillary lymph node metastases are encountered in about 30% of patients with tubulolobular carcinoma who undergo an axillary dissection (15). Affected lymph nodes are usually in the low axilla (level 1), and only rarely are more than three lymph nodes involved (10). Metastases in lymph nodes tend to reproduce the tubular growth pattern of the primary tumor, but less well-differentiated or solid metastases may be encountered. The presence of multifocal carcinoma at the primary site appears to predispose patients with tubular and tubulolobular carcinoma to the development of axillary lymph node metastases, perhaps because of the greater tumor volume associated with multifocality (15).

REFERENCES

1. World Health Organization. *Histological typing of breast tumours,* 2nd ed. International histological classification of tumours No. 2. Geneva: World Health Organization, 1981;19.
2. Rosen PP, Saigo PE, Braun DW Jr, Weathers E, DePalo A. Predictors of recurrence in stage I ($T_1N_0M_0$) breast carcinoma. *Ann Surg* 1981; 193:15–25.
3. Rosen PP, Saigo PE, Braun DW Jr, Weathers E, Kinne DW. Prognosis in stage II ($T_1N_1M_0$) breast cancer. *Ann Surg* 1981;194:576–584.
4. Beahrs O, Shapiro S, Smart C. Report of the Working Group to Review the National Cancer Institute-American Cancer Society Breast Cancer Detection Demonstration Projects. *J Natl Cancer Inst* 1979;62: 640–709.
5. Elson BC, Helvie MA, Frank TS, Wilson TE, Adler DD. Tubular carcinoma of the breast: mode of presentation, mammographic appearance, and frequency of nodal metastases. *AJR Am J Roentgenol* 1993; 161:1173–1176.
6. Leibman AJ, Lewis M, Kruse B. Tubular carcinoma of the breast: mammographic appearance. *AJR Am J Roentgenol* 1993;160:263–265.
7. Vega A, Garijo. Radial scar and tubular carcinoma. Mammographic and sonographic findings. *Acta Radiol* 1993;34:43–47.
8. Frouge C, Tristant H, Guinebretière J-M, et al. Mammographic lesions suggestive of radial scars: microscopic findings in 40 cases. *Radiology* 1995;195:623–625.
9. Peters GN, Wolff M, Haagensen CD. Tubular carcinoma of the breast. Clinical pathologic correlations based on 100 cases. *Ann Surg* 1981; 193:138–149.
10. McDivitt RW, Boyce W, Gersell D. Tubular carcinoma of the breast. Clinical and pathological observations concerning 135 cases. *Am J Surg Pathol* 1982;6:401–410.
11. Winchester DJ, Sahin AA, Tucker SL, Singletary SE. Tubular carcinoma of the breast. Predicting axillary nodal metastases and recurrence. *Ann Surg* 1996;223:342–347.
12. Rosen PP. Microglandular adenosis. A benign lesion simulating invasive mammary carcinoma. *Am J Surg Pathol* 1983;7:137–144.
13. Joshi MG, Lee AKC, Pedersen CA, Schnitt S, Camus MG, Hughes KS. The role of immunocytochemical markers in the differential diagnosis of proliferative and neoplastic lesions of the breast. *Mod Pathol* 1996; 9:57–62.
14. Ekblom P, Miettinen M, Forsman L, Andersson LC. Basement membrane and apocrine epithelial antigens in differential diagnosis between tubular carcinoma and sclerosing adenosis of the breast. *J Clin Pathol* 1984;37:357–363.
15. Green I, McCormick B, Cranor M, Rosen PP. A comparative study of pure tubular and tubulolobular carcinoma of the breast. *Am J Surg Pathol* 1997;21:653–657.
16. Boppana S, Erroll M, Reiches E, Hoda SA. Cytologic characteristics of tubulolobular carcinoma of the breast. *Acta Cytol* 1996;40:465–471.
17. Tremblay G. Elastosis in tubular carcinoma of the breast. *Arch Pathol* 1974;98:302–307.
18. Goldstein NS, O'Malley BA. Cancerization of small ectatic ducts of the breast by ductal carcinoma *in situ* cells with apocrine snouts. A lesion associated with tubular carcinoma. *Am J Clin Pathol* 1997;107: 561–566.
19. Rosen PP, Groshen S, Saigo PE, Kinne DW, Hellman S. A long-term follow-up study of survival in stage I ($T_1N_0M_0$) and stage II ($T_1N_1M_0$) breast carcinoma. *J Clin Oncol* 1989;7:355–366.

CHAPTER 11

Papillary Carcinoma

About 1% to 2% of breast carcinomas can be classified as papillary in women, and a slightly greater percentage of male breast carcinomas are papillary. A distinction should be made between invasive and noninvasive papillary carcinoma (1). Intracystic carcinoma is a variant of papillary carcinoma that may have an invasive component (2).

Women with solid or cystic papillary carcinoma of the breast are reportedly older than patients with other types of carcinoma, with a mean age ranging from 63 to 67 years (1,3). Nearly 50% of papillary carcinomas arise in the central part of the breast, and as a consequence, nipple discharge has been described in at least one third of patients. Bleeding from the nipple occurs in a higher percentage of patients with papillary carcinoma than in those with a papilloma. The average size of papillary carcinoma clinically is 2 to 3 cm. Papillary carcinomas are usually rich in estrogen and progesterone receptors (4), and they tend to have a low growth rate when measured by thymidine labeling (5).

Papillary carcinomas often appear as rounded, circumscribed mass lesions on mammography (6,7). If part of the contour lacks circumscription, an invasive component may be present (7,8). Examination by ultrasound can suggest a papillary tumor when a solid area is detected in a hypoechoic cystic lesion (7–9). When present, calcifications tend to be punctate and associated with intraductal papillary carcinoma (9). Coarse, pleomorphic calcifications may develop in areas of sclerosis or resolved hemorrhage. Needle core biopsy can be used effectively for the diagnosis of papillary carcinoma. A series of 26 papillary lesions diagnosed by needle core biopsy included 7 classified as papillary carcinoma *in situ* (10). Invasive carcinoma was found in three (43%) of subsequent excisional biopsy specimens.

The term papillary applies to carcinomas in which the underlying microscopic pattern is predominantly frond-forming. Many papillary carcinomas have cystic areas, but this is not necessary for the diagnosis. When cyst formation is minimal or absent, separate fronds may be inconspicuous, and the papillary character is appreciated because the epithelium is supported by a network of fibrovascular stroma. These tumors are referred to as *solid papillary carcinomas*.

The epithelium on the papillae in papillary carcinomas is composed of cells arranged in the patterns typically found in intraductal carcinoma, which include papillary, micropapillary, cribriform, reticular, and solid appearances (Fig. 1). The epithelial proliferation fills the space between neighboring fibrovascular stromal cores and contributes to the formation of complex patterns of papillae, glandular spaces, and solid areas within the lesion.

Fibrovascular stroma is present to some extent in virtually all papillary carcinomas, but it tends to be inconspicuous and less evenly distributed in carcinomas than in benign papillary lesions (Figs. 1,2). A minority of papillary carcinomas have areas in which there are relatively broad fibrous stalks with extensive sclerosis (Fig. 3). The epithelial cells in papillary carcinomas generally grow in a less orderly fashion than in papillomas. This is manifested by uneven stratification and loss of polarity with respect to the basement membrane of the fibrovascular stroma (Fig. 4). Nuclei are characteristically hyperchromatic regardless of cytologic grade, and there is usually a high nuclear-to-cytoplasmic ratio. Mitotic figures are variably present and more numerous in lesions that exhibit the most severe cytologic atypia. The tumor cells sometimes have secretory "snouts" at the luminal surface (Fig. 5). Intracytoplasmic mucin vacuoles may be conspicuous (Fig. 6). Mucin may accumulate between papillary fronds (Fig. 7). Apocrine areas in a papillary carcinoma exhibit cytologic atypia consistent with the rest of the tumor and therefore differ from the bland foci of apocrine metaplasia sometimes encountered in papillomas. When present, microcalcifications are more often found in glandular portions of the lesion than in the stroma (Fig. 8).

Myoepithelial cells, which are distributed relatively uniformly and proportionately with the epithelium of benign papillary lesions, persist to a variable extent in papillary carcinomas (Figs. 1,5,9). Myoepithelial cells are characteristically absent from areas of papillary carcinoma, but they can be present as a discontinuous layer or even be hyperplastic in carcinomatous areas (11,12).

Lefkowitz et al. (3) drew attention to papillary carcinomas containing cuboidal cells with abundant clear or faintly eosinophilic cytoplasm located mainly near the basement membrane, either singly, in small clusters, or in broad sheets. In some instances, the polygonal cells with pale cytoplasm become quite numerous, creating solid and cribriform regions beneath a superficial layer of columnar epithelium

Text continues on page 139

135

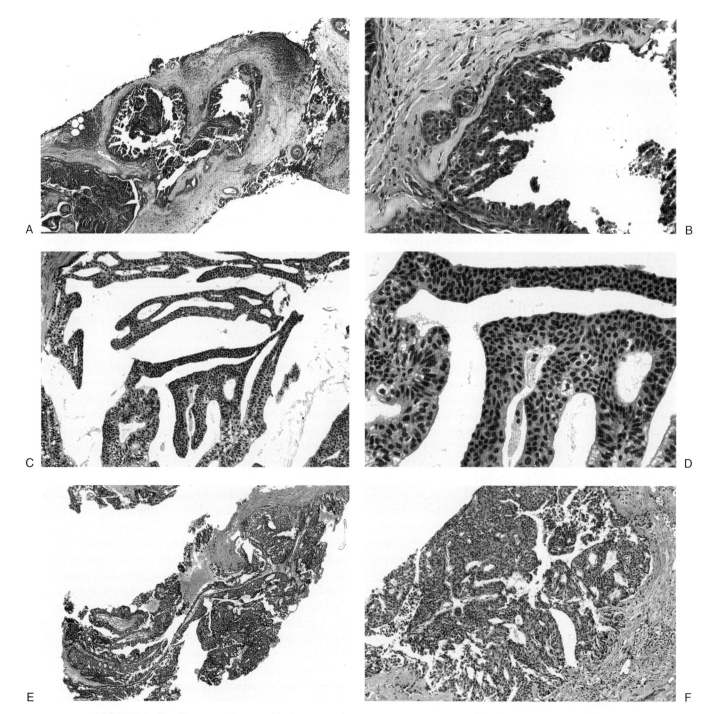

FIGURE 1. Papillary carcinoma. Various growth patterns are represented in these needle core biopsy specimens. **A,B:** Papillary and micropapillary intraductal carcinoma. Myoepithelial cells represented by oval nuclei arranged parallel to the basement membrane are seen beneath the micropapillary carcinoma in (B). **C,D:** Arborizing cribriform and micropapillary intraductal carcinoma with well-differentiated nuclear grade. Residual columnar epithelium is apparent on some papillary fronds. **E,F:** Cribriform areas.

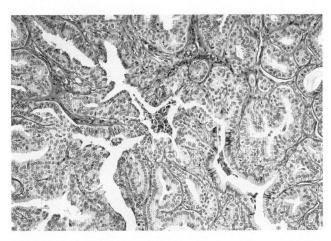

FIGURE 2. Papillary carcinoma. The fibrovascular stroma forms slender, branching strands in this orderly lesion with foci of residual papilloma represented by regular columnar epithelium, seen mainly near the lower right corner.

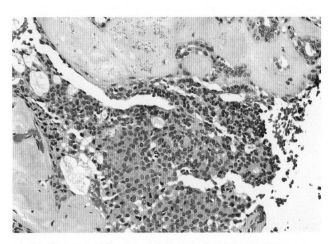

FIGURE 3. Papillary carcinoma. Dense collagenization with finely granular basophilic calcification (*upper center*) is present in this lesion.

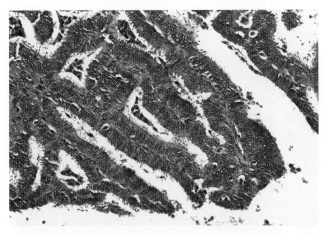

FIGURE 4. Papillary carcinoma. The columnar carcinoma cells in this orderly tumor are closely arrayed along the basement membrane. There is a high nuclear-to-cytoplasmic ratio and loss of nuclear polarity with respect to the basement membrane.

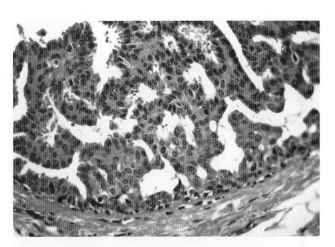

FIGURE 5. Papillary carcinoma. Papillary intraductal carcinoma was present in this needle core biopsy specimen of a circumscribed, nonpalpable tumor detected by mammography. Many carcinoma cells have cytoplasmic "snouts" at their apical surface. A myoepithelial cell layer is present at the periphery of the lesion.

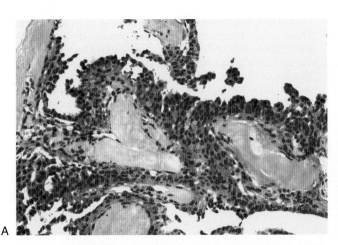

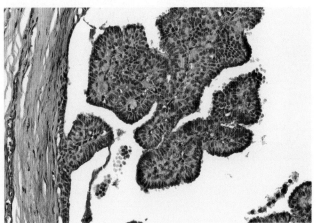

A   B

FIGURE 6. Papillary carcinoma with intracytoplasmic mucin. A: Intracytoplasmic mucin is represented by discrete, pale blue vacuoles. **B:** The mucin is stained magenta by the mucicarmine stain.

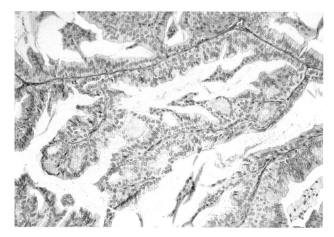

FIGURE 7. Papillary carcinoma with extracellular mucin. This papillary carcinoma with apocrine differentiation has a micropapillary structure and unusually abundant mucin secretion between papillary fronds.

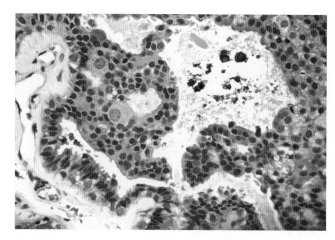

FIGURE 8. Papillary carcinoma with calcification. Granular calcifications are present in a glandular lumen in this needle core biopsy specimen. The picture shows micropapillary carcinoma and the columnar epithelium of a papilloma (*lower left corner*) in which the carcinoma arose.

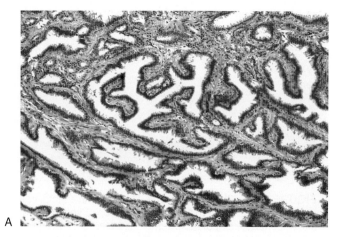

A

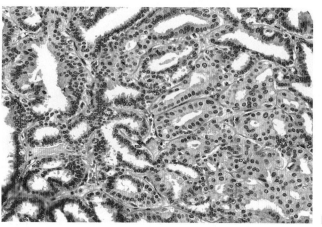

B

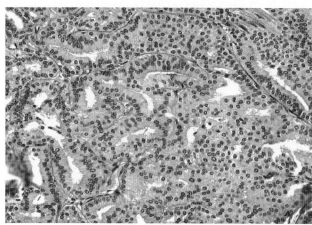

C

FIGURE 9. Papillary carcinoma arising in a papilloma. Three areas in a single tumor are shown. **A:** This papilloma has a thin, uniform layer of cuboidal and low columnar cells overlying prominent myoepithelial cells and broad strands of stroma. **B:** An enlarged view from another region shows hyperplastic epithelium on the left merging with atypical glandular hyperplasia on the right composed of cells with eosinophilic cytoplasm. Note the loss of myoepithelial cells and more slender stromal strands on the right. **C:** Carcinoma with a cribriform structure. Note the persisting inconspicuous arborizing stroma and virtual absence of myoepithelial cells.

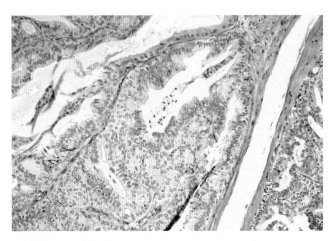

FIGURE 10. Papillary carcinoma with dimorphic differentiation. Polygonal cells form clusters surmounted by columnar cells.

(Fig. 10). Despite the difference in cytoplasmic features between the clear cells and the columnar carcinomatous cells, the nuclei of the two cells types are similar, and both cell types are immunoreactive for CAM5.2, which stains myoepithelial cells weakly or not at all. There is no reactivity for S-100 protein or smooth-muscle actin in the polygonal cells. On the basis of this immunoprofile, Lefkowitz et al. (3) con-

cluded that both cell types are of epithelial origin, and they referred to this pattern as dimorphic carcinoma.

The solid variant of papillary carcinoma is not widely recognized (13). These tumors are formed by ducts nearly or completely filled by a neoplastic proliferation supported by an arborizing fibrovascular stroma (Fig. 11). The epithelium generally has a solid structure, which can be so densely cellular that the stroma is obscured (Fig. 12). When cribriform and papillary patterns are present, the stroma is more apparent. Solid areas may be divided into ribbons or trabeculae of neoplastic cells by prominent fibrovascular stroma (Fig. 13). Comedo necrosis is very infrequent. Collagenization of stroma around and among the ducts occurs to a variable degree, in some cases producing the appearance of a radial sclerosing lesion. Intraductal carcinoma can be present in ducts surrounding a solid papillary carcinoma.

The diagnosis of a papillary carcinoma that has arisen in a papilloma can be a problem even with sections of the entire lesion in hand, a difficulty compounded by the limited and often noncontiguous sampling in needle core biopsy specimens. Foci of papilloma in such lesions should not impede recognition of the carcinomatous element (see Fig. 9). Papillary lesions that have been characterized as "borderline" have modest or substantial areas of benign papillary proliferation as well as more cellular and atypical components. To make a diagnosis of carcinoma in this setting, it is necessary to find one

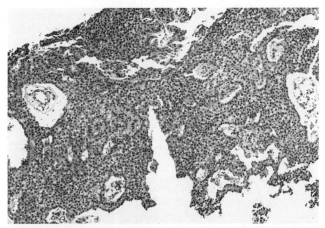

A

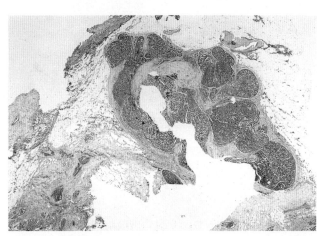

B

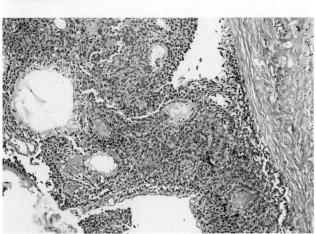

C

FIGURE 11. Solid papillary carcinoma. A: A needle core biopsy specimen shows solid areas of *in situ* carcinoma arranged around fibrovascular stromal cores. The tumor cells have vacuolated amphophilic cytoplasm and well-differentiated, round nuclei. This specimen could be mistaken for invasive carcinoma if the basic papillary structure were not appreciated. **B:** A low-magnification view of the tumor in the excisional biopsy specimen. **C:** An area at the periphery of the excised tumor duplicating the appearance of the needle core biopsy specimen.

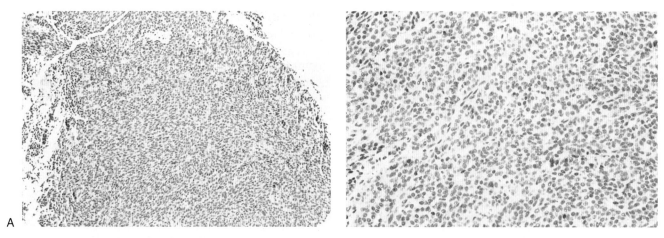

FIGURE 12. Solid papillary carcinoma. A: In this needle core biopsy specimen, the dense *in situ* epithelial proliferation has greatly obscured the fibrovascular stroma. This type of material could be mistaken for invasive carcinoma if the fundamental papillary character of the specimen were not appreciated. **B:** Delicate fibrovascular strands can be seen at higher magnification.

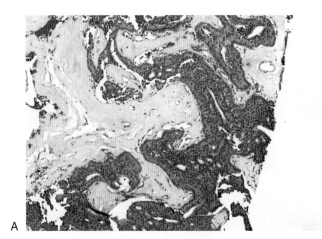

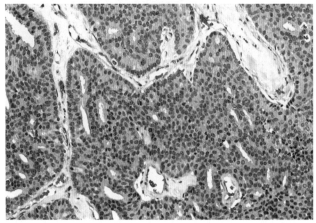

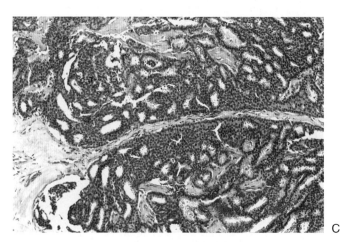

FIGURE 13. Solid papillary carcinoma. A: Collagenized stroma in this needle core biopsy specimen has distorted the structure of an *in situ* solid papillary carcinoma. This pattern might be mistaken for invasive carcinoma with a trabecular pattern if the papillary character of the lesion were not appreciated. Spaces formed by separation of the epithelium from the stroma are not uncommon in solid papillary carcinoma. **B:** This part of the lesion has a cribriform structure. **C:** Cribriform intraductal carcinoma is apparent in the excisional biopsy specimen of the papillary tumor. *Figure continues*

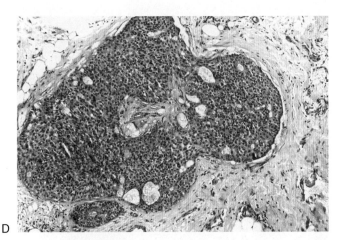
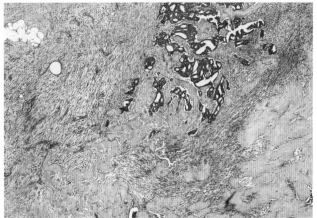

D   E

FIGURE 13. *Continued* **D:** Solid papillary carcinoma is present in a duct at the periphery of the excised tumor. **E:** An area in the center of the excised tumor with reactive stromal proliferation resulting from the prior needle core biopsy. The disrupted glands in granulation tissue are difficult to distinguish from invasive carcinoma.

or more low-power microscopic fields where the growth pattern and cytologic appearance of the epithelium between neighboring fibrovascular cores have the pattern of one of the established forms of intraductal carcinoma. Some authors have illustrated focal intraductal carcinoma in papillomas but classified these lesions as "papillomas with atypical ductal hyperplasia" (14,15). In one of these studies, the relative risk for subsequent carcinoma in women with such papillomas was more than four times that of women with papillomas that lacked atypical hyperplasia or intraductal carcinoma (15).

Histochemical and immunohistochemical studies can be helpful for evaluating difficult lesions. Intracytoplasmic mucin indicative of carcinoma is demonstrable with the mucicarmine, alcian blue, and periodic acid–Schiff stains (see Fig. 6). In the majority of cases, intracytoplasmic mucin secretion is not prominent, and therefore a negative stain result does not rule out carcinoma. A small number of papillary carcinomas exhibit abundant, diffuse intracellular mucin secretion that can be manifested by signet-ring cell formation and the accumulation of extracellular mucin. The cells in a minority of papillary carcinomas contain Grimelius- and chromogranin-positive cytoplasmic granules, which have not been demonstrated by histochemical methods in the cells of papillomas. These tumors typically have a solid papillary growth pattern with mucinous differentiation. They are usually immunoreactive for synaptophysin, neuron-specific enolase, have mucin-positive cells, and are usually estrogen receptor-positive (16) (Fig. 14).

The microscopic diagnosis of invasive papillary carcinoma may be difficult. Many papillary carcinomas are bounded by zones of fibrosis, recent or resolved hemorrhage, and chronic inflammation. Similar alterations may also occur within the lesion. Papillary or glandular clusters of epithelial cells within these areas are difficult to interpret. It is not possible to rule out invasion in a needle core biopsy specimen because the sample may not include this aspect of the lesion (Figs. 15,16). The most reliable evidence of invasion is extension of carcinoma beyond the border of the tumor and the adjacent stromal reaction. Cytologically, the invasive component tends to resemble the *in situ* portion of the lesion. There is usually also an appreciable change in growth pattern between the *in situ* and invasive components (see Fig. 16). Invasive carcinoma arising in solid papillary carcinoma with mucinous differentiation is often mucinous carcinoma (see Fig. 15). Invasive tubular, cribriform, solid, and papillary carcinoma can be encountered.

An unusual pattern of true invasion observed in solid papillary carcinomas simulates epithelial displacement associated with needling procedures. This type of invasion is characterized by the presence of one or more irregularly shaped cohesive sheets of carcinoma cells surrounding fat or stroma without the reactive stromal changes that ordinarily accompany invasive carcinoma. These invasive carcinomatous foci abut sharply on normal fat cells, or less often on collagenous stroma, in a fashion suggesting on superficial inspection that they were "pushed" or artifactually displaced to this location (see Fig. 16). Features that favor true invasion include the absence at this site of evidence of needling, such as hemorrhage or tissue disruption. Intimate mingling of carcinoma and normal tissue occurs in these foci, especially in fat, where individual adipose cells are found in the sheet of carcinoma cells.

Whether cystic or solid, papillary carcinoma without invasion is a form of intraductal carcinoma. If treated by mastectomy and axillary dissection, the patients ordinarily are cured by the procedure (2). Invasive papillary carcinomas may be relatively large tumors if a bulky, cystic component is present. The low frequency of axillary lymph node metastases encountered in these patients (1,3) is consistent with the actual sizes of the invasive elements as well as the histologically low-grade character of most of the carcinomas. When axillary nodal metastases occur, they rarely involve

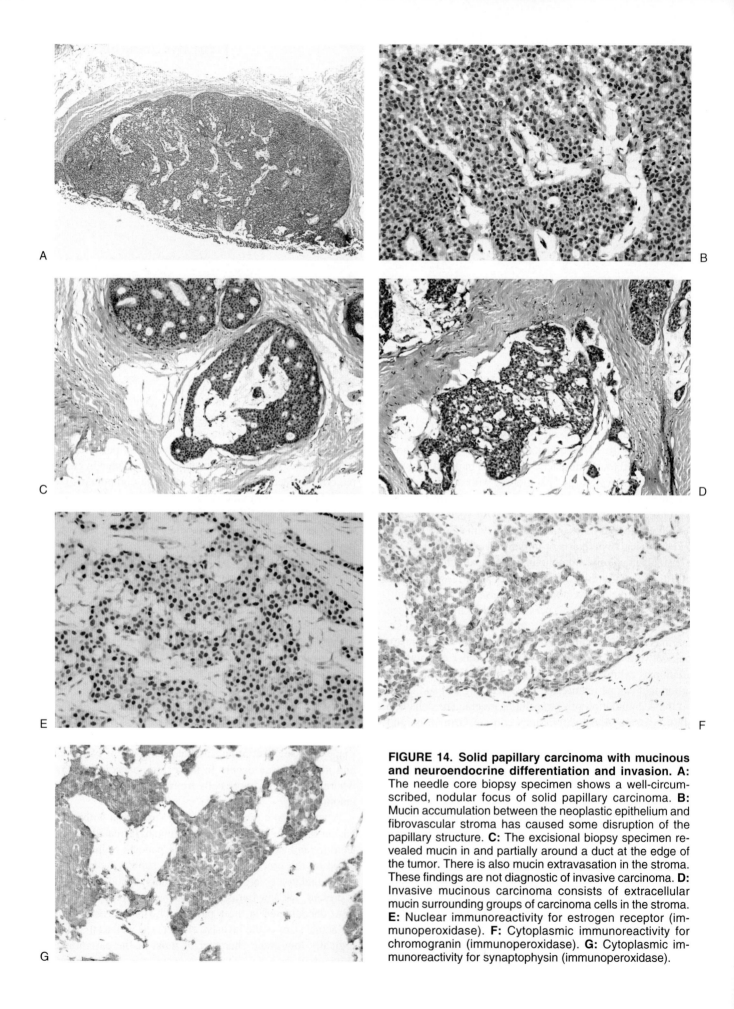

FIGURE 14. Solid papillary carcinoma with mucinous and neuroendocrine differentiation and invasion. A: The needle core biopsy specimen shows a well-circumscribed, nodular focus of solid papillary carcinoma. **B:** Mucin accumulation between the neoplastic epithelium and fibrovascular stroma has caused some disruption of the papillary structure. **C:** The excisional biopsy specimen revealed mucin in and partially around a duct at the edge of the tumor. There is also mucin extravasation in the stroma. These findings are not diagnostic of invasive carcinoma. **D:** Invasive mucinous carcinoma consists of extracellular mucin surrounding groups of carcinoma cells in the stroma. **E:** Nuclear immunoreactivity for estrogen receptor (immunoperoxidase). **F:** Cytoplasmic immunoreactivity for chromogranin (immunoperoxidase). **G:** Cytoplasmic immunoreactivity for synaptophysin (immunoperoxidase).

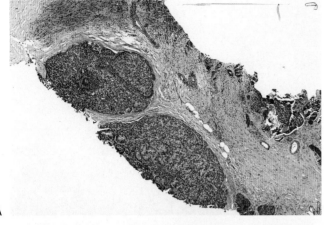

**FIGURE 15. Solid papillary carcinoma with invasion.
A,B:** A needle core biopsy specimen showing solid papillary carcinoma with signet-ring cells that were positive with the mucicarmine stain. Some glandular areas in the lower left of (B) have uneven borders, but invasion is not evident. **C:** The subsequent excisional biopsy specimen contained this area of invasive carcinoma. Note the distinctly different growth patterns of the *in situ* and invasive components.

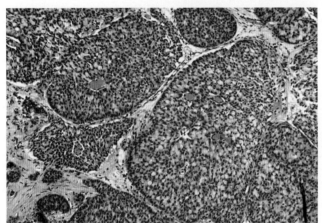

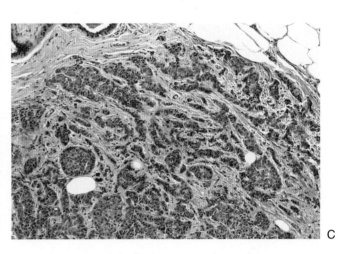

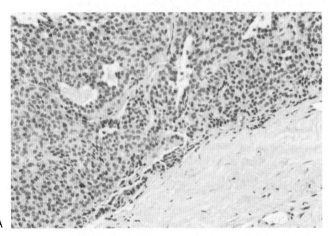

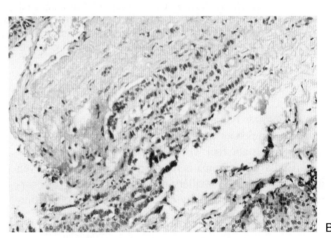

FIGURE 16. Solid papillary carcinoma with invasion. A: This needle core biopsy specimen shows solid papillary carcinoma. **B:** Another part of the specimen contained this fragment of tissue, in which were seen infiltrating carcinoma cells with a linear pattern suggestive of lobular carcinoma. *Figure continues*

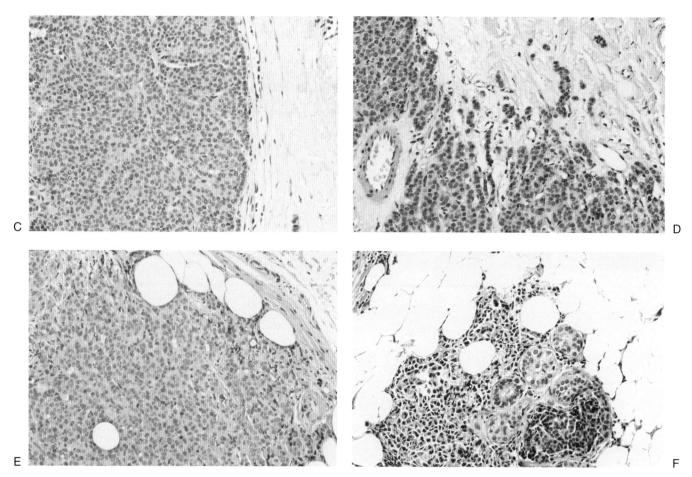

FIGURE 16. *Continued* **C:** Solid papillary carcinoma as it appeared in the excisional biopsy specimen. **D:** Infiltrating carcinoma at the edge of the excised lesion with the same appearance as in the needle core biopsy specimen in (B). **E:** An area of excised tumor in which there is invasion of fat with a solid growth pattern. **F:** Carcinoma in fat around a lobule in another biopsy specimen of solid papillary carcinoma. The loss of cohesion and poorly preserved cytology of some carcinoma cells are features suggesting that this could be epithelium displaced by a needle core biopsy. The absence of hemorrhage or fat necrosis and the delicate manner in which the carcinoma cells surround lipocytes support interpreting this as true invasive carcinoma.

more than three lymph nodes (1). The growth pattern of the invasive component of the primary tumor is usually duplicated in metastatic foci. The prognosis of patients with invasive papillary carcinoma is reportedly very favorable, even in women who have axillary nodal metastases (1). Recurrences of invasive papillary carcinoma often become clinically apparent more than 5 years after diagnosis.

REFERENCES

1. Fisher ER, Palekar AS, Redmond C, Barton B, Fisher B. Pathologic findings from the National Surgical Adjuvant Breast Project (Protocol No. 4). VI. Invasive papillary cancer. *Am J Clin Pathol* 1980;73: 313–320.
2. Carter D, Orr SL, Merino MJ. Intracystic papillary carcinoma of the breast after mastectomy, radiotherapy or excisional biopsy alone. *Cancer* 1983;52:14–19.
3. Lefkowitz M, Lefkowitz W, Wargotz ES. Intraductal (intracystic) papillary carcinoma of the breast and its variants: a clinicopathological study of 77 cases. *Hum Pathol* 1994;25:802–809.
4. Masood S, Barwick K. Estrogen receptor expression of the less common breast carcinomas. *Am J Clin Pathol* 1990;93:437.
5. Meyer JS, Bauer WC, Rao BR. Subpopulations of breast carcinoma defined by S-phase fraction, morphology and estrogen receptor content. *Lab Invest* 1978;39:225–235.
6. Estabrook A, Asch T, Gump F, Kister SJ, Geller P. Mammographic features of intracystic papillary lesions. *Surg Gynecol Obstet* 1990;170: 113–116.
7. Schneider JA. Invasive papillary breast carcinoma: mammographic and sonographic appearance. *Radiology* 1989;171:377–379.
8. Silva R, Ferrozi F, Paties C. Invasive papillary carcinoma in elderly women: sonographic and mammographic features. *AJR Am J Roentgenol* 1992;159:898–899.
9. Soo MS, Williford ME, Walsh R, Bentley RC, Kornguth PJ. Papillary carcinoma of the breast: imaging findings. *AJR Am J Roentgenol* 1995; 164:321–326.
10. Liberman L, Bracero N, Vuolo M, et al. Percutaneous large core biopsy of papillary breast lesions *Am J Roentgenol* (in press).
11. Papotti M, Gugliotta P, Eusebi V, Bussolati G. Immunohistochemical analysis of benign and malignant papillary lesions of the breast. *Am J Surg Pathol* 1983;7:451–461.
12. Papotti M, Gugliotta P, Ghiringhello B, Bussolati G. Association of breast carcinoma and multiple intraductal papillomas: an histological

and immunohistochemical investigation. *Histopathology* 1984;8: 963–975.

13. Rosen PP, Oberman HA. Papillary carcinoma. In: *Tumors of the mammary gland*. Washington, DC: Armed Forces Institute of Pathology, 1993:217 (fasc. 7, 3rd series).

14. Raju U, Vertes D. Breast papillomas with atypical ductal hyperplasia: a clinicopathologic study. *Hum Pathol* 1996;27:1231–1238.

15. Page DL, Salhany KE, Jensen RA, Dupont WD. Subsequent breast carcinoma risk after biopsy with atypia in a breast papilloma. *Cancer* 1996;78:258–266.

16. Cross AS, Azzopardi JG, Krausz T, Van Noorden S, Polak JM. A morphologic and immunocytochemical study of a distinctive variant of ductal carcinoma *in situ* of the breast. *Histopathology* 1985;9:21–37.

CHAPTER 12

Medullary Carcinoma

Medullary carcinoma is a "well-circumscribed carcinoma composed of poorly differentiated cells with scant stroma and prominent lymphoid infiltration" (1). It accounts for fewer than 5% of breast carcinomas (2–4). Patients with medullary carcinoma tend to be relatively young, and it constitutes up to 10% of carcinomas diagnosed in women 35 years of age or less. The mean age in several series ranged from 45 to 54 years (5–8). Bilateral carcinoma is uncommon in patients with medullary carcinoma, and synchronous or metachronous medullary carcinoma involving both breasts is rare event (3,6,9). The size distribution of medullary carcinomas is not appreciably different from that of infiltrating duct carcinomas, with a median size of 2 to 3 cm (5,6).

Because they have circumscribed margins and a firm consistency, medullary carcinomas can be mistaken clinically and radiologically for fibroadenomas (10). There are no ultrasound or mammographic criteria specific for medullary carcinoma or for distinguishing medullary from circumscribed nonmedullary carcinoma (10,11).

Ipsilateral axillary lymph nodes tend to be enlarged in patients with medullary carcinoma, even when no nodal metastases are present, a phenomenon that may complicate clinical staging (12). The average number of lymph nodes recovered from the axillary dissection specimen of a patient with medullary carcinoma is greater than for other types of carcinoma. This difference probably results from the greater ease of finding enlarged, hyperplastic lymph nodes that exhibit reactive changes when examined microscopically.

The typical intact medullary carcinoma is a moderately firm, discrete tumor. A distinct margin usually outlines the tumor when it is bisected and distinguishes it from the surrounding breast tissue, but some small medullary carcinomas have poorly circumscribed borders that result from an intense lymphoplasmacytic reaction extending beyond the immediate perimeter of the tumor (5). The tumor has a lobulated or nodular structure, occasionally with secondary nodules at the periphery. Necrosis is not unusual. As the amount of necrosis increases, there is a greater likelihood that the tumor will have cystic foci.

Medullary carcinoma is defined by a constellation of histopathologic features: prominent lymphoplasmacytic reaction, microscopic circumscription, growth of tumor cells in sheets (syncytial pattern), poorly differentiated nuclear grade, and high mitotic rate. When most but not all of these components are present, the tumor may be termed an *atypical medullary carcinoma*. A medullary carcinoma is classified as atypical if it has one or more of the following features: invasive growth at the periphery of the tumor, a diminished lymphoplasmacytic reaction, nuclear cytology that is not poorly differentiated, a low frequency of mitoses, or conspicuous glandular or papillary growth. The major contribution of the term atypical medullary carcinoma has been to draw attention to the existence of a subset of infiltrating duct carcinomas that may be misdiagnosed as medullary carcinoma.

The diagnosis of medullary carcinoma cannot be made conclusively by needle core biopsy because of the limited sample provided by such materials. It is appropriate to report that the findings are suggestive of medullary carcinoma and that the final classification depends on complete evaluation of the excised tumor.

The *lymphoplasmacytic reaction* involves the periphery and is present diffusely in the substance of the tumor. The internal lymphoplasmacytic infiltrate tends to be sharply limited to fibrovascular stroma between syncytial zones of tumor cells, but in a minority of tumors, the lymphoplasmacytic infiltrate mingles intimately with carcinoma cells (Fig. 1). The lymphoplasmacytic reaction usually encompasses surrounding ducts and lobules occupied by *in situ* carcinoma and more remote ducts and lobules not involved by carcinoma. It may be composed almost entirely of either lymphocytes or plasma cells or a mixed population of these cell types. Intense lymphoplasmacytic infiltrates can occur in nonmedullary infiltrating duct carcinomas, but when plasma cells predominate, the tumor is more likely to be a medullary carcinoma. Rarely, the lymphocytic infiltrate gives rise to germinal centers within or around the tumor.

Microscopic circumscription describes the edge of the carcinoma, which should have a well-defined contour rather than infiltrate the breast parenchyma (Fig. 2). Glandular or fatty breast tissue should not be found within the substance of the invasive tumor, but ducts, lobules, or islands of fat cells may be trapped in the surrounding lymphoplasmacytic reaction or between nodular components of the tumor.

A *syncytial growth pattern* is present as broad irregular sheets or islands in which the borders of individual cells are

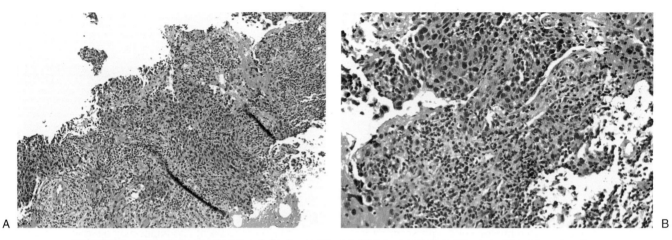

FIGURE 1. Medullary carcinoma. A,B: A needle core biopsy specimen shows a diffuse lymphoplasmacytic infiltrate between syncytial masses of poorly differentiated carcinoma cells. Excisional biopsy revealed a typical medullary carcinoma.

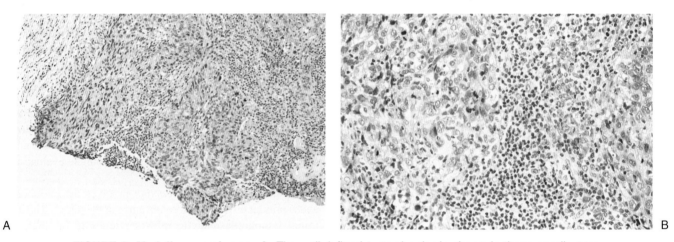

FIGURE 2. Medullary carcinoma. A: The well-defined tumor border is shown in these needle core biopsy samples from a medullary carcinoma. **B:** The round cell infiltrate is lymphoplasmacytic, and the tumor cells have poorly differentiated nuclei.

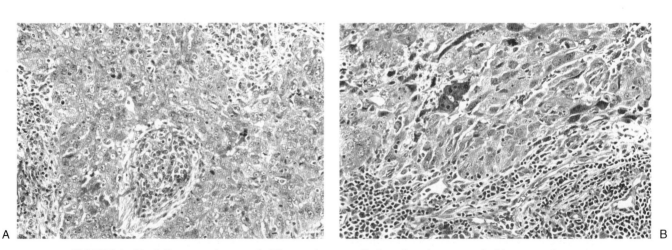

FIGURE 3. Medullary carcinoma. A: The carcinoma cells form bands surrounded by a reaction composed predominantly of plasma cells. The borders of individual cells are indistinct, and they have poorly differentiated nuclei. **B:** A multinucleated giant cell is present.

indistinct (13) (Figs. 2,3). A tumor that is otherwise characteristic may be accepted as a medullary carcinoma if it has minor components of trabecular, glandular, alveolar, or papillary growth. Epidermoid differentiation is not unusual in medullary carcinomas, and about 15% of these tumors have fully developed foci of squamous metaplasia. Necrosis is more common in medullary carcinomas with squamous elements. Osseous, cartilaginous, and spindle-cell metaplasia is much less common, and bizarre epithelial giant cells can be found in an otherwise typical medullary carcinoma (see Fig. 3). The tumor cells have a poorly differentiated nuclear grade and a high mitotic rate (see Figs. 2,3). Pyknotic nuclei of degenerating cells are easily found, as are mitotic figures.

Intraductal carcinoma with lobular extension is found at the periphery of many medullary carcinomas. Foci of intraductal carcinoma occur more frequently with increasing tumor size, and they are accompanied by the same prominent mononuclear cell infiltrate that one finds in the main tumor. The *in situ* carcinoma is composed of cells with the same poorly differentiated nuclei as the invasive portion of the medullary carcinoma. It has a comedo or solid growth pattern and can contain calcifications.

The majority of medullary carcinomas exhibit nuclear expression of p53, and membrane reactivity for HER2/neu is usually lacking. The characteristic immunophenotype of medullary carcinoma is p53(+) HER2/neu(−) (14). Vimentin expression was reported to be more frequent in medullary carcinomas and in duct carcinomas with medullary features than in ordinary invasive duct carcinomas (15). Fewer than 10% of medullary carcinomas have nuclear immunoreactivity for estrogen and progesterone receptors (16).

Patients with medullary carcinoma have axillary lymph node metastases less often than do patients with atypical medullary or infiltrating duct carcinoma, and when present, metastases usually involve no more than three lymph nodes (3,5,6,17). Tumor size and nodal status are significant determinants of disease-free survival. The prognosis of patients with node-negative medullary carcinoma treated by mastectomy is particularly favorable if the tumor is not larger than 3 cm in diameter, with a disease-free survival of 90% or better (5,6,18). The survival results for stage II ($T_1N_1M_0$) medullary carcinoma have also been exceptionally good after 20 years of follow-up (18). Recurrences tend to appear early in the clinical course of patients with medullary carcinoma, and recurrence is rare 5 years or more after diagnosis. Patients whose tumors are larger than 3 cm with four or more involved lymph nodes have high recurrence rates that are not appreciably different from the recurrence rates of patients with infiltrating duct carcinoma.

There is presently little reported experience with breast-conserving primary radiotherapy of medullary carcinoma. In one study of 27 women with medullary carcinoma treated by primary radiotherapy, the mammary recurrence rate was 4%, the 5-year overall survival was 90%, and relapse-free survival was 92% at 5 years (19). Haffty et al. (20) reported that the 10-year actuarial breast recurrence-free survival was lower for medullary carcinoma (75%) than for infiltrating duct carcinoma (85%), but metastatic disease developed in none of 17 patients with medullary carcinoma treated by breast-conserving therapy.

REFERENCES

1. World Health Organization. Histological typing of breast tumors. *Tumori* 1982;68:181–198.
2. Bloom HJG, Richardson WW, Fields JR. Host resistance and survival in carcinoma of breast: a study of 104 cases of medullary carcinoma in a series of 1511 cases of breast cancer followed for 20 years. *Br Med J [Clin Res]* 1970;3:181–188.
3. Rapin V, Contesso G, Mouriesse H, et al. Medullary carcinoma. A re-evaluation of 95 cases of breast cancer with inflammatory stroma. *Cancer* 1988;61:2503–2510.
4. Rosen PP, Saigo PE, Braun DW Jr, Weathers E, DePalo A. Predictors of recurrence in stage 1 ($T_1N_0M_0$) breast carcinoma. *Ann Surg* 1981;193:15–25.
5. Ridolfi R, Rosen P, Port A, Kinne D, Mike V. Medullary carcinoma of the breast. A clinicopathologic study with 10-year follow-up. *Cancer* 1977;40:1365–1385.
6. Wargotz ES, Silverberg SG. Medullary carcinoma of the breast. A clinicopathologic study with appraisal of current diagnostic criteria. *Hum Pathol* 1988;19:1340–1346.
7. Rosen PP, Lesser ML, Senie RT, Duthie K. Epidemiology of breast carcinoma. IV. Age and histologic tumor type. *J Surg Oncol* 1982;19:44–47.
8. Rosen PP, Lesser ML, Kinne DW. Breast carcinoma at the extremes of age: a comparison of patients younger than 35 years and older than 75 years. *J Surg Oncol* 1985;28:90–96.
9. Lesser ML, Rosen PP, Kinne DW. Multicentricity and bilaterality in invasive breast carcinoma. *Surgery* 1982;1:234–240.
10. Meyer JE, Amin E, Lindfors KK, Lipman JC, Stomper PC, Genest D. Medullary carcinoma of the breast: mammographic and US appearance. *Radiology* 1989;170:79–82.
11. Kopans DB, Rubens J. Medullary carcinoma of the breast. *Radiology* 1989;171:876.
12. Neuman ML, Homer MJ. Association of medullary carcinoma with reactive axillary adenopathy. *AJR Am J Roentgenol* 1996;167:185–186.
13. Pedersen L, Schiodt T, Holck S, Zedeler K. The prognostic importance of syncytial growth pattern in medullary carcinoma of the breast. *APMIS* 1990;98:921–926.
14. Rosen PP, Lesser ML, Arroyo CD, Cranor M, Borgen P, Norton L. Immunohistochemical detection of HER2/neu in patients with axillary lymph node negative breast carcinoma: a study of epidemiologic risk factors, histologic features and prognosis. *Cancer* 1995;75:1320–1326.
15. Holck S, Pedersen L, Schiodt T, Zedeler K, Mouridsen H. Vimentin expression in 98 breast cancers with medullary features and its prognostic significance. *Virchows Arch [A]* 1993;422:475–479.
16. Rosen PP, Menendez-Botet CJ, Nisselbaum JS, et al. Pathological review of breast lesions analyzed for estrogen receptor protein. *Cancer Res* 1975;35:3187–3194.
17. Reinfuss M, Stelmach A, Mitus J, Rys J, Duda K. Typical medullary carcinoma of the breast: a clinical and pathological analysis of 52 cases. *J Surg Oncol* 1995;60:89–94.
18. Rosen PP, Groshen S, Saigo PE, Kinne DW, Hellman S. A long-term follow-up study of survival in stage I ($T_1N_0M_0$) and stage II ($T_1N_1M_0$) breast carcinoma. *J Clin Oncol* 1989;7:355–366.
19. Kurtz JM, Jacquemier J, Torhorst J, et al. Conservation therapy for breast cancers other than infiltrating ductal carcinoma. *Cancer* 1989;63:1630–1635.
20. Haffty BG, Perrotta PL, Ward B, et al. Conservatively treated breast cancer: outcome by histologic subtype. *Breast J* 1997;3:7–14.

CHAPTER 13

Carcinoma with Metaplasia

The term metaplasia has traditionally been reserved for neoplasms that exhibit microscopic structural changes that diverge from glandular differentiation. In the breast, these phenotypic structural alterations are the expression of genotypic properties not manifested by the normal epithelium of the breast. Hence, metaplasia represents patterns of gene expression rather than histogenesis.

The frequency of metaplastic change in mammary carcinoma is probably underreported because inconspicuous foci of such change are easily overlooked or ignored (Fig. 1). Squamous metaplasia was present in 3.7% of 1,665 invasive carcinomas reviewed by Fisher et al. (1). Heterologous or sarcomatoid metaplasia was detected in 26 of 12,045 (0.2%) breast carcinomas in another study (2). Carcinomas with metaplasia usually have low levels of estrogen receptor and are classified as receptor-negative when studied by biochemistry or immunohistochemistry (3–5).

The range of age at diagnosis and the clinical features of metaplastic mammary carcinoma are not appreciably different from those of invasive mammary carcinoma generally (2,5). The first symptom is typically a palpable tumor. The patient usually describes rapid growth and short duration before diagnosis (5). There are no specific features to the radiologic appearance of metaplastic carcinoma except that bone formation in tumors with osseous metaplasia may be detectable by mammography. The tumors tend to have circumscribed contours radiologically and grossly. The mean or median size (3 to 4 cm) reported in various series tends to be greater than that of ordinary infiltrating duct carcinomas.

The precise cell type that gives rise to metaplastic carcinomas remains uncertain. The concurrent presence of ordinary intraductal and invasive duct carcinoma in many of these tumors and transitions observed from carcinomatous foci to metaplastic components has led to the conclusion that these neoplasms are carcinomas derived from mammary glandular epithelial cells. Immunohistochemical studies that revealed coexpression of S-100, vimentin, and cytokeratin in components with epithelial and sarcomatoid phenotypes have been interpreted as evidence for the epithelial origin of both elements by some investigators (6). Others have interpreted these same observations as suggesting myoepithelial origin (3).

It has been customary to subdivide metaplastic carcinomas into two categories: squamous and heterologous or pseudosarcomatous. These distinctions are somewhat arbitrary because some tumors exhibit both types of growth. A common pattern of metaplastic carcinoma is focal squamous metaplasia in an otherwise typical invasive duct carcinoma. A spectrum of differentiation may be found in squamous metaplasia. Mature keratinizing epithelium, sometimes with keratohyaline granules, may be associated with poorly differentiated carcinoma or spindle-cell, pseudosarcomatous areas (Fig. 2). Spindle-cell carcinoma of the breast comprises a subset of carcinomas with squamous metaplasia in which most or virtually all of the neoplasm has assumed a pseudosarcomatous growth pattern that resembles fibrosarcoma or fibromatosis (5,7) (Fig. 3). In some instances, the nature of the lesion can be obscured by an inflammatory reaction that may suggest a non-neoplastic condition, such as inflammatory pseudotumor or fasciitis (Fig. 4). Another variant is characterized by dense, keloid-like areas of fibrosis in which the spindle cells and stroma often have a storiform pattern (Fig. 5).

Low-grade adenosquamous carcinoma is an unusual form of metaplastic duct carcinoma that is morphologically similar to adenosquamous carcinoma of the skin (8). These tumors are typically smaller than other varieties of metaplastic carcinoma (0.5 to 3.4 cm; average, about 2.0 cm). They form hard nodules with grossly ill-defined borders. Microscopically, the invasive carcinoma exhibits variable amounts of epidermoid and glandular differentiation in collagenous stroma. Foci of lymphocytic reaction are often present. A tendency to grow between and around ducts and lobules is most prominent at the periphery of the lesion, and it is not unusual to find a central area of sclerosing proliferation, such as a radial scar or sclerosing adenosis. Conventional intraductal carcinoma is inconspicuous. Squamous metaplasia is found in varying patterns, including extensive epidermoid growth, syringoma-like differentiation (Fig. 6), and isolated inconspicuous squamous foci (Fig. 7). Large keratinizing cysts are uncommon. Microcysts that may contain keratotic debris with calcification are more often present.

The distinction between spindle-cell carcinoma and primary sarcoma of the breast may be difficult, and the neoplasm may be mistaken for a sarcoma, especially in a needle core biopsy specimen (9). Extensive sampling of the excised

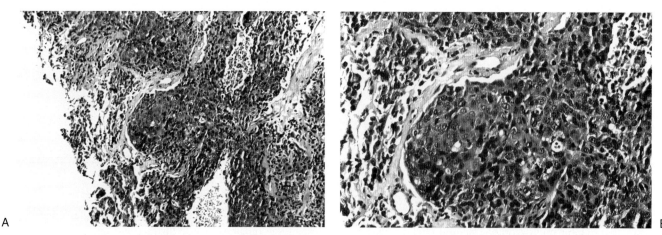

A

B

FIGURE 1. Carcinoma with squamoid traits. This tumor is not classified as metaplastic carcinoma. **A,B:** A needle core biopsy specimen showing poorly differentiated infiltrating duct carcinoma. An area suggestive of squamous metaplasia, shown magnified in (B), has cells with dense eosinophilic cytoplasm and vague keratin pearl formation.

tumor is sometimes necessary to identify areas of squamous differentiation and to search for foci of intraductal or invasive adenocarcinoma at the periphery. An unusual variant of spindle-cell mammary carcinoma with squamous metaplasia has been described as pseudoangiosarcomatous or acantholytic carcinoma (10,11) (Fig. 8). The resemblance to angiosarcoma is a consequence of degeneration of the squamous epithelial component, resulting in a pseudovascular pattern of anastomosing spaces. Cells lining these spaces are immunoreactive for cytokeratin and other epithelial markers, and they do not stain for factor VIII or CD34, which characterize endothelial cells.

Metaplastic carcinoma must be considered in the differential diagnosis of virtually any spindle lesion encountered in a needle core biopsy specimen. Immunohistochemistry should be employed to detect evidence of epithelial differentiation. If this effort is not successful, the report given for the needle core biopsy sample should indicate the need to study the excised tumor to establish a specific diagnosis. The distinction between a sarcoma and metaplastic carcinoma has important implications for therapy.

Heterologous metaplasia is most commonly encountered as bone and/or cartilage (Fig. 9). These foci often coexist with areas composed of undifferentiated round or spindle cells. Zones of spindle-cell metaplasia usually intervene between the adenocarcinomatous and heterologous elements (Fig. 10). Metaplastic carcinomas that have multinucleated giant cells resembling osteoclasts usually exhibit osseous or

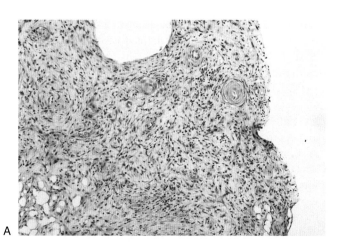

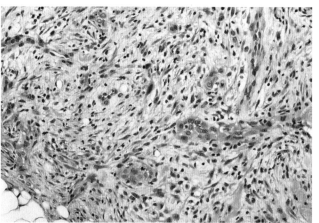

A

B

FIGURE 2. Metaplastic carcinoma, spindle-cell and squamous type. This lesion might be misinterpreted as fibromatosis or as an inflammatory tumor. **A:** The needle core biopsy specimen shows a moderately cellular spindle-cell lesion infiltrating fat with scattered lymphocytes. The spindle cells have bland cytologic features. Discrete foci of squamous cells are present. **B:** Indistinct cords and nests of polygonal carcinoma cells.

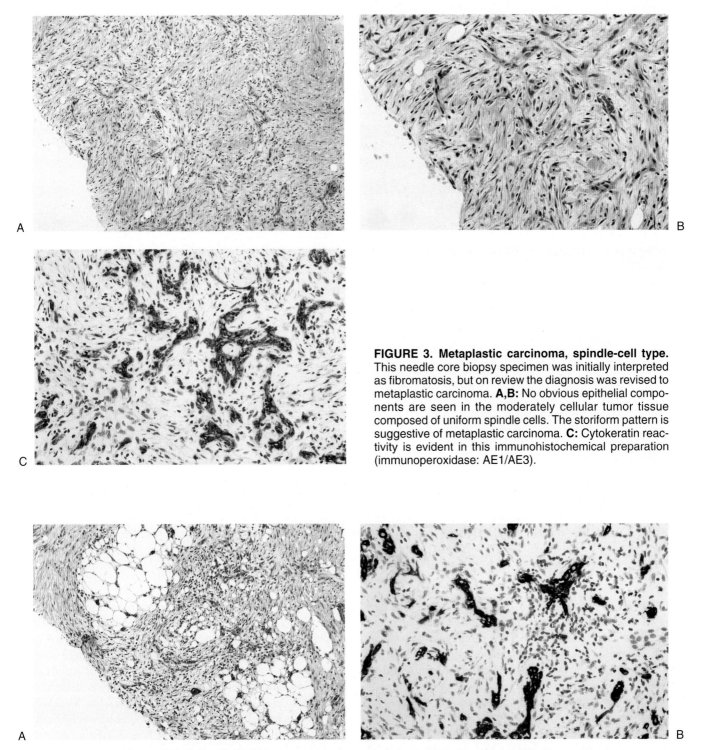

FIGURE 3. Metaplastic carcinoma, spindle-cell type. This needle core biopsy specimen was initially interpreted as fibromatosis, but on review the diagnosis was revised to metaplastic carcinoma. **A,B:** No obvious epithelial components are seen in the moderately cellular tumor tissue composed of uniform spindle cells. The storiform pattern is suggestive of metaplastic carcinoma. **C:** Cytokeratin reactivity is evident in this immunohistochemical preparation (immunoperoxidase: AE1/AE3).

FIGURE 4. Metaplastic carcinoma, spindle-cell type. A tumor with features that resemble those of an inflammatory lesion. **A:** The pattern of infiltration into fat and lymphocytic reaction in this needle core biopsy specimen was mistaken for fat necrosis. **B:** Cytokeratin expression is demonstrated in some of the spindle cells (immunoperoxidase: 34BE12).

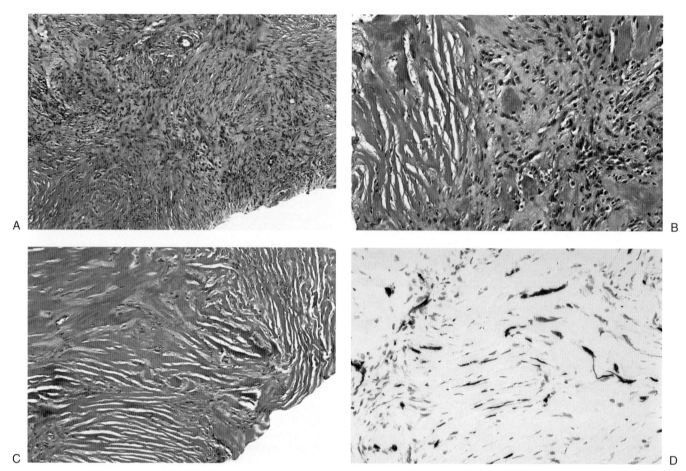

FIGURE 5. Metaplastic carcinoma, spindle-cell type. A: This area in the needle core biopsy specimen has a storiform pattern. **B:** Another region with a component that resembles (A) is on the right. A keloid-like area composed of dense collagen and a pseudoangiomatous appearance is on the left. These findings resemble an area of scarring. **C:** A fully developed keloid-like area with prominent spaces between collagen bands. **D:** Some spindle cells among the collagen bands are immunoreactive for cytokeratin (immunoperoxidase: 34BE12).

cartilaginous metaplasia (2,4). This type of metaplastic carcinoma does not have the diffuse stromal hemorrhage and prominent adenocarcinoma found in carcinomas with osteoclast-like giant cells. *Matrix-producing carcinoma* is a variant of heterologous metaplastic carcinoma composed of "overt carcinoma with direct transition to a cartilaginous and/or osseous stromal matrix without an intervening spindle-cell zone or osteoclastic cells" (12) (Fig. 11). The majority of the tumors are circumscribed or nodular. The carcinomatous element is a moderately to poorly differentiated adenocarcinoma. Mucin positivity is demonstrated in the carcinomatous areas, but matrix-forming cells do not contain mucin. The chondroid matrix has the histochemical properties of a sulfated acid mucopolysaccharide, consistent with chondroitin sulfate.

Immunohistochemical studies have attempted to elucidate the relationship between epithelial and heterologous elements in metaplastic carcinomas, but the reported results have been inconsistent. It is very likely that there are intrin-

sic differences in the phenotypic expression of these markers that reflect the variable nature of genetic alterations in individual tumors. Rather than a single pattern of cytokeratin expression, these neoplasms appear to have a range of cytoskeletal phenotypes that express differing proportions and types of cytofilaments. A series of markers is usually required to detect evidence of epithelial expression. Most helpful in this regard are low- and high-molecular-weight cytokeratins, including CAM5.2, CK7, 34BE12, and the AE1/AE3 combination. In a given tumor, one marker will stain more strongly and more diffusely than the others, but the pattern of expression tends to be unpredictable in a given tumor.

Prognostic data thus far have been based on patients treated by mastectomy, usually with axillary dissection. Because of the rarity of metaplastic carcinomas and the relatively low frequency of axillary metastases, especially in patients with heterologous metaplastic tumors, it is difficult to assemble a sufficient number of cases to stratify them by ma-

Text continues on page 158

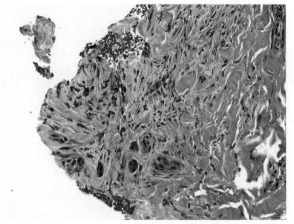

FIGURE 6. Metaplastic carcinoma, low-grade adenosquamous type. A: This needle core biopsy sample of a mammographically detected nonpalpable stellate tumor revealed infiltrating carcinoma in fibrous stroma. The small oval nests of tumor cells have squamoid traits. **B,C:** The excisional biopsy specimen revealed cords and clusters of cells similar to those in (A) surrounded by spindle-cell carcinoma. Glandular and squamoid differentiation are evident. The lymphocytic aggregate shown in (C) is a characteristic feature of low-grade adenosquamous carcinoma.

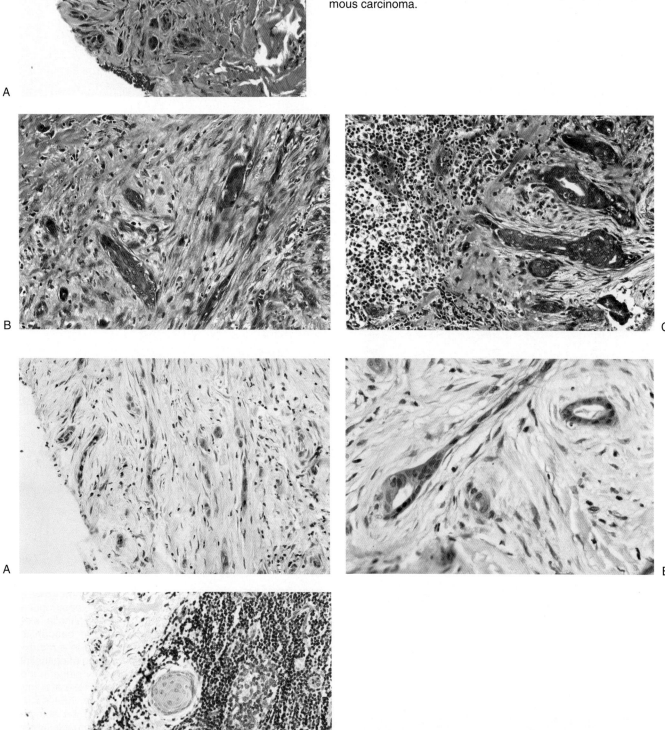

FIGURE 7. Metaplastic carcinoma, low-grade adenosquamous type. A: Epithelial strands are shown in moderately cellular stroma in this needle core biopsy specimen. **B:** Syringoma-like epithelial elements are also present. **C:** In another area of the specimen, a squamous pearl is surrounded by lymphocytes.

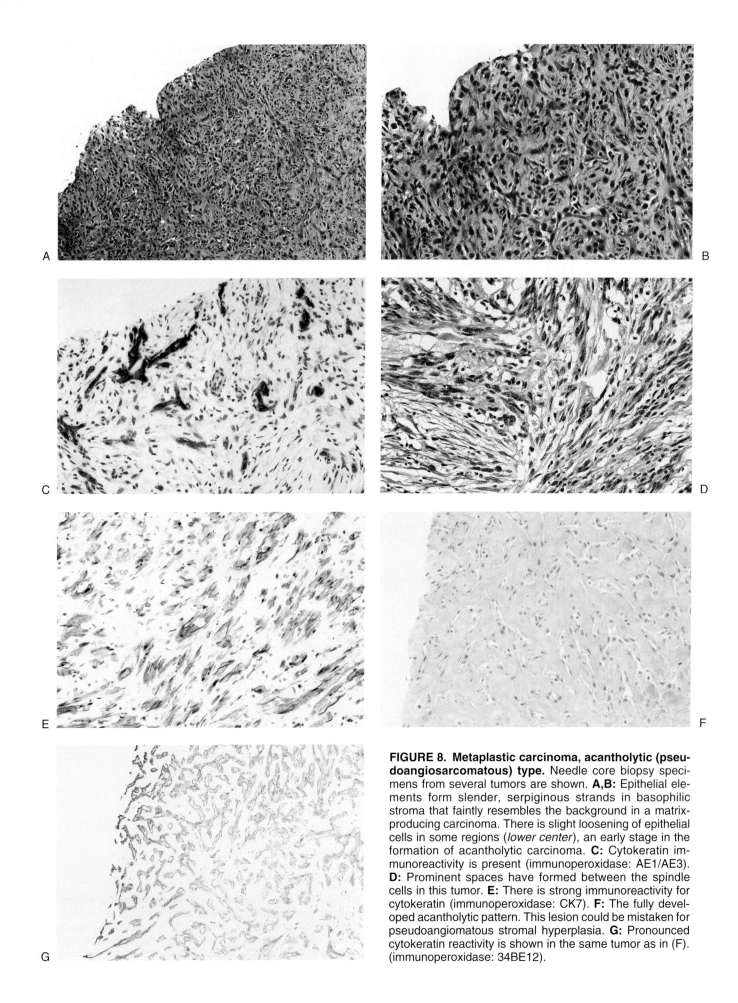

FIGURE 8. Metaplastic carcinoma, acantholytic (pseudoangiosarcomatous) type. Needle core biopsy specimens from several tumors are shown. **A,B:** Epithelial elements form slender, serpiginous strands in basophilic stroma that faintly resembles the background in a matrix-producing carcinoma. There is slight loosening of epithelial cells in some regions (*lower center*), an early stage in the formation of acantholytic carcinoma. **C:** Cytokeratin immunoreactivity is present (immunoperoxidase: AE1/AE3). **D:** Prominent spaces have formed between the spindle cells in this tumor. **E:** There is strong immunoreactivity for cytokeratin (immunoperoxidase: CK7). **F:** The fully developed acantholytic pattern. This lesion could be mistaken for pseudoangiomatous stromal hyperplasia. **G:** Pronounced cytokeratin reactivity is shown in the same tumor as in (F). (immunoperoxidase: 34BE12).

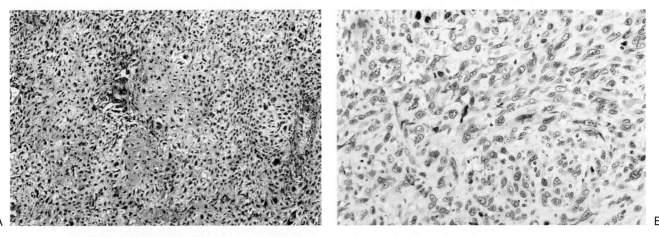

FIGURE 9. Metaplastic carcinoma, osteocartilaginous metaplasia. A: The tumor has poorly formed osteoid and chondroid matrix. **B:** Cytokeratin expression is demonstrated in a few spindle and round cells (immunoperoxidase: CAM5.2).

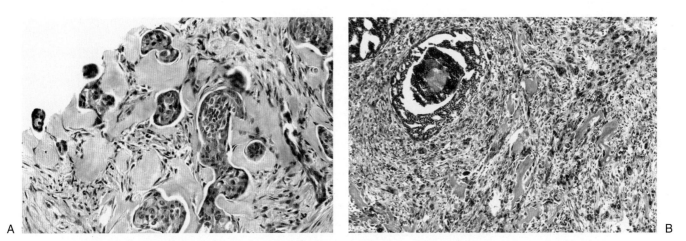

FIGURE 10. Metaplastic carcinoma with osteosarcomatous differentiation. A: The needle core biopsy specimen shows poorly differentiated carcinoma and osteoid. **B:** Intraductal carcinoma was found in the midst of the tumor in the excisional biopsy specimen.

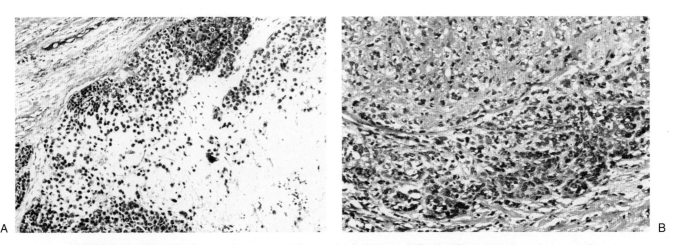

FIGURE 11. Metaplastic carcinoma, matrix-producing type. A,B: Undifferentiated carcinoma cells are seen blending with matrix material. The lacunar structure of cartilage is not present.

jor prognostic factors, such as tumor size, nodal status, and pattern of metaplasia. The frequency of positive axillary lymph nodes associated with heterologous metaplastic carcinoma, including so-called matrix-producing tumors, ranges from 6% (12) to 31% (9). Disease-free survival, generally reported for 5 or more years of follow-up, has been as high as 67% (9). Axillary lymph node metastases were reported in 6% to 14% of patients with squamous and spindle-cell metaplasia. Squamous metaplasia does not seem to influence prognosis, but extensive spindle-cell metaplasia associated with squamous foci may have an adverse influence on outcome.

REFERENCES

1. Fisher ER, Gregorio RM, Palekar AS, Paulson JD. Mucoepidermoid and squamous cell carcinomas of breast with reference to squamous metaplasia and giant cell tumors. *Am J Surg Pathol* 1984;7:15–27.
2. Kaufman MW, Marti JR, Gallager HS, Hoehn JL. Carcinoma of the breast with pseudosarcomatous metaplasia. *Cancer* 1984;53: 1908–1917.
3. Wargotz ES, Norris HJ. Metaplastic carcinoma of the breast. IV. Squamous cell carcinoma of ductal origin. *Cancer* 1990;65:272–276.
4. Wargotz ES, Norris HJ. Metaplastic carcinomas of the breast. V. Metaplastic carcinoma with osteoclastic giant cells. *Hum Pathol* 1990;21: 1142–1150.
5. Oberman HA. Metaplastic carcinoma of the breast. A clinicopathologic study of 29 patients. *Am J Surg Pathol* 1987;11:918–929.
6. Palmer JO, Ghiselli RW, McDivitt RW. Immunohistochemistry in the differential diagnosis of breast diseases. *Pathol Annu* 1990;25(Pt 2): 287–315.
7. Gersell DJ, Katzenstein A-L. Spindle cell carcinoma of the breast. A clinicopathologic and ultrastructural study. *Hum Pathol* 1981;12: 550–561.
8. Rosen PP, Ernsberger D. Low-grade adenosquamous carcinoma. A variant of metaplastic mammary carcinoma. *Am J Surg Pathol* 1987;11: 351–358.
9. Pitts WC, Rojas VA, Gaffey MJ, et al. Carcinomas with metaplasia and sarcomas of the breast. *Am J Clin Pathol* 1991;95:623–632.
10. Banerjee SS, Eyden BP, Wells S, McWilliam LJ, Harris M. Pseudoangiosarcomatous carcinoma: a clinicopathological study of seven cases. *Histopathology* 1992;21:13–23.
11. Eusebi V, Lamovec J, Cattani MC, Fedeli F, Millis RR. Acantholytic variant of squamous cell carcinoma of the breast. *Am J Surg Pathol* 1986;10:855–861.
12. Wargotz ES, Norris HJ. Metaplastic carcinomas of the breast. I. Matrix-producing carcinoma. *Hum Pathol* 1989;20:628–636.

CHAPTER 14

Squamous Carcinoma

The term squamous carcinoma should be used for lesions in which more than 90% of the neoplasm is composed of keratinizing squamous carcinoma or one of its variant forms. Squamous carcinoma of the breast is a form of metaplastic carcinoma, as the mammary glandular epithelium is not normally keratinizing. Benign metaplastic squamous epithelium is a potential precursor of pure squamous carcinoma. Squamous metaplasia occurs in the epithelium of cysts, fibroepithelial tumors, and duct hyperplasia (Fig. 1). Extensive benign squamous metaplasia of duct and lobular epithelium has been described in association with fat necrosis and other lesions (1). When squamous metaplasia occurs in an inflamed cyst, metaplastic epithelium may be embedded in a reactive process, resulting in a pattern that is difficult to distinguish from invasive squamous carcinoma.

There are no clinical features that are specific for squamous carcinoma of the breast. The tumors have indistinct or partially distinct margins on mammography, but no specific mammographic findings have been described (2,3). Calcifications in necrotic squamous tissue can sometimes be seen radiographically. Involvement of the skin makes it difficult to distinguish between cutaneous origin and secondary skin involvement by an underlying mammary lesion. When the bulk of the tumor is in the breast and the clinical history indicates that a breast mass preceded skin ulceration, the lesion may be considered to be a mammary carcinoma. Most of these tumors are estrogen receptor–negative.

Squamous carcinomas tend to be somewhat larger than other types of breast carcinoma. Reported sizes vary from 1 to 10 cm, with nearly half of the cases 5 cm or more in diameter (4). Central cystic degeneration is especially common in tumors larger than 2 cm, the cavity being filled with necrotic squamous debris.

Squamous carcinomas of the breast are differentiated sufficiently to form keratinized cells, and keratohyaline granules may be seen in the neoplastic epithelium (Fig. 2). Conversion of the squamous epithelium to spindle-cell pseudosarcomatous growth can be found at least focally in most squamous carcinomas of the breast. Extensive sampling of the lesion following excisional biopsy is necessary to determine if the tumor is a metaplastic carcinoma with squamous differentiation or a pure squamous carcinoma. The latter diagnosis is made if there is extensive squamous differentiation of the epithelium with little or no spindle-cell element and no detectable adenocarcinoma.

When squamous carcinoma is found in the breast, it is necessary to consider the possibility that the tumor is metastatic from an extramammary primary. The most common sources of metastatic squamous carcinoma in the breast are the lung, esophagus, uterine cervix, and urinary bladder. The distinction between a primary tumor and metastatic squamous carcinoma is unlikely to be resolved with a needle core biopsy.

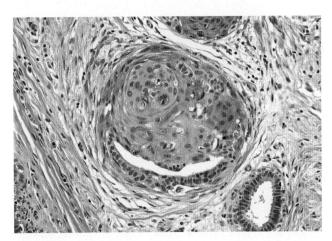

FIGURE 1. Squamous metaplasia in a hyperplastic duct. Benign metaplastic foci such as this may be the source of primary squamous carcinoma in the breast.

159

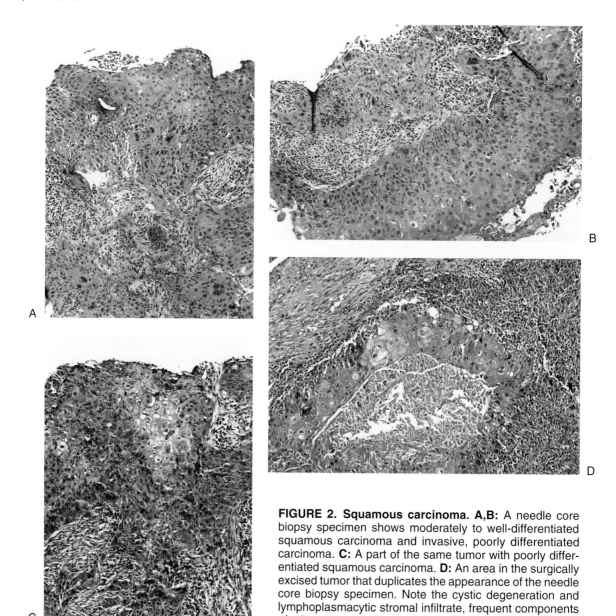

FIGURE 2. Squamous carcinoma. A,B: A needle core biopsy specimen shows moderately to well-differentiated squamous carcinoma and invasive, poorly differentiated carcinoma. **C:** A part of the same tumor with poorly differentiated squamous carcinoma. **D:** An area in the surgically excised tumor that duplicates the appearance of the needle core biopsy specimen. Note the cystic degeneration and lymphoplasmacytic stromal infiltrate, frequent components of primary squamous carcinoma of the breast.

REFERENCES

1. Hurt MA, Diaz-Arias AA, Rosenholtz MJ, Havey AD, Stephenson HF Jr. Posttraumatic lobular squamous metaplasia of breast. An unusual pseudocarcinomatous metaplasia resembling squamous (necrotizing) sialometaplasia of the salivary gland. *Mod Pathol* 1988;1:385–390.
2. Tashjian J, Kuni CC, Bohn LE. Primary squamous cell carcinoma of the breast: mammographic findings. *Can Assoc Radiol J* 1989;40:228–229.
3. Samuels TH, Miller NA, Manchul LA, DeFreitas G, Panzarella T. Squamous cell carcinoma of the breast. *Can Assoc Radiol J* 1996;47: 177–182.
4. Eggers JW, Chesney TM. Squamous cell carcinoma of the breast: a clinicopathologic analysis of eight cases and review of the literature. *Hum Pathol* 1984;15:526–531.

CHAPTER 15

Mucinous Carcinoma

When the diagnosis is restricted to tumors consisting of pure or nearly pure mucinous carcinoma, not more than 2% of mammary carcinomas fall into this category (1–3). Focal mucinous differentiation occurs in up to 2% of other carcinomas, which are termed infiltrating duct carcinoma with mucinous differentiation, or mixed mucinous carcinoma (3,4). Mucinous carcinoma occurs throughout the age range of breast carcinoma generally. Some studies found the mean age of women with mucinous carcinoma to be older than that of patients with nonmucinous carcinoma (2,3,5). Mucinous carcinoma constitutes about 7% of carcinomas in women 75 years or older and only 1% among those younger than 35 years (6). Immunohistochemical studies have shown nuclear estrogen receptor activity in nearly 90% of cases (7).

The initial symptom is a breast mass in the majority of patients. Mixed mucinous carcinomas tend to have irregular margins mammographically because of fibrosis and an infiltrative growth pattern (8). A spiculated contour is associated with a lesser mucinous component and a higher frequency of lymph node metastases. Mammographically detected calcifications occur in about 40% of the tumors and involve the invasive portion of approximately 20% of mucinous carcinomas (9,10). Calcifications may be localized in associated intraductal carcinoma.

Mucinous carcinomas have been described ranging from less than 1 cm to more than 20 cm in diameter. In 1987, a nationwide study of Danish breast cancer patients found that only 16% of mucinous carcinomas were larger than 5 cm (1), and a report from Japan found that 53.6% of tumors were 2.0 cm or less (T_1) and 37.8% were 2.1 to 5.0 cm (T_2) (4).

Pure mucinous carcinoma features the accumulation of extracellular mucin around invasive tumor cells (Fig. 1). The proportions of mucin and neoplastic epithelium vary from case to case, but the distribution within a given tumor is fairly constant. Multiple sections can be necessary to detect carcinoma cells if a tumor is composed almost entirely of extracellular mucin. The proportion of the lesion that consists of extracellular mucin in tumors classified as pure mucinous carcinomas varies from less than 40% to 99.8%, with a mean percentage of 83.5 ± 14.3 (4) (Fig. 2).

Intraductal carcinoma found associated with about 75% of the lesions, generally at the periphery, can have any of the conventional patterns (cribriform, papillary, micropapillary,

comedo) (Fig. 3). Occasionally, intracytoplasmic and extracellular mucin are evident in the intraductal component. One of the most infrequent variants is a cystic papillary mucinous carcinoma composed of multiple cysts distended by mucinous secretion and lined by micropapillary, papillary, and cribriform intraductal carcinoma.

Several patterns of epithelial distribution can be found in mucinous carcinomas (11). Lesions with epithelium arranged in clusters, trabeculae, or festoons have been associated with a younger age at diagnosis than tumors in which the carcinoma cells form larger clumps (Figs. 1,2,4). The latter lesions tend to have more abundant intracytoplasmic mucin and granular cytoplasm, and some of these tumors cells are argyrophilic. Areas with a cribriform structure are present in many mucinous carcinomas, and a subset of the lesions exhibits mixed growth patterns consisting of ribbons and clumps of cells. The margin of mucinous carcinoma is determined by the extent of the mucinous component, which can be devoid of epithelial cells in the peripheral zone. The border is characterized as a pushing in more than 70% of cases, but the actual contour may be irregular or knobby (10). It is difficult to recognize lymphatic tumor emboli in mucinous carcinomas because carcinoma cells suspended in mucin resemble intralymphatic carcinoma (Fig. 5).

Argyrophilic granules are present in the cells of 25% to 50% of mucinous carcinomas (1–3,11). Mucinous carcinomas that contain these granules occur frequently in elderly women. The granules of some mucinous carcinomas contain immunohistochemically detectable serotonin, somatostatin, gastrin, and neuron-specific enolase (12). The presence or absence of argyrophilic granules is not prognostically significant in pure mucinous tumors or in infiltrating duct carcinomas with focal mucinous differentiation (1,2,13).

Mucocele-like lesions must be considered in the differential diagnosis of mucinous carcinoma (14). The final classification of a mucocele-like tumor depends on the pattern of epithelial growth, which may include duct hyperplasia with or without atypia, intraductal carcinoma, or invasive mucinous carcinoma (15,16). Mucocele-like lesions present as palpable tumors, or they are detected by mammography as well-circumscribed, lobulated tumors. Large and granular calcifications formed in many mucocele-like lesions lead to mammographic detection. The finding of this type of calcifi-

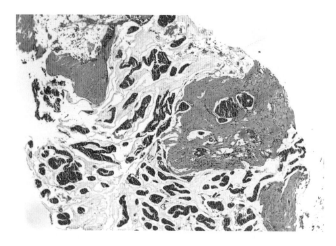

FIGURE 1. Mucinous carcinoma. In this needle core biopsy specimen, trabecular groups of carcinoma cells are distributed in mucin.

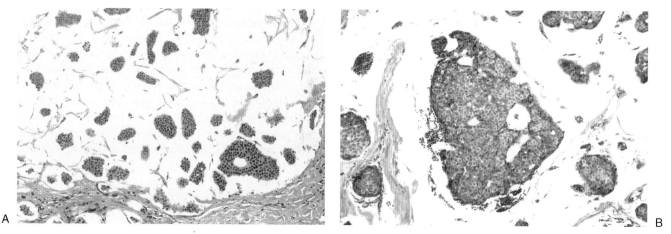

FIGURE 2. Mucinous carcinoma. A,B: Needle core biopsy specimens show varying proportions of extracellular mucin and carcinoma cells. The epithelium forms small nests and glands.

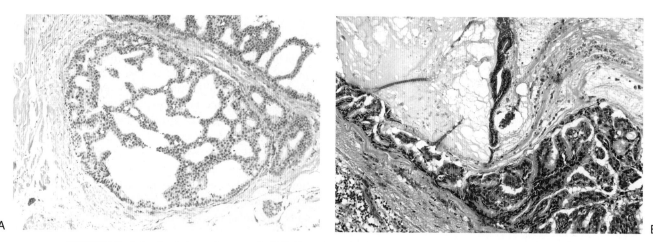

FIGURE 3. Intraductal carcinoma. A: Cribriform intraductal carcinoma that was present in the needle core biopsy specimen in Fig. 2A. Invasive mucinous carcinoma is present in the lower right corner. **B:** Papillary intraductal carcinoma with mucin formation in the duct.

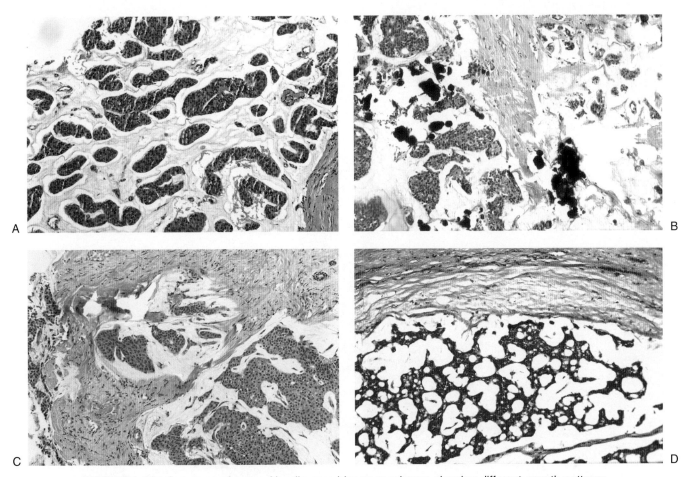

FIGURE 4. Mucinous carcinoma. Needle core biopsy specimens showing different growth patterns. **A:** Trabecular pattern. **B:** Irregular clusters of carcinoma cells and calcification in the mucin. **C:** Festoon growth pattern. **D:** Cribriform mucinous carcinoma.

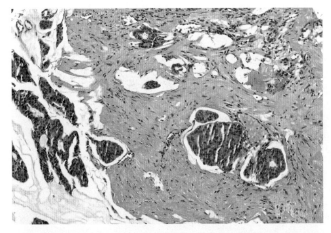

FIGURE 5. Mucinous carcinoma simulating lymphatic tumor emboli. A magnified view of a needle core biopsy specimen shows carcinoma cells surrounded by mucin in the stroma. This appearance simulates carcinoma in lymphatic spaces. Note the absence of endothelial cell nuclei around the mucin-filled spaces and infiltration into the collagenous stroma beyond the edge of the predominantly mucinous part of the tumor on the left.

cation in a needle core biopsy specimen is sufficient evidence to suggest the diagnosis of a mucocele-like tumor, especially if mucin is also present (Fig. 6).

A mucocele-like tumor is composed of mucin-containing cysts, which may rupture and discharge the secretion into the adjacent stroma. The epithelium lining the cysts in a typical benign mammary mucocele-like tumor is flat or cuboidal, but low columnar and minor papillary elements may be present (Figs. 7,8). Detached epithelial cells are almost never found in the secretion within the cysts or in secretion extruded into the stroma, but histiocytes and inflammatory cells may be present in the extruded mucin. Atypical duct hyperplasia is present in some mucocele-like lesions (Fig. 9).

Hamele-Bena et al. (16) reviewed 49 examples of mucocele-like lesions. Four patients had bilateral tumors; these were both benign in two cases and both carcinomatous in the other two patients. Overall, 25 of the lesions were classified as benign and 28 as carcinomatous. In 13 tumors, the carcinoma was entirely *in situ*, growing largely as micropapillary or focally cribriform intraductal carcinoma (Fig. 10). Twenty-five tumors had invasive carcinoma of the mucinous

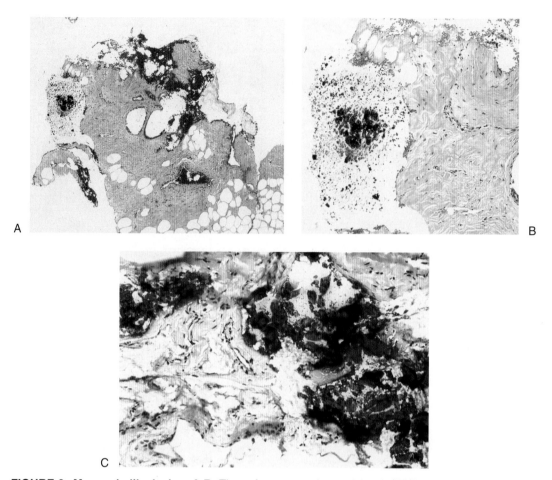

FIGURE 6. Mucocele-like lesion. A,B: These fragments of granular calcification with mucin in a needle core biopsy specimen are highly suggestive of a mucocele-like tumor and are an indication for excisional biopsy. Portions of small cysts are present in (A). **C:** This needle core biopsy specimen from a benign mucocele-like lesion consists of mucin, coarse calcifications, and fragments of cysts virtually devoid of epithelium.

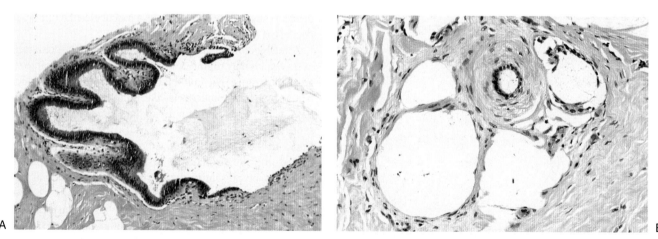

FIGURE 7. Benign mucocele-like lesion. A: This cystically dilated, partially disrupted duct was present in the specimen from a needle core biopsy performed for nonpalpable calcifications. The duct is lined by benign, low columnar epithelium. Note the epithelium curled back toward the duct lumen near the upper border at the site of disruption. This is a characteristic feature of mucocele-like lesions. **B:** Another area in the specimen has intact and partially disrupted ducts and extruded mucin in the stroma.

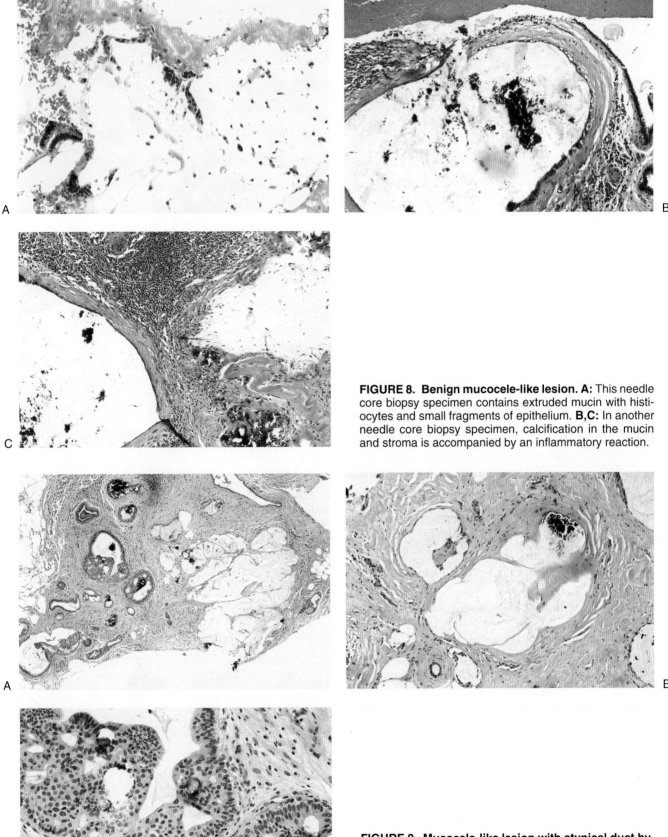

FIGURE 8. Benign mucocele-like lesion. A: This needle core biopsy specimen contains extruded mucin with histiocytes and small fragments of epithelium. **B,C:** In another needle core biopsy specimen, calcification in the mucin and stroma is accompanied by an inflammatory reaction.

FIGURE 9. Mucocele-like lesion with atypical duct hyperplasia. A: Ductal hyperplasia with calcifications and extruded mucin are evident at low magnification. **B:** Extruded mucin with calcification in the stroma. **C:** Atypical micropapillary and cribriform hyperplasia with calcifications. Note the regular, low columnar epithelium focally present at the periphery of the ducts.

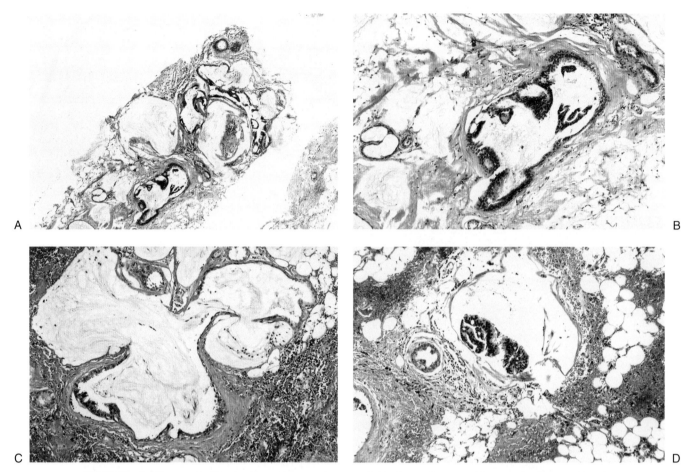

FIGURE 10. Mucocele-like lesion with carcinoma. A,B: A needle core biopsy specimen with micropapillary intraductal carcinoma in one duct. **C:** Excisional biopsy revealed disruption of ducts with extrusion of mucin. **D:** Invasive mucinous carcinoma is manifested by clusters of carcinomatous epithelial cells in the mucin.

type (Figs. 10,11). The age range for the entire group was 24 to 79 years (mean, 48 years), without significant differences in the age distribution of patients with benign and malignant lesions. Malignant mucocele-like lesions tended to have coarse calcifications more often than the benign tumors and were therefore more frequently detected by mammography. Breast recurrences developed in one patient with a benign and one with a carcinomatous lesion. There were no instances of systemic metastases and no deaths from carcinoma associated with a mucocele-like lesion.

Women with pure mucinous carcinoma have had a better relapse-free survival 5 and 10 years after mastectomy than those with mixed mucinous carcinoma containing infiltrating duct carcinoma components and those with infiltrating duct carcinoma (2,5,17). Pure mucinous carcinomas tend to be smaller than tumors with a mixed pattern, and these patients have a lower frequency of axillary lymph node metastases (2,4,17,18). The frequency of negative axillary lymph nodes in patients with pure mucinous carcinoma is about 75%, and about 50% in patients with mixed mucinous carci-

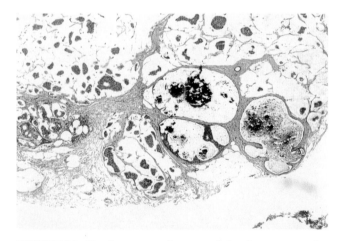

FIGURE 11. Mucinous carcinoma arising in a mucocele-like lesion. This needle core biopsy specimen demonstrates mucinous carcinoma surrounding a central area of extruded mucin that contains a prominent basophilic calcification. A duct with micropapillary intraductal carcinoma, cysts with mucin and finely granular calcification, typical of a mucocele-like lesion, are present.

nomas (2–4,17). Recurrence is least likely with smaller tumors and in the absence of lymph node metastases (3,19). Komaki et al. (4) described a 90% 10-year survival for patients with pure mucinous carcinoma and a 60% 10-year survival for those with mixed duct and mucinous carcinoma. In another report, the 15-year disease-free survival rates were 85% and 63% for patients with pure mucinous and mixed mucinous-duct carcinoma, respectively (3). A series of 1,008 women treated by breast conservation with radiotherapy at Yale University from 1970 to 1990 included 16 patients with mucinous carcinoma (20). After a median follow-up of 11.2 years, there were no breast recurrences, and a systemic recurrence developed in one patient 11 years after initial therapy.

REFERENCES

1. Rasmussen BB, Rose C, Christensen I. Prognostic factors in primary mucinous breast carcinoma. *Am J Clin Pathol* 1987;87:155–160.
2. Scopsi L, Andreola S, Pilotti S, et al. Mucinous carcinoma of the breast. A clinicopathologic, histochemical and immunocytochemical study with special reference to neuroendocrine differentiation. *Am J Surg Pathol* 1994;18:702–711.
3. Toikkanen S, Kujari H. Pure and mixed mucinous carcinomas of the breast: a clinicopathologic analysis of 61 cases with long-term follow-up. *Hum Pathol* 1989;20:758–764.
4. Komaki K, Sakamoto G, Sugano H, Morimoto T, Monden Y. Mucinous carcinoma of the breast in Japan. A prognostic analysis based on morphologic features. *Cancer* 1988;61:989–996.
5. Rosen PP, Wang T-Y. Colloid carcinoma of the breast. Analysis of 64 patients with long-term follow-up. *Am J Clin Pathol* 1980;73:30.
6. Rosen PP, Lesser ML, Kinne DW. Breast carcinoma at the extremes of age: a comparison of patients younger than 35 years and older than 75 years. *J Surg Oncol* 1985;28:90–96.
7. Shousha S, Coady AT, Stamp T, James KR, Alaghband-Zadeh J. Oestrogen receptors in mucinous carcinoma of the breast: an immunohistochemical study using paraffin wax sections. *J Clin Pathol* 1989; 42:902–905.
8. Wilson TE, Helvie MA, Oberman HA, Joynt LK. Pure and mixed mucinous carcinoma of the breast: pathologic basis for differences in mammographic appearance. *AJR Am J Roentgenol* 1995;165:285–289.
9. Ruggieri AM, Scola FH, Schepps B, Esparza AR. Mucinous carcinoma of the breast: mammographic findings. *Breast Dis* 1995;8:353–361.
10. Goodman DNF, Boutross-Tadross O, Jong RA. Mammographic features of pure mucinous carcinoma of the breast with pathological correlation. *Can Assoc Radiol J* 1995;46:296–301.
11. Capella C, Eusebi V, Mann B, Azzopardi JG. Endocrine differentiation in mucoid carcinoma of the breast. *Histopathology* 1980;4:613–630.
12. Hull MT, Warfel KA. Mucinous breast carcinomas with abundant intracytoplasmic mucin and neuroendocrine features: light microscopic, immunohistochemical and ultrastructural study. *Ultrastruct Pathol* 1987;11:29–38.
13. Coady AT, Shousha S, Dawson PM, Moss M, James KR, Bull TB. Mucinous carcinoma of the breast: further characterization of its three subtypes. *Histopathology* 1989;15:617–626.
14. Rosen PP. Mucocele-like tumors of the breast. *Am J Surg Pathol* 1986; 10:464–469.
15. Ro JY, Sneige N, Sahin AA, Silva EG, delJunco GW, Ayala AG. Mucocele-like tumor of the breast associated with atypical duct hyperplasia or mucinous carcinoma. A clinicopathologic study of seven cases. *Arch Pathol Lab Med* 1991;115:137–140.
16. Hamele-Bena D, Cranor ML, Rosen PP. Mammary mucocele-like lesions: benign and malignant. *Am J Surg Pathol* 1996;20:1081–1085.
17. Andre S, Cunha F, Bernardo M, Sousa JME, Cortez F, Soares J. Mucinous carcinoma of the breast: a pathologic study of 82 cases. *J Surg Oncol* 1995;58:162–167.
18. Rasmussen BB. Human mucinous carcinomas and their lymph node metastases. A histological review of 247 cases. *Pathol Res Pract* 1985; 180:377–382.
19. Rosen PP, Groshen S, Saigo PE, Kinne DW, Hellman S. A long-term follow-up study of survival in stage I ($T_1N_0M_0$) and stage II ($T_1N_1M_0$) breast carcinoma. *J Clin Oncol* 1989;7:355–366.
20. Haffty BG, Perrotta PL, Ward B, et al. Conservatively treated breast cancer: outcome by histologic subtype. *Breast J* 1997;3:7–14.

CHAPTER 16

Apocrine Carcinoma

Most apocrine carcinomas probably arise from preexisting apocrine metaplasia (Fig. 1). Apocrine metaplasia is particularly abundant and often atypical in the breasts of women with apocrine carcinoma (Fig. 2). Transitions from atypical hyperplastic apocrine lesions to carcinoma are evident in some but not all examples of apocrine carcinoma (1) (Fig. 3).

The diagnosis of apocrine carcinoma should be reserved for neoplasms in which all or nearly all of the epithelium has apocrine cytologic features, in which case, 1% to 2% of breast carcinomas qualify as true apocrine carcinomas. Apocrine carcinomas are usually classified as ductal, but an apocrine variant of lobular carcinoma has been described (2,3).

There are no specific clinical or mammographic features associated with apocrine duct carcinomas (4). The reported age at diagnosis ranges from 19 to 86 years, with a distribution not significantly different from that of patients with non-apocrine duct carcinoma. In rare instances, the mammogram in a patient with extensive intraductal apocrine carcinoma displays diffuse "mixed form" linear and punctate calcifications "characterized by a strikingly wild, chaotic appearance with profuse deposition of calcium" (5). Patients who have invasive apocrine carcinoma usually present with a mass. The frequency of bilaterality in patients with apocrine carcinoma in one breast is not exceptional. Apocrine carcinoma of the male breast is very uncommon. One unusual apocrine male mammary carcinoma had a glandular structure and psammoma bodies (6). When studied by immunohistochemistry, 98% of 102 apocrine lesions, including benign conditions and carcinomas, were estrogen receptor– and progesterone receptor–negative (7); in this latter series, androgen receptors were present in 94% of benign lesions and 72% of carcinomas with apocrine differentiation.

The distinction between atypical apocrine hyperplasia and apocrine intraductal carcinoma is sometimes difficult (Figs. 3,4). Carter and Rosen (8) described sclerosing breast lesions with atypical apocrine epithelium characterized by nuclear atypia, varying degrees of cytoplasmic clearing, and rare mitoses. *In situ* apocrine carcinoma is diagnosed only when neoplastic epithelial proliferation is sufficient to produce one of the characteristic growth patterns of intraductal carcinoma (Fig. 5).

The characterization of atypical apocrine lesions on the basis of size as well as cytologic and structural criteria has been suggested. For example, Tavassoli and Norris (9) considered apocrine ductal lesions that occupied an area of less than 2 mm to be atypical apocrine hyperplasia, regardless of cytologic and structural features. Larger histologically identical foci qualified as apocrine intraductal carcinoma. O'Malley et al. (10) used a combination of cytologic criteria and lesional diameter to define a "borderline" group of apocrine lesions. Foci with borderline cytologic features were considered to be apocrine intraductal carcinoma if larger than 8 mm. Borderline or atypical apocrine hyperplasias were proliferative foci smaller than 8 mm with nuclear atypia lacking the characteristic irregular nuclear membranes, coarse chromatin, and large, often multiple nucleoli of apocrine carcinoma.

The diagnosis of apocrine lesions on the basis of size is not readily applicable to needle core biopsies. The requisite measurements are imprecise and subject to many uncontrolled variables. A cluster of closely connected duct cross sections with little intervening stroma could occupy an area less than 2 mm, leading to a diagnosis of atypical apocrine hyperplasia on the basis of the 2-mm "rule," whereas the same group of duct sections separated by more stroma would encompass an area greater than 2 mm and qualify as intraductal carcinoma. Because these microscopic lesions are rarely appreciated grossly, there is no assurance that the tissue is oriented in a paraffin block so that the plane of section represents the maximum diameter. These issues are further compounded in a needle core biopsy specimen if the lesion is seen in more than one tissue core because the spatial relationship of the pieces is indeterminate. Consequently, these so-called criteria cannot be accepted as precise guidelines for the interpretation of surgical or needle core biopsy specimens.

Cytologic features of *in situ* and invasive apocrine carcinomas are manifested in the nuclei and cytoplasm. The nuclei are enlarged and pleomorphic when compared with the nuclei of benign apocrine cells. They usually contain large, prominent, and eosinophilic nucleoli, although they occasionally exhibit basophilia (Figs. 3,6). Nuclear membranes tend to be hyperchromatic and irregular. Some apocrine car-

Text continues on page 173

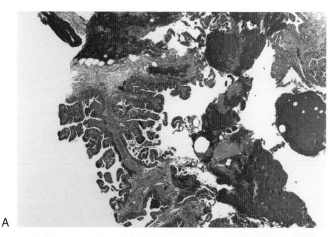

A

FIGURE 1. Apocrine metaplasia. Needle core biopsy specimens show two different lesions. **A,B:** Cystic papillary apocrine metaplasia is composed of cells with abundant eosinophilic cytoplasm and small, round nuclei with punctate nucleoli. The nuclei are regularly and evenly distributed with respect to the basement membrane. **C:** These small glands are lined by cuboidal and columnar cells with evenly spaced, basally oriented nuclei. The eosinophilia seen in (A) and (B) and the basophilia in (C) reflect different staining properties encountered in apocrine lesions.

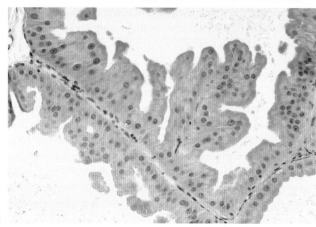

B

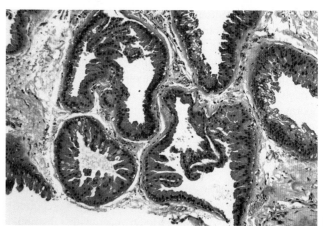

C

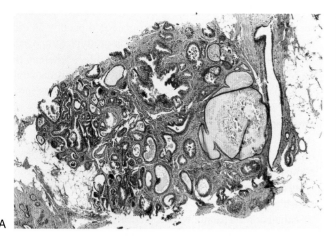

A

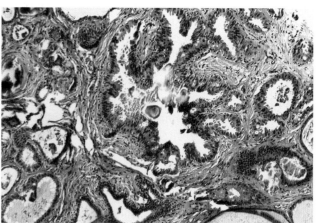

B

FIGURE 2. Apocrine metaplasia with atypia. A,B: This needle core biopsy sample was obtained from a nonpalpable focus of mammographically detected calcifications. Some of the columnar and cuboidal apocrine epithelial cells have pleomorphic and hyperchromatic nuclei.

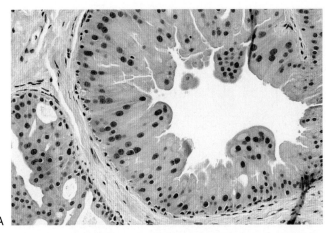

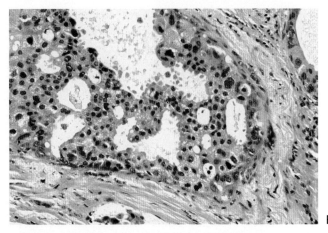

A
B

FIGURE 3. Apocrine metaplasia with atypia and apocrine intraductal carcinoma. A: Hyperplastic apocrine epithelium arranged in micropapillary fronds is composed of cells with abundant eosinophilic cytoplasm and unevenly distributed nuclei with punctate nucleoli. **B:** Apocrine intraductal carcinoma in the same needle core biopsy specimen is characterized by cells with less abundant, partially vacuolated cytoplasm and pleomorphic nuclei arranged in a cribriform pattern.

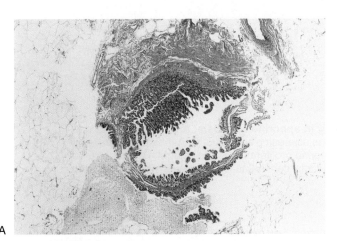

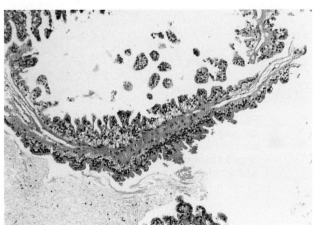

A
B

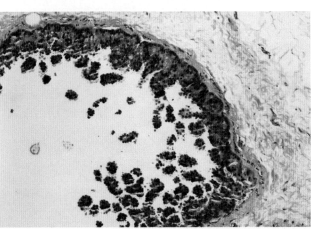

C

FIGURE 4. Cystic micropapillary apocrine metaplasia and cystic micropapillary apocrine intraductal carcinoma. A,B: A needle core biopsy specimen shows parts of the wall of a cystic apocrine lesion. A view of the epithelium in a perpendicular section is provided in (B). The hyperplastic cells have small, round, regularly spaced nuclei distributed almost entirely in a single line that follows the contour of the epithelium, especially on the lower surface. Cytoplasmic tufting is apparent at the apical cell borders, and there is subnuclear cytoplasmic clearing. **C:** Apocrine intraductal carcinoma with a micropapillary structure in a different needle core biopsy specimen is characterized by a disorderly distribution of atypical hyperchromatic nuclei and uneven cytoplasmic vacuolization.

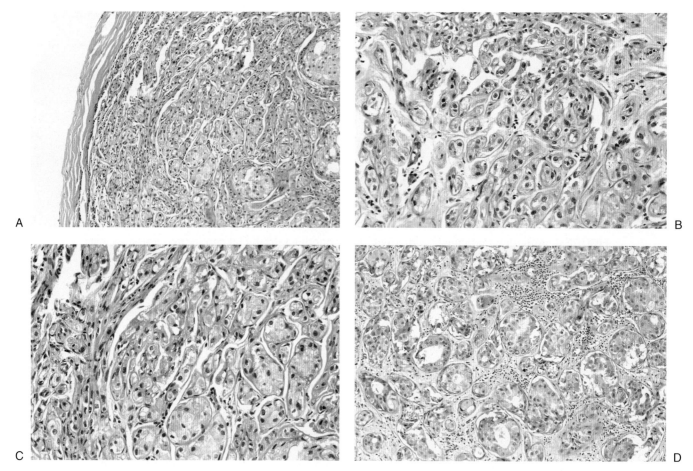

FIGURE 5. Apocrine intraductal carcinoma arising in apocrine adenosis. A,B: This part of a needle core biopsy specimen shows apocrine metaplasia in sclerosing adenosis. **C:** A transitional area with apocrine adenosis is on the left, and a more florid apocrine proliferation is on the right. **D:** Markedly enlarged adenosis glands are occupied by apocrine intraductal carcinoma. There is nuclear pleomorphism, and lymphocytes are present in the stroma.

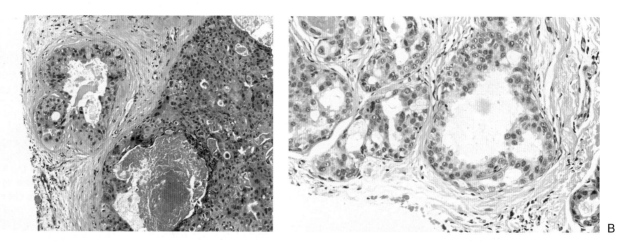

FIGURE 6. Apocrine intraductal carcinoma. Two different needle core biopsy specimens are shown. **A:** Solid intraductal carcinoma with necrosis. **B:** Cribriform intraductal carcinoma with extension into lobular glands on the left.

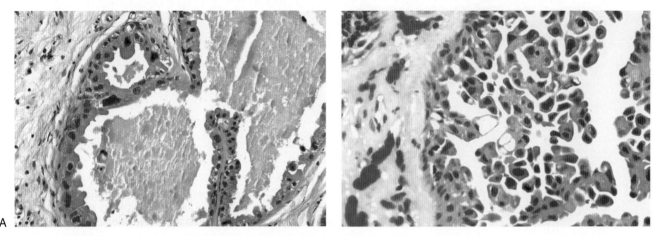

FIGURE 7. Apocrine intraductal carcinoma. A,B: Micropapillary and papillary foci of apocrine intraductal carcinoma with pleomorphic, deeply basophilic nuclei.

cinomas have pleomorphic, deeply basophilic nuclei in which little or no internal structure can be discerned, whereas in other instances, the chromatin is coarse (Fig. 7). Nucleoli are usually obscured when the chromatin is dense and hyperchromatic. The cytoplasm commonly exhibits eosinophilia that may be homogeneous or granular. Cytoplasmic vacuolization and clearing are features associated with atypical apocrine proliferations as well as apocrine carcinoma (Fig. 8).

The architecture of apocrine intraductal carcinoma exhibits the same structural patterns as non-apocrine intraductal carcinomas, including comedocarcinoma, micropapillary, solid, and cribriform configurations (11) (see Figs. 3–8). Calcifications are sometimes present in the affected ducts. Periductal fibrosis with inflammation is a common reactive change around the ducts, and "foamy" histiocytes with vacuolated cytoplasm in the reactive process can be mistaken for invasive carcinoma cells (12). Atypical apoc-

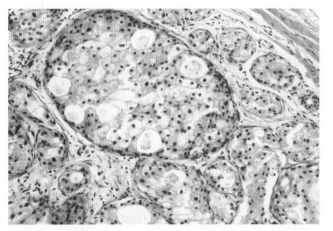

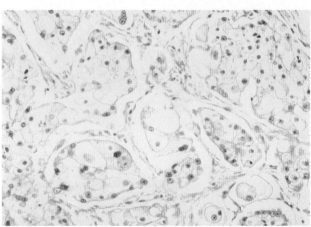

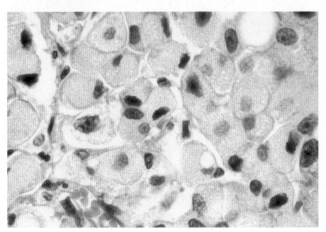

FIGURE 8. Apocrine intraductal carcinoma, clear-cell type. A: Cribriform intraductal carcinoma. **B:** An invasive apocrine carcinoma with marked cytoplasmic clearing. The tumor cells have prominent nucleoli. **C:** Intracytoplasmic mucin is a magenta spot in one cell (mucicarmine stain).

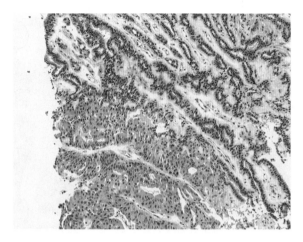

FIGURE 9. Apocrine metaplasia in a papilloma. Hyperplastic apocrine epithelium is present in part of this needle core biopsy specimen from a papillary lesion.

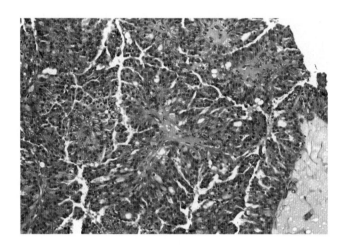

FIGURE 10. Papillary apocrine carcinoma. Apocrine carcinoma supported by fibrovascular stroma is present in this needle core biopsy sample of a solid papillary carcinoma.

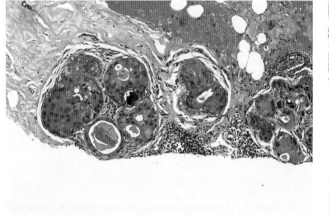

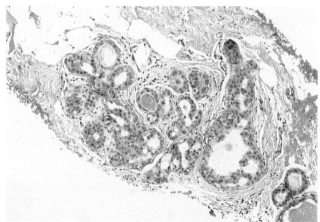

A

B

FIGURE 11. Apocrine intraductal carcinoma with lobular extension. Two different needle core biopsy specimens are shown. **A:** Microcalcification is present in a lobular gland. **B:** A low-magnification view of the lesion shown in Fig. 6B.

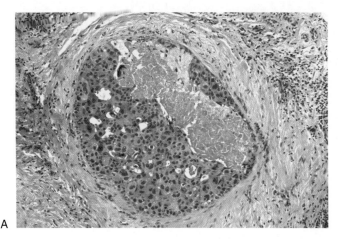
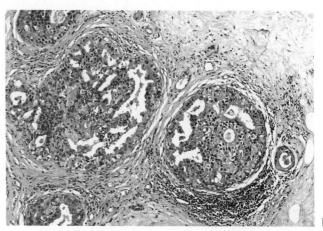

FIGURE 12. Apocrine intraductal carcinoma with stromal fibrosis and lymphocytic reaction. A: Solid intraductal carcinoma with necrosis. **B:** Cribriform intraductal carcinoma. Cytoplasmic vacuolization is apparent in some cells.

rine metaplasia may occupy part of a complex papillary lesion that has fully developed apocrine carcinoma in other areas (Fig. 9). The criteria for the diagnosis of carcinoma are the same as those outlined for the diagnosis of non-apocrine carcinoma in a papilloma. Pure cystic papillary apocrine carcinoma is infrequent (Fig. 10). Extension of carcinoma into the epithelium of lobules is more common in apocrine intra-

ductal carcinoma than in other types of intraductal carcinoma, with the possible exception of non-apocrine comedocarcinoma (Fig. 11). Fibrosis and chronic inflammation are often present around ducts in foci of apocrine intraductal carcinoma (Fig. 12).

Infiltrating apocrine carcinomas may assume any of the growth patterns of infiltrating duct carcinoma (Figs. 13,14),

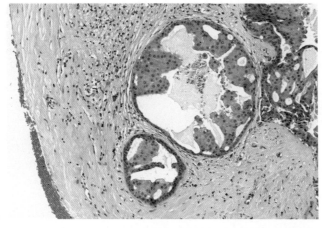
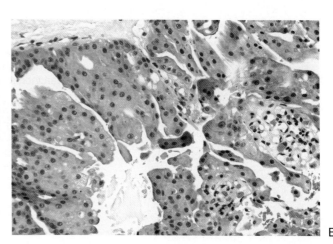
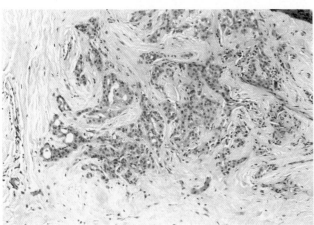

FIGURE 13. Apocrine carcinoma, intraductal and invasive. A: A needle core biopsy specimen shows micropapillary intraductal carcinoma. Note the disorderly distribution of nuclei, degenerated cells in the larger duct, and the periductal reaction consisting of lymphocytes and histiocytes. **B:** Magnified view of the microscopic field contiguous with the right border of (A). **C:** Moderately differentiated invasive apocrine carcinoma in the same needle core biopsy specimen.

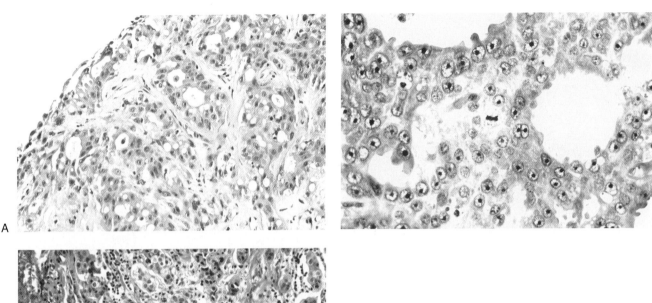

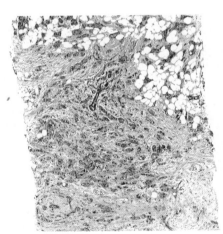

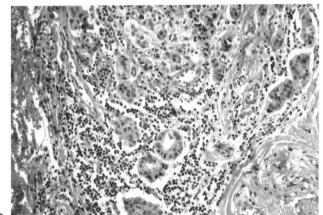

FIGURE 14. Apocrine carcinoma, invasive. Three different needle core biopsy specimens are shown. **A:** Invasive apocrine duct carcinoma with a cribriform pattern and intermediate nuclear grade. **B:** Invasive apocrine duct carcinoma with a cribriform pattern and poorly differentiated nuclear grade. **C:** Invasive apocrine duct carcinoma forming small glands. A stromal lymphocytic reaction is evident.

FIGURE 15. Apocrine carcinoma, invasive. A,B: The carcinoma in this needle core biopsy specimen is composed of cords and strands of cells without gland formation. The magnified view in (B) reveals the poorly differentiated nuclear grade. **C:** In another needle core biopsy specimen, the carcinoma cells are arrayed in clusters and have slightly basophilic cytoplasm.

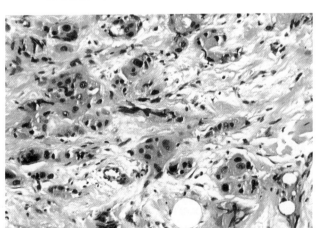

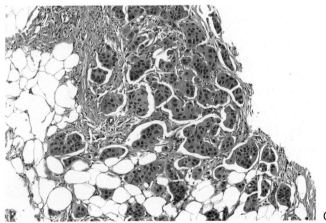

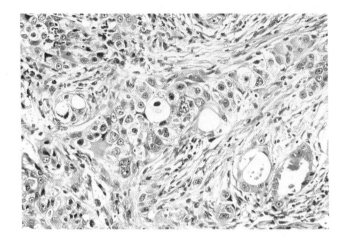

FIGURE 16. Apocrine carcinoma with histiocytoid features. The tumor cells have abundant vacuolated and granular cytoplasm with pleomorphic, poorly differentiated nuclei. Traces of gland formation are evident.

but they are often structurally poorly differentiated (Fig. 15). An uncommon variant of infiltrating apocrine carcinoma is composed of large polygonal cells with abundant foamy or granular cytoplasm (Fig. 16). Loss of cohesion is a characteristic feature of these carcinomas when a diffuse growth pattern is present. This type of apocrine carcinoma has been referred to as myoblastomatoid or histiocytoid (13). The expression of gross cystic disease fluid protein (GCDFP) has been demonstrated in these lesions by immunohistochemistry and by *in situ* hybridization (13). Follow-up information is insufficient to define the prognosis of this type of apocrine carcinoma.

Invasive apocrine carcinomas are prone to the development of lymphatic tumor emboli (14). This may be manifested by clinical presentation as inflammatory carcinoma and in some cases predisposes to locally recurrent carcinoma with an inflammatory pattern. D'Amore et al. (14) found dermal invasion in 7 of 34 (21%) of their cases, and 4 cases (12%) had associated lymphatic invasion within the breast.

Most apocrine carcinomas are negative for mucin, or only

a few cells contain mucicarmine-positive secretion (see Fig. 8) (15). In exceptional cases, extensive intracytoplasmic mucin accumulation can result in numerous, sometimes substantially enlarged cells of the signet-ring type (Fig. 17). Benign and malignant apocrine cells are strongly immunoreactive for GCDFP-15. Staining for GCDFP-15 also occurs in nearly 25% of carcinomas that lack apocrine features (2,3).

Patients with intraductal apocrine carcinoma have generally had the same clinical course as women with non-apocrine intraductal carcinoma. Comparison of patients with invasive apocrine and non-apocrine carcinomas has revealed no statistically significant differences in recurrence-free and overall survival between the two groups (11,14). The prognosis of apocrine carcinoma, whether intraductal or invasive, is determined mainly by conventional prognostic factors, such as grade, tumor size, and nodal status (9,11,14). Apocrine differentiation should be mentioned as a descriptive feature, but presently it does not seem to be an important determinant of prognosis or treatment (16).

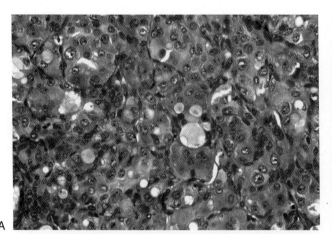
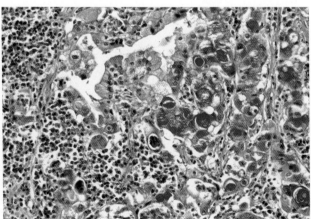

A   B

FIGURE 17. Apocrine carcinoma with signet-ring cells. A: Many of the cells in this apocrine carcinoma have discrete intracytoplasmic vacuoles that contain secretion. **B:** The secretion appears red with the mucicarmine stain.

REFERENCES

1. Yates AJ, Ahmed A. Apocrine carcinoma and apocrine metaplasia. *Histopathology* 1988;13:228–231.
2. Mossler J, Barton TK, Brinkhous AD, McCarty KS, Moylan JA, McCarty KS Jr. Apocrine differentiation in human mammary carcinoma. *Cancer* 1980;46:2463–2471.
3. Eusebi V, Betts C, Haagensen DE, Gugliotta P, Bussolati G, Azzopardi JG. Apocrine differentiation in lobular carcinoma of the breast: a morphologic, immunologic and ultrastructural study. *Hum Pathol* 1984;15:134–140.
4. Gilles R, Lasnik A, Guinebretière J-M, et al. Apocrine carcinoma: clinical and mammographic features. *Radiology* 1994;190:495–497.
5. Kopans DB, Nguyen PL, Koerner FC, et al. Mixed form, diffusely scattered calcifications in breast cancer with apocrine features. *Radiology* 1990;177:807–811.
6. Bryant J. Male breast cancer: a case of apocrine carcinoma with psammoma bodies. *Hum Pathol* 1981;12:751–753.
7. Tavassoli FA, Purcell CA, Bratthauer GL, Man Y-G. Androgen receptor expression along with loss of bcl-2, ER, and PR expression in benign and malignant apocrine lesions of the breast: implications for therapy. *Breast J* 1996;2:261–269.
8. Carter D, Rosen PP. Atypical apocrine metaplasia in sclerosing lesions of the beast: a study of 51 patients. *Mod Pathol* 1991;4:1–5.
9. Tavassoli FA, Norris HJ. Intraductal apocrine carcinoma: a clinicopathologic study of 37 cases. *Mod Pathol* 1994;7:813–818.
10. O'Malley FP, Page DL, Nelson EH, Dupont WD. Ductal carcinoma *in situ* of the breast with apocrine cytology: definition of a borderline category. *Hum Pathol* 1994;25:164–168.
11. Abati AD, Kimmel M, Rosen PP. Apocrine mammary carcinoma: a clinicopathologic study of 72 patients. *Am J Clin Pathol* 1990;94:371–377.
12. Shousha S, Bull TB, Southall PJ, Mazoujian G. Apocrine carcinoma of the breast containing foam cells. An electron microscopic and immunohistochemical study. *Histopathology* 1987;11:611–620.
13. Eusebi V, Foschini MP, Bussolati G, Rosen PP. Myoblastomatoid (histiocytoid) carcinoma of the breast. A type of apocrine carcinoma. *Am J Surg Pathol* 1995;19:553–562.
14. d'Amore ESG, Terrier-Lacombe MJ, Travagli JP, Friedman S, Contesso G. Invasive apocrine carcinoma of the breast: a long-term follow-up study of 34 cases. *Breast Cancer Res Treat* 1988;12:37–44.
15. Bussolati G, Cattani MG, Gugliotta P, Patriarca E, Eusebi V. Morphologic and functional aspects of apocrine metaplasia in dysplastic and neoplastic breast tissue. *Ann N Y Acad Sci* 1986;464:262–274.
16. Bundred NJ, Walker RA, Everington D, White GK, Stewart HJ, Miller WR. Is apocrine differentiation in breast carcinoma of prognostic significance? *Br J Cancer* 1990;62:113–117.

CHAPTER 17

Adenoid Cystic Carcinoma

Fewer than 0.1% of mammary carcinomas have an adenoid cystic growth pattern. The term cylindroma, previously used interchangeably with adenoid cystic carcinoma, refers to the histologic appearance, which suggests entwined cylinders of stroma and epithelial cells. Adenoid cystic carcinoma occurs in adult women throughout the age distribution of mammary carcinoma, with patients between 25 and 80 years of age and a reported mean age that varies from 50 to 63 years. Isolated cases have been encountered in men and children (1,2). Adenoid cystic carcinoma shows no tendency to develop bilaterally, but other types of carcinoma may develop in the contralateral breast (3,4), or in rare instances, another carcinoma may be found elsewhere in the same breast (5).

Adenoid cystic carcinoma usually presents as a discrete, firm mass. Calcifications occur in these tumors, but few have been detected by mammography, and in some instances, the mammogram result was reportedly negative (4). The typical mammographic image is that of a lobulated mass (6). Pain or tenderness has been described in a minority of cases. The median duration of a symptomatic mass in one series was 24 months (4). Most adenoid cystic carcinomas have been described as hormone receptor-negative by biochemical and immunohistochemical analysis, with occasional tumors positive for estrogen and/or progesterone receptors at relatively low levels (7–9).

Gross size of the lesions varies from 2 mm to 12 cm, with the majority between 1 and 3 cm. Low-grade tumors tend to be smaller (mean, 1.6 cm) than high-grade tumors (mean, 3.5 cm). Many adenoid cystic carcinomas are circumscribed or nodular grossly, but about 50% of adenoid cystic carcinomas have an invasive growth pattern microscopically (Fig. 1). Microcystic areas formed by the coalescent spaces in dilated glands are seen in about 25% of tumors.

Adenoid cystic carcinoma consists of a mixture of proliferating glands (adenoid component) and stromal or basement membrane elements ("pseudoglandular" or cylindromatous component). These elements are usually not distributed homogeneously in a given tumor (Fig. 2). Some regions may consist only of the adenoid elements, resembling cribriform carcinoma (10). Abundant stromal material in other parts of the tumor can produce a pattern that is easily mistaken for scirrhous carcinoma. Because of this intra-

tumoral heterogeneity, adenoid cystic carcinoma may be difficult to recognize in a needle core biopsy specimen if a characteristic sample has not been obtained (Fig. 3). Inspissated secretion and stromal fragments from benign lesions or other forms of carcinoma may be mistaken for cylindromatous material in needle core biopsy samples.

The microscopic growth patterns of mammary adenoid cystic carcinoma have been described as cribriform, solid, glandular (tubular), reticular (trabecular), and basaloid. Focal sebaceous or adenosquamous differentiation is variably present (4). Adenomyoepitheliomatous and syringomatous areas are further evidence of structural diversity. Perineural invasion is found in a minority of tumors, and lymphatic tumor emboli are extremely uncommon. Shrinkage artifacts, a relatively frequent occurrence in histologic sections of adenoid cystic carcinoma, may be mistaken for lymphatic tumor emboli.

Ro et al. (11) proposed stratifying adenoid cystic carcinomas into three grades on the basis of the proportion of solid growth within the lesion (1, no solid elements; 2, less than 30% solid; 3, more than 30% solid). High-grade lesions are composed of poorly differentiated cells that have relatively large, hyperchromatic nuclei and sparse cytoplasm (Fig. 4). Intraductal carcinoma is sometimes a prominent feature of high-grade tumors with extensive intralobular and intraductal growth, whereas low-grade adenoid cystic carcinoma rarely has a distinct *in situ* component. Areas of cribriform and nearly confluent solid growth as well as typical adenoid cystic components may be present in a high-grade tumor. Prominent basaloid features are seen in some instances. Tumors with a solid component (grades 2 and 3) tend to be larger than those without a solid element (grade 1), and tumors with a solid element are more likely to recur (11). The Ki67 labeling index when the Mib1 antibody is used is greater in high-grade than in low-grade tumors, but proliferative activity has not proved to be prognostically significant (12).

Some conventional forms of mammary carcinoma may be incorrectly diagnosed as adenoid cystic carcinoma (10,13). When reexamined, about half of the cases recorded by the Connecticut Tumor Registry as adenoid cystic carcinoma were duct carcinomas with a prominent cribriform compo-

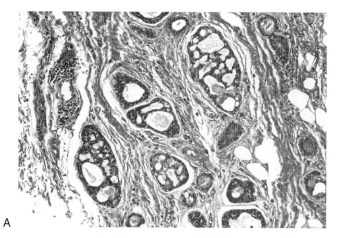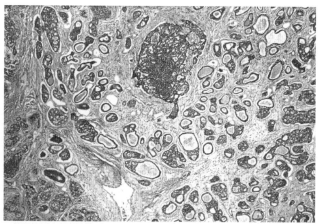

A   B

FIGURE 1. Adenoid cystic carcinoma. A: A needle core biopsy specimen shows nests of invasive carcinoma consisting of glands and cylindromatous elements. **B:** The surgically excised tumor has a more heterogeneous growth pattern than the sample obtained by needle biopsy.

nent (13). Problems have occurred in distinguishing adenoid cystic from papillary and mucinous carcinomas. Because cribriform areas may be found in an adenoid cystic carcinoma, their presence does not exclude this diagnosis, and this heterogeneity can complicate the interpretation of needle core biopsy specimens (see Fig. 3). Collagenous spherulosis must be considered in the differential diagnosis of adenoid cystic carcinoma (14). This stromal alteration, usually found in benign papillary duct hyperplasia, consists of nodular deposits of basement membrane components with myoepithelial cells between the glandular elements, a combination that mimics adenoid cystic carcinoma (Chapter 4).

Mucicarmine or alcian blue stains identify the secretion within glands, whereas laminin and fibronectin, noncollage-

nous glycoproteins associated with basal lamina, and type IV collagen can be demonstrated by immunohistochemistry in the cylindromatous elements (7). The carcinomatous glands are invested by a ring of reticulin-positive fibers.

Data on the prognosis of adenoid cystic carcinoma are based almost entirely on patients usually treated by mastectomy (1–4,11,13,15). Mastectomy has been curative in virtually all cases. There have been a few isolated instances of systemic metastases after mastectomy (3,16–18). Most patients with metastases have had pulmonary involvement; recurrences in the lung were detected as late as 6 to 12 years after initial treatment in patients who had had negative axillary lymph nodes (17,18). Axillary nodal metastases were present at mastectomy in two other cases (11,19).

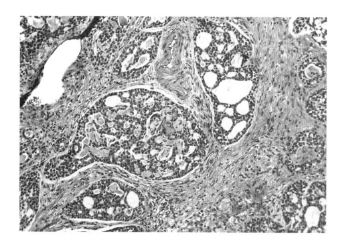

FIGURE 2. Adenoid cystic carcinoma. Some areas have prominent cylindromatous elements, whereas cribriform growth is accented in other foci.

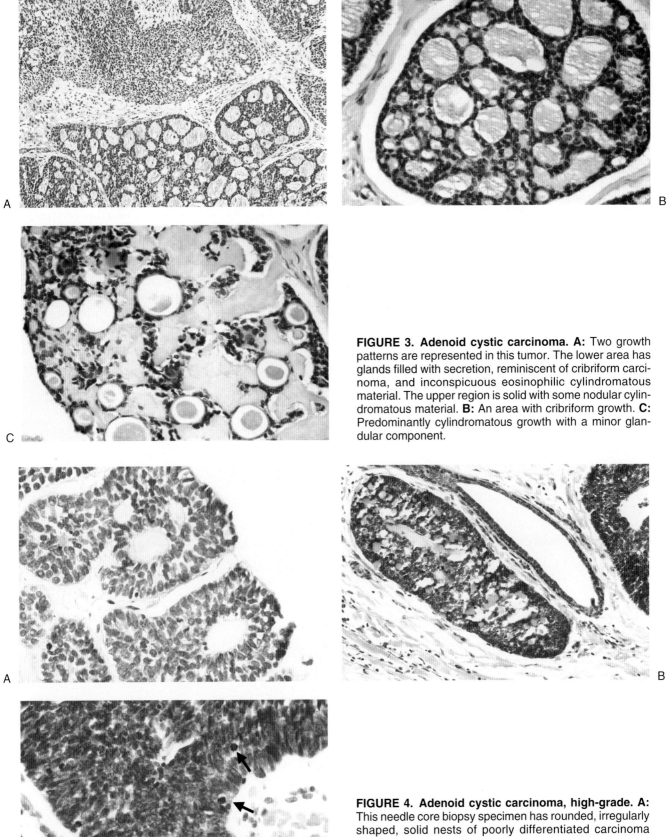

FIGURE 3. Adenoid cystic carcinoma. A: Two growth patterns are represented in this tumor. The lower area has glands filled with secretion, reminiscent of cribriform carcinoma, and inconspicuous eosinophilic cylindromatous material. The upper region is solid with some nodular cylindromatous material. **B:** An area with cribriform growth. **C:** Predominantly cylindromatous growth with a minor glandular component.

FIGURE 4. Adenoid cystic carcinoma, high-grade. A: This needle core biopsy specimen has rounded, irregularly shaped, solid nests of poorly differentiated carcinoma cells. Nodular cylindromatous material is evident in some tumor masses. Peripheral palisading of cells with a basaloid appearance is evident. **B,C:** Another needle core biopsy specimen shows more pronounced basophilia in the carcinoma cells. Carcinoma surrounds a normal duct in (B). Mitoses are shown in (C) (*arrows*).

REFERENCES

1. Hjorth S, Magnusson PH, Blomquite P. Adenoid cystic carcinoma of the breast. *Acta Chir Scand* 1977;143:155–158.
2. Quizilbash AH, Patterson MC, Oliveira KF. Adenoid cystic carcinoma of the breast. *Arch Pathol Lab Med* 1977;101:302–306.
3. Peters GN, Wolff M. Adenoid cystic carcinoma of the breast; report of 11 new cases. *Cancer* 1982;52:680–686.
4. Rosen PP. Adenoid cystic carcinoma of the breast. A morphologically heterogeneous neoplasm. *Pathol Annu* 1989;24(Pt 2):237–254.
5. Koss LG, Brannan CD, Ashikari R. Histologic and ultrastructural features of adenoid cystic carcinoma of the breast. *Cancer* 1970;26:1271–1279.
6. Bourke AG, Metcalf C, Wylie EJ. Mammographic features of adenoid cystic carcinoma. *Australas Radiol* 1994;38:324–325.
7. Düe W, Herbst H, Loy V, Stein H. Characterization of adenoid cystic carcinoma of the breast by immunohistology. *J Clin Pathol* 1989;42:470–476.
8. Lamovec J, Us-krasovec M, Zidar A, Kjun A. Adenoid cystic carcinomas of the breast: a histologic, cytologic and immunohistochemical study. *Semin Diagn Pathol* 1989;6:153–164.
9. Pastolero G, Hanna W, Zbieranowski I, Kahn HJ. Proliferative activity and p53 expression in adenoid cystic carcinoma of the breast. *Mod Pathol* 1996;9:215–219.
10. Harris, M. Pseudoadenoid cystic carcinoma of the breast. *Arch Pathol Lab Med* 1977;101:307–309.
11. Ro JY, Silva EG, Gallager HS. Adenoid cystic carcinoma of the breast. *Hum Pathol* 1987;18:1276–1281.
12. Kloer CG, Oberman HA. Adenoid cystic carcinoma of the breast: value of histologic grading and proliferative activity. *Mod Pathol* 1997;10:21A.
13. Sumpio BE, Jennings TA, Merino MJ, Sullivan PD. Adenoid cystic carcinoma of the breast. Data from the Connecticut Tumor Registry and a review of the literature. *Ann Surg* 1987;205:295–301.
14. Clement PB, Young RH, Azzopardi JG. Collagenous spherulosis of the breast. *Am J Surg Pathol* 1987;11:411–417.
15. Zaloudek C, Oertel YC, Orenstein JM. Adenoid cystic carcinoma of the breast. *Am J Clin Pathol* 1984;81:297–307.
16. Nayer HR. Cylindroma of the breast with pulmonary metastases. *Dis Chest* 1957;31:324–327.
17. Herzberg AJ, Bossen EH, Walter PJ. Adenoid cystic carcinoma of the breast metastatic to the kidney. A clinically symptomatic lesion requiring surgical management. *Cancer* 1991;68:1015–1020.
18. Lim SK, Kovi J, Warner OG. Adenoid cystic carcinoma of breast with metastasis: a case report and review of the literature. *J Natl Med Assoc* 1979;71:329–330.
19. Wells CA, Nicoll S, Ferguson DJP. Adenoid cystic carcinoma of the breast: a case with axillary lymph node metastasis. *Histopathology* 1986;10:415–424.

CHAPTER 18

Secretory Carcinoma

Secretory carcinoma was first described in children (1), but the majority of cases have been reported in adults (2). More than 40 adult cases have been described. There have been reports of secretory carcinoma in children before age 5 (3) and in a 6-year-old boy (4). There is a dearth of cases of secretory carcinoma in girls 10 to 15 years of age, and with the rare exceptions of two men, male patients have been younger than 10 years (5). The name secretory is preferable to juvenile, a term used in early descriptions of the tumor. The microscopic appearance of the lesion is the same regardless of patient age.

In most cases, the patient has a painless, circumscribed mass that may have been present for years before biopsy (2,3). Coexistence of juvenile papillomatosis and secretory carcinoma has been reported (6). The majority of tumors examined by biochemistry or immunohistochemistry have been negative for estrogen receptors, with only a few lesions positive for estrogen and progesterone receptors (2).

Secretory carcinoma is usually a circumscribed, firm mass; it may be lobulated, but rarely, the tumor has infiltrative margins. The tumors tend to be 3 cm or less in diameter, with larger lesions up to 12 cm found mainly in adults.

Secretory carcinoma has an intraductal component that exhibits the growth patterns associated with more conventional types of duct carcinoma. Most commonly, the intraductal carcinoma is papillary or cribriform, but solid foci and, rarely, comedo necrosis may be found (2,7). The invasive areas are relatively compact, with papillary, microcystic, and cribriform patterns. Microcalcifications are rarely seen in the neoplastic glands or in the stroma.

The tumor consists of cells with abundant, pale-to-clear, pink or amphophilic cytoplasm and small, round, cytologically low-grade nuclei (Fig. 1). Signet-ring cell forms may be present. Rarely, portions of the lesion may have more granular or eosinophilic cytoplasm and the nuclear cytology of apocrine differentiation (Fig. 2). The glands and microcystic spaces contain abundant, pale pink or amphophilic secretion that is often vacuolated or "bubbly." Strong staining of cells but not the secretion has been reported for alpha-lactalbumin as well as for S-100 protein and carcinoembryonic antigen (polyclonal) (4,5). No reactivity was observed for gross cystic disease fluid protein or for monoclonal carcinoembryonic antigen (4).

Surgical biopsy is usually necessary for the diagnosis of secretory carcinoma, although the lesion may be suspected in a needle core biopsy specimen. Local excision is the preferred initial treatment in children. Consideration should be

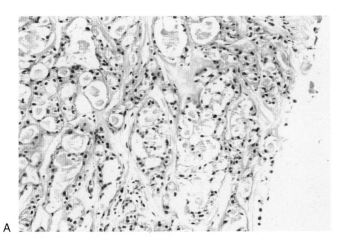
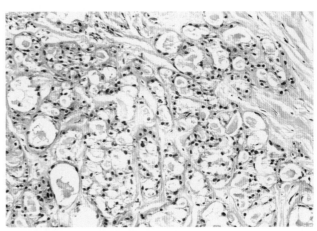

A   B

FIGURE 1. Secretory carcinoma. A needle core biopsy specimen from a circumscribed 2-cm tumor in a 68-year-old woman. **A,B:** The carcinoma has a characteristic microcystic architecture. In this example, the tumor cells have small, low-grade nuclei.

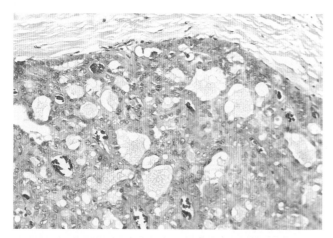

FIGURE 2. Secretory carcinoma with apocrine cytology. The lesion has a well-circumscribed border and microcystic growth pattern. The nuclei in the tumor cells have prominent nucleoli typically associated with apocrine differentiation.

given to preserving the breast bud in prepubertal patients, but this cannot always be accomplished, and breast development may be impaired or abolished.

In the majority of patients, secretory carcinoma has a low-grade clinical course with a very favorable prognosis. Most children and adults have been treated by mastectomy. Data on treatment by breast conservation therapy are lacking. Axillary metastases have been described, and they rarely involve more than three lymph nodes. The risk for nodal involvement is at least as great in children as in adults (2).

REFERENCES

1. McDivitt RW, Stewart FW. Breast carcinoma in children. *JAMA* 1966; 195:388–390.
2. Rosen PP, Cranor ML. Secretory carcinoma of the breast. *Arch Pathol Lab Med* 1991;115:141–144.
3. Romdhane KB, Ayed B, Labbane N, et al. Carcinome sécrétant juvénile du sein. A propos d'une observation chez une fille de 4 ans. *Ann Pathol* 1987;3:227–230.
4. Hartman AW, Magrish P. Carcinoma of breast in children. Case report: six-year-old boy with adenocarcinoma. *Ann Surg* 1955;141:792–797.
5. Lamovec J, Bracko M. Secretory carcinoma of the breast: light microscopical, immunohistochemical and flow cytometric study. *Mod Pathol* 1994;7:475–479.
6. Rosen PP, Holmes G, Lesser ML, Kinne DW, Beattie EJ. Juvenile papillomatosis and breast carcinoma. *Cancer* 1985;55:1345–1352.
7. Oberman HA, Stephens PJ. Carcinoma of the breast in childhood. *Cancer* 1972;30:420–474.

CHAPTER 19

Cystic Hypersecretory Carcinoma

This variant of duct carcinoma was first described in 1984 (1). The majority of cases have been intraductal carcinomas. A benign proliferative lesion that resembles cystic hypersecretory carcinoma has been termed cystic hypersecretory hyperplasia (2). The age distribution of cystic hypersecretory carcinoma ranges from 34 to 79 years, with a mean of 56 years (2). The presenting symptom is usually a palpable mass. Mammography in one case revealed a prominent ductal pattern and an irregular density in the breast (3). Among 10 tumors studied biochemically, 8 were negative for estrogen and progesterone receptors. Two specimens were positive for both receptors.

The distinctive feature of cystic hypersecretory carcinoma is the presence of numerous cysts measuring up to 1.5 cm. Secretion within cysts has been described as sticky, mucinous, gelatinous, or resembling thyroid colloid. It is usually not possible to distinguish grossly between cystic hypersecretory intraductal carcinoma and cystic hypersecretory hyperplasia. An invasive component associated with cystic hypersecretory carcinoma produces a distinct, solid mass.

The microscopic hallmark of a cystic hypersecretory lesion is the presence of cysts containing eosinophilic secretion that resembles thyroid colloid (Fig. 1). The homogeneous and virtually acellular secretion often retracts from the surrounding epithelium, resulting in a smooth or scalloped margin that duplicates the contour of the epithelial proliferation. Folds, linear cracks, or small, "punched-out" holes are features of the secretion. There are no appreciable differences in the character of the secretion between cystic hypersecretory carcinoma and cystic hypersecretory hyperplasia. Positive reactions for carcinoembryonic antigen, alpha-lactalbumin, period acid–Schiff, and mucin have been observed in the cyst contents, which are consistently negative for thyroglobulin. Disruption results in spillage of cyst contents into the stroma, eliciting an intense inflammatory reaction that consists of lymphocytes and histiocytes.

The cysts in benign cystic hypersecretory lesions are lined by inconspicuous flat cells or a single layer of cuboidal-to-columnar cells (see Fig. 1) (2). The cells in such lesions have uniform, cytologically bland nuclei and scant cytoplasm. Atypical features in this setting are epithelial crowding sometimes resulting in micropapillary hyperplasia, hyper-

chromasia, and enlargement of nuclei, which may contain nucleoli (Fig. 2). Lesions that lack fully developed intraductal carcinoma are diagnosed as *cystic hypersecretory hyperplasia* or *cystic hypersecretory hyperplasia with atypia*.

Lobules in and around the lesional areas in women with benign and carcinomatous cystic hypersecretory lesions often exhibit hypersecretory changes that include the accumulation of secretion in lobular gland lumina (Fig. 3). This lobular abnormality may occur as an isolated finding in the absence of a fully developed cystic hypersecretory lesion, an observation suggesting that the process may originate in such foci. The finding of cystic hypersecretory change in lobules in a needle core biopsy sample should prompt consideration of excisional biopsy.

In cystic hypersecretory carcinoma, the epithelium of some cysts and ducts grows as micropapillary intraductal carcinoma (Fig. 4). The spectrum of epithelial patterns ranges from short, knobby epithelial tufts to complex branching fronds that may extend across the duct lumen. The so-called Roman arch, or bridging pattern, commonly seen in other forms of micropapillary carcinoma, is uncommon in these lesions. Fibrovascular stroma is rarely found within the micropapillary fronds. Cytologically, the cells of the micropapillary carcinoma have crowded and overlapping hyperchromatic nuclei with sparse cytoplasm. There is no secretion within the cytoplasm, but frayed, apical cell borders and cytoplasmic blebs are consistent with some degree of secretory activity. There are usually foci of cystic hypersecretory hyperplasia scattered in an area of cystic hypersecretory carcinoma. A few examples of intraductal cystic hypersecretory carcinoma have been encountered that were characterized by pronounced vacuolization of the cytoplasm of the carcinoma cells and secretion, a pattern reminiscent of pseudolactational hyperplasia (Chapter 1). Cystic hypersecretory cysts are rarely a feature of pseudolactational hyperplasia.

Invasive cystic hypersecretory carcinoma consists of cystic hypersecretory intraductal carcinoma accompanied by an invasive component. Most invasive carcinomas encountered in this setting have been poorly differentiated duct carcinomas with a solid growth pattern. Nuclei in the invasive carcinoma cells usually have an "open" appearance, similar to those of cells found in papillary thyroid carcinoma.

Text continues on page 188

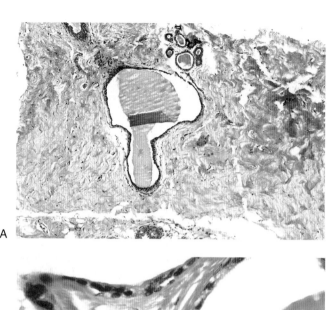

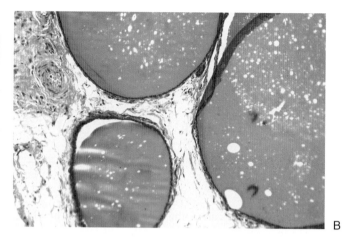

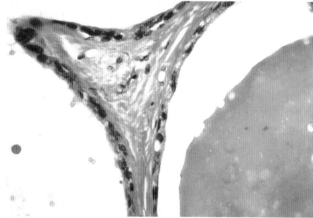

FIGURE 1. Cystic hypersecretory hyperplasia. A,B: The cystically dilated ducts in two different needle core biopsy specimens contain dense eosinophilic secretion that retracts from the inconspicuous epithelium. The secretion has developed parallel cracks and small punctate holes. **C:** The cystic spaces are lined by flat and cuboidal cells distributed in a single layer.

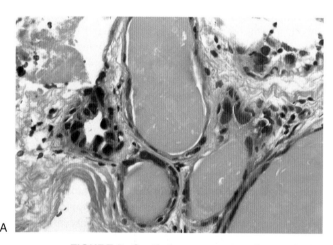

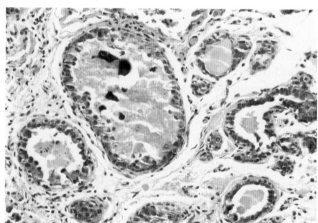

FIGURE 2. Cystic hypersecretory hyperplasia with atypia. A: The cells in this cystic hypersecretory lesion have hyperchromatic and pleomorphic nuclei. **B:** Cells with hyperchromatic, enlarged nuclei form blunt mounds in this atypical cystic hypersecretory lesion. Calcification, shown in one cyst, is not often present in this condition.

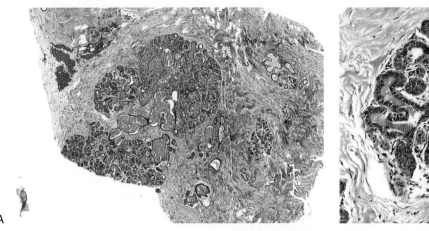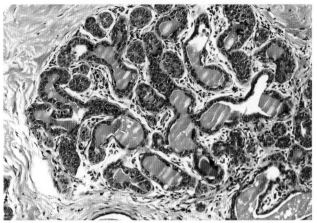

FIGURE 3. Cystic hypersecretory hyperplasia in lobules. A,B: Characteristic eosinophilic secretion is present in the terminal ducts and lobular glands of this needle core biopsy specimen.

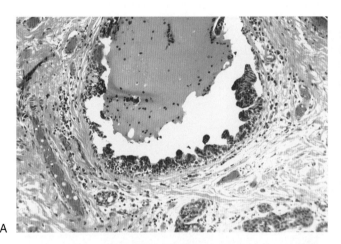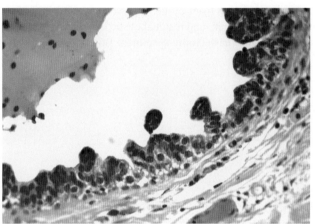

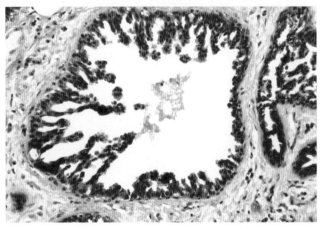

FIGURE 4. Cystic hypersecretory intraductal carcinoma. A,B: Low micropapillary fronds are present at the border of this cystically dilated duct. The retracted eosinophilic secretion has a scalloped border. **C:** Micropapillary intraductal carcinoma with diverse structural patterns ranging from flat growth to elongated micropapillary fronds. The almost complete absence of secretion, as seen here, can be encountered in foci with florid cystic hypersecretory intraductal carcinoma.

Excisional biopsy is required if cystic hypersecretory hyperplasia is present in a needle core biopsy specimen because it is not possible to exclude focal carcinoma on this basis. Some lesions have been misclassified as "cystic disease," with the true nature of the process becoming apparent after a recurrence (1,3).

The finding of areas with the typical features of cystic hypersecretory hyperplasia, sometimes with atypia, associated with cystic hypersecretory carcinoma suggests that these processes are related, but convincing evidence of progression through these stages has not yet been observed. Review of prior biopsy findings from women later found to have cystic hypersecretory carcinoma has disclosed various lesions, including seemingly unrelated common proliferative changes, cystic hypersecretory hyperplasia, and cystic hypersecretory carcinoma. Follow-up of eight patients with cystic hypersecretory hyperplasia revealed subsequent breast carcinoma in two cases. In one woman, a fatal contralateral invasive duct carcinoma developed that lacked cystic hypersecretory features. The other patient had intraductal carcinoma separate from cystic hypersecretory hyperplasia in a biopsy specimen, and residual cystic hypersecretory hyperplasia in the mastectomy specimen. Bogomoletz (4) described a 55-year-old woman who was well without recurrence 6 years after excisional biopsy of a 7-cm example of cystic hypersecretory hyperplasia.

The clinical course of cystic hypersecretory intraductal carcinoma does not differ from that of other forms of intraductal carcinoma. There have been no recurrences in women treated by mastectomy after a mean follow-up of 8 years, extending in one case to 23 years. All had negative lymph nodes. Two of four women with invasive cystic hypersecretory carcinoma had metastases in axillary lymph nodes, and a third patient presented with locally advanced or inflammatory carcinoma. Thus far, the one reported death from cystic hypersecretory carcinoma occurred in this latter patient.

REFERENCES

1. Rosen PP, Scott M. Cystic hypersecretory duct carcinoma of the breast. *Am J Surg Pathol* 1984;8:31–41.
2. Guerry P, Erlandson RA, Rosen PP. Cystic hypersecretory hyperplasia and cystic hypersecretory duct carcinoma of the breast. Pathology, therapy and follow-up of 39 patients. *Cancer* 1988;61:1611–1620.
3. Colandrea JM, Shmookler BM, O'Dowd GJ, Cohen MH. Cystic hypersecretory duct carcinoma of the breast. Report of a case with fine needle aspiration. *Arch Pathol Lab Med* 1988;112:560–563.
4. Bogomoletz W-V. Hyperplasie hypersécrétoire cystique du sein. Un diagnostic rare en pathologie mammaire. *Ann Pathol* 1994;14:131–132.

CHAPTER 20

Other Special Types of Invasive Duct Carcinoma

MAMMARY CARCINOMA WITH OSTEOCLAST-LIKE GIANT CELLS

Fewer than 100 examples of this type of breast carcinoma have been reported since the first series was published in 1979 (1). The clinical features are similar to those of breast carcinoma generally. Patients ranged in age from 28 to 88 years, with an average age at diagnosis in three reviews of 53 years (1–3). Mammographically, the well-circumscribed margin of most tumors suggests a benign lesion, such as a cyst or fibroadenoma (2). The gross appearance is quite striking owing to the dark brown or red-brown color of the bisected tumor. Reported diameters range from 0.5 to 10 cm, with most measuring 3 cm or less.

Most of these lesions are moderately or poorly differentiated invasive duct carcinomas (Fig. 1). A cribriform growth pattern is present relatively more often than among duct carcinomas generally. Osteoclast-like giant cells have been encountered in well-differentiated or tubular, infiltrating lobular, squamous, papillary, apocrine, mucinous, and metaplastic carcinomas (1–3) (Fig. 2). Rarely, the carcinoma has a glandular pattern, reminiscent of the infiltrating colonic carcinoma. The giant cells are located close to the edges of carcinomatous glands, as well as in stroma between glands, and they may be found in the glandular lumina. Extravasated erythrocytes and hemosiderin are invariably present in the intervening, highly vascular stroma. Erythrophagocytosis by the giant cells is uncommon, and they contain scant hemosiderin that is detectable by light microscopy. Fibroblastic reaction, collagenization, and lymphocytic infiltration are variably present. Mammary carcinoma with osteoclast-like giant cells may be a variant of metaplastic carcinomas that have giant cells in areas of osseous and cartilaginous differentiation (4).

The giant cells are stained by a variety of antibodies that react with macrophages and osteoclasts, exhibiting strong reactivity with acid phosphatase (5,6), alpha$_1$-antitrypsin, KP-1 (CD68), and lysozyme (7,8). The tumors have had low levels of estrogen receptor, but many had remarkably high levels of progesterone receptors (2).

Axillary lymph node metastases have been reported in approximately a third of cases. Osteoclast-like giant cells are found in some but not all metastases in axillary lymph nodes or other sites and within intralymphatic tumor emboli (1,2).

Nearly two thirds of patients have been reported to be alive and well with follow-up rarely reaching beyond 5 years (1,2,8).

CRIBRIFORM CARCINOMA

Invasive carcinomas with a cribriform pattern are termed classic cribriform carcinomas. Some of these tumors have cribriform and tubular components. The diagnosis of mixed invasive cribriform carcinoma has been reserved for tumors in which less than 50% of the lesion has a cribriform pattern and the remainder of the tumor is composed of nontubular, less well-differentiated areas. Fewer than 6% of invasive mammary carcinomas have a cribriform component, with nearly equal proportions of pure and mixed lesions (9,10).

A mammographic study of eight cases revealed spiculated masses measuring 20 to 35 mm in four of the patients (11). Two of these lesions contained a few punctate calcifications. Four other tumors were not visualized radiographically. Venable et al. (12) reported that 16 classic and mixed cribriform carcinomas were estrogen receptor–positive and that 11 (69%) of the tumors were also progesterone receptor–positive. There was no appreciable difference in progesterone receptor positivity between classic and mixed cribriform tumors. When present, nodal metastases from classic tumors usually also have a cribriform structure, whereas those derived from mixed tumors are more likely to have a non-cribriform pattern (9,12).

A small proportion of cribriform carcinomas occur as multifocal lesions (9,10). The invasive component of cribriform carcinoma duplicates the sievelike growth pattern of conventional cribriform intraductal carcinoma (Fig. 3). The rounded and angular masses of uniform, well-differentiated tumor cells are embedded in variable amounts of collagenous stroma (Fig. 4). Some tumors have areas of tubular growth that comprise up to 50% of the tumor. Page et al. (9) found tubular areas in 6 of 35 classic cribriform tumors (17%). Mucin-positive secretion is present in varying amounts within these lumina, and they may contain microcalcifications (13,14). The intraductal component has a cribriform pattern in most but not all classic cribriform carcinomas.

Cribriform carcinoma should be distinguished morphologically from adenoid cystic carcinoma. Cribriform growth

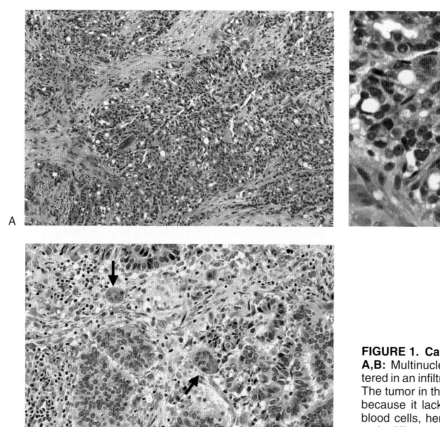

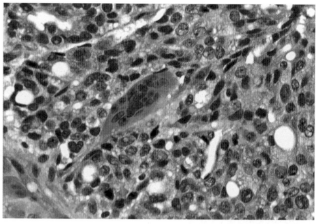

FIGURE 1. Carcinoma with osteoclast-like giant cells.
A,B: Multinucleated osteoclast-like giant cells are scattered in an infiltrating, poorly differentiated duct carcinoma. The tumor in this needle core biopsy specimen is unusual because it lacks typical stromal elements, including red blood cells, hemosiderin, and lymphocytes. **C:** A moderately differentiated duct carcinoma with osteoclast-like giant cells (*arrows*) in stroma that contains red blood cells, lymphocytes, plasma cells, and hemosiderin.

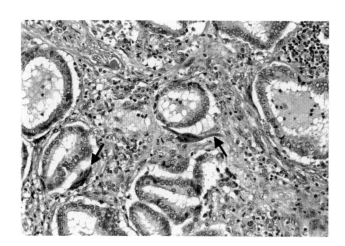

FIGURE 2. Carcinoma with osteoclast-like giant cells. Infiltrating duct carcinoma with a well-differentiated glandular pattern and characteristic stroma. The giant cells (*arrows*) are attenuated and apposed to the outer surfaces of the glands.

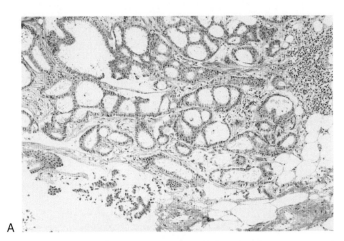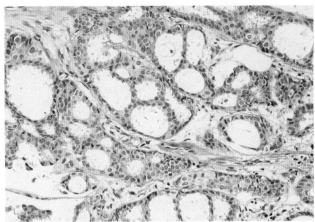

A   B

FIGURE 3. Invasive cribriform carcinoma. A,B: The invasive carcinoma in this needle core biopsy specimen has a cribriform structure composed of round or oval glandular spaces separated by thin, rigid bands of tumor cells with low-grade nuclei.

produces a fenestrated structural pattern that lacks the cylindromatous components composed of basal lamina material characteristic of adenoid cystic carcinoma. However, cribriform areas may be found in adenoid cystic carcinomas in which gland formation is more prominent than cylindromatous elements (15).

The majority of patients have been treated by mastectomy and axillary dissection (9,12). Two studies concluded that axillary lymph node metastases were less likely to develop in patients with classic cribriform carcinoma than in women with mixed cribriform (9) or ordinary invasive duct carcinoma (12). No deaths from classic cribriform carcinoma occurred among 34 patients studied by Page et al. (9) with follow-up of 10 to 21 years. Among 16 women with mixed cribriform carcinoma followed for an average of 12.5 years, there were six deaths resulting from the breast carcinoma. Venable et al. (12) reported a disease-free survival of 100%

among 45 patients with classic cribriform carcinoma followed for 1 to 5 years.

SMALL-CELL (OAT-CELL) CARCINOMA

Carcinoma with neuroendocrine features that resembles small-cell (oat-cell) carcinoma of the lung is one of the most uncommon variants of breast carcinoma (16,17). The diagnosis of primary small-cell mammary carcinoma can be made with confidence only if a nonmammary site is excluded clinically or if an *in situ* component can be demonstrated histologically in the breast. These criteria have not been met in all published descriptions of this rare neoplasm.

Intraductal carcinoma associated with small-cell carcinoma may exhibit various growth patterns, including cribriform, solid, and micropapillary (Fig. 5). The tumor cells are immunoreactive for cytokeratin (CAM5.2) and may also be immunoreactive for synaptophysin, neuron-specific enolase, and the Grimelius stain. Small-cell carcinoma can occur as part of a dimorphic intraductal carcinoma in which the small tumor cells in the center of the duct are surrounded at the periphery by large cells with abundant cytoplasm. Squamous metaplasia may occur in such lesions. Scattered neurosecretory granules were detected by electron microscopy in one tumor (16).

Metastatic pulmonary oat-cell carcinoma can involve the breast (18,19). In most cases, the existence of a pulmonary primary was previously documented, but the mammary metastasis may be the first manifestation of an occult pulmonary carcinoma.

LIPID-RICH CARCINOMA

This rare variant of infiltrating duct carcinoma is composed of cells containing abundant lipid that is extracted when the tissue is processed for histologic sections, so that vacuolated cytoplasm is left (20–22) (Fig. 6). The tumor

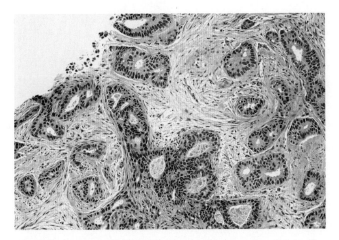

FIGURE 4. Invasive cribriform carcinoma. Small microlumina are separated by slender bands of cells in this example of cribriform carcinoma in a needle core biopsy specimen.

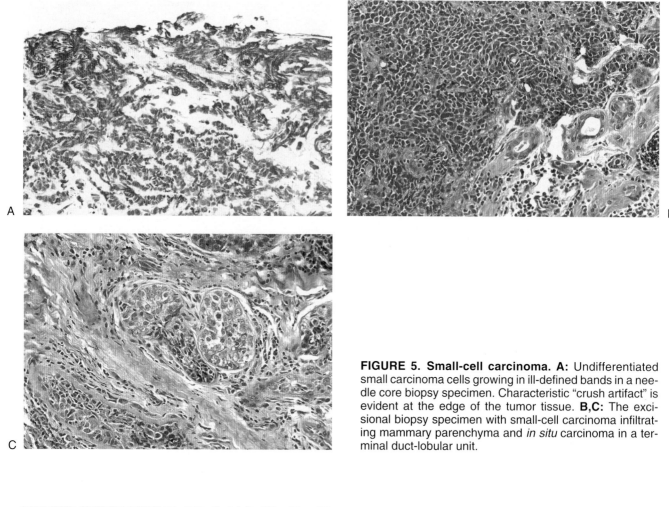

FIGURE 5. Small-cell carcinoma. A: Undifferentiated small carcinoma cells growing in ill-defined bands in a needle core biopsy specimen. Characteristic "crush artifact" is evident at the edge of the tumor tissue. **B,C:** The excisional biopsy specimen with small-cell carcinoma infiltrating mammary parenchyma and *in situ* carcinoma in a terminal duct-lobular unit.

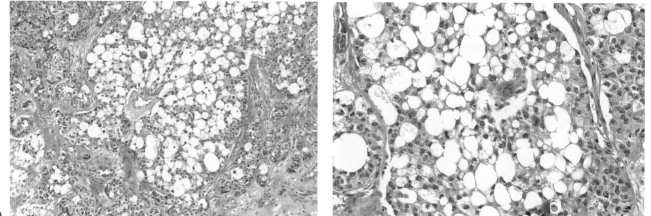

FIGURE 6. Lipid-rich carcinoma. A,B: Prominent cytoplasmic vacuoles are present after extraction of cytoplasmic lipid during tissue processing. (Courtesy of Dr. Frank Braza.)

cells have small, dark nuclei (23). The presence of lipid can be demonstrated in frozen sections of fresh tissue, by electron microscopy, or in tissue prepared by processes that preserve cytoplasmic lipids. The carcinoma is immunoreactive for epithelial membrane antigen, cytokeratin, and alpha-lactalbumin.

Ramos and Taylor (21) described 13 cases that had the growth pattern of lipid-rich carcinoma in routine histologic sections, but they were able to demonstrate lipid only in 4 cases that were available as unfixed specimens. The other 9 tumors were identified retrospectively among 900 tumors on the basis of histologic pattern alone. Eleven of the 12 patients treated by radical mastectomy had axillary lymph node metastases. Follow-up revealed that six patients died of metastatic carcinoma and two were alive with recurrence. The remainder were alive and recurrence-free, with the majority followed less than 2 years.

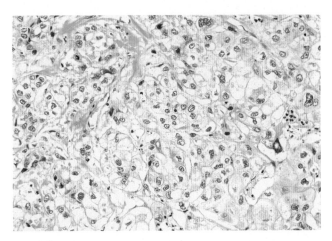

FIGURE 7. Glycogen-rich carcinoma. Prominent clear vacuoles were created during tissue processing because glycogen was dissolved from the tumor cells.

GLYCOGEN-RICH CARCINOMA

Carcinomas that accumulate abundant cytoplasmic glycogen can arise in the breast. Extraction of the water-soluble glycogen during histologic processing causes the cytoplasm in these tumor cells to have a clear, vacuolated appearance in routine sections. In one series, 3% of 1,555 carcinomas were classified as clear-cell, glycogen-rich carcinomas (24). These investigators were able to find lesser amounts of intracytoplasmic glycogen in 58% of non–clear-cell carcinomas. Others reported that glycogen-rich clear-cell carcinomas accounted for fewer than 1% of mammary duct carcinomas (25).

The patients range in age from 37 to 78 years and present with a mass. Intraductal and invasive glycogen-rich lesions have been detected by mammography (26–28). Hormone receptor analysis revealed that approximately 50% of tumors were estrogen receptor–positive, but all lesions studied have been negative for progesterone receptor (26–29).

The lesions have the basic structural features of conventional intraductal carcinoma alone or of intraductal and infiltrating duct carcinoma. The intraductal component has a compact solid, comedocarcinoma, cribriform, or papillary growth pattern (28). In invasive areas, the tumor cells form cords, solid nests, or papillary structures. A linear pattern consisting of strands of cells resembling invasive lobular carcinoma may be seen.

Cytologically, the tumor cells have sharply defined borders and polygonal contours. The cytoplasm is clear and less often finely granular or foamy. The central or eccentrically placed nuclei are hyperchromatic, sometimes exhibiting clumped chromatin and nucleoli (Fig. 7). Mitotic figures are infrequent. The differential diagnosis includes lipid-rich carcinoma of the breast and metastatic clear-cell renal carcinoma. Apocrine cytologic features are identified focally in a majority of the tumors, and it has been suggested that glycogen-rich carcinoma may be a variant of apocrine carcinoma (28). The cytoplasm gives a positive, diastase-labile reaction with the periodic acid–Schiff (PAS) stain. The cells stain only focally with alcian blue or mucicarmine (25,27), and do not stain with the oil red O stain for lipid (27).

Approximately 30% of the reported patients had metastatic tumor in their axillary lymph nodes. In one series (25), 50% of the patients treated by mastectomy died of metastatic mammary carcinoma 1 to 175 months (median, 15 months) after diagnosis, and one patient was alive with recurrent carcinoma 36 months after local excision and lymph node dissection.

INVASIVE MICROPAPILLARY CARCINOMA

Invasive micropapillary carcinoma is a histologically distinctive form of duct carcinoma in which the tumor cells are arranged in morule-like clusters, referred to as an "exfoliative" appearance (30). This growth pattern may be found throughout the lesion (pure invasive micropapillary carcinoma) or as part of an otherwise conventional invasive duct carcinoma (mixed invasive micropapillary carcinoma). Luna-Moré et al. (31) found micropapillary differentiation in 27 of 986 (2.7%) consecutive breast carcinomas. In 15 of the tumors, the micropapillary component occupied more than 50% of the lesion. The distinction between pure and mixed invasive micropapillary carcinoma cannot be made with certainty in the limited sample obtained by needle core biopsy.

The reported age range at diagnosis was 36 to 81 years in one series, with a median age of 62 years (32). Patients with lesions composed of more than 50% micropapillary carcinoma tend to be older than patients with less extensive micropapillary involvement (31). The majority of patients present with a palpable mass, but an occasional lesion has been detected mammographically as a soft-tissue density or as a result of microcalcifications (32). Tumors with more than 50% of micropapillary growth tend to be larger (mean size, 6 cm) than those with a lesser amount of this pattern (mean size, 3.5 cm).

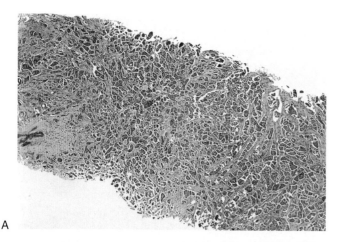

A

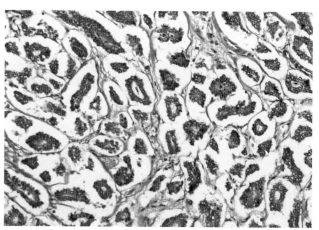

B

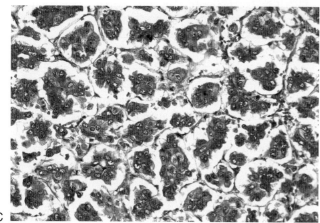

C

FIGURE 8. Invasive micropapillary carcinoma. A: This needle core biopsy specimen shows small nests of carcinoma cells outlined by a clear space. **B:** In one part of the lesion, the tumor cells are arranged around glandular lumina. Secretion is not evident in the spaces between carcinomatous glands and the slender bands of stroma. **C:** This area exhibits the "inside-out" pattern consisting of morulelike solid clusters of tumor cells with a serrated outer border. The tumor cells show apocrine differentiation. Spaces between the carcinoma cells and the stroma are devoid of secretion.

The carcinoma cells are cuboidal to columnar, containing finely granular or dense eosinophilic cytoplasm. They are arranged in small clusters that have a serrated peripheral border or may sometimes surround a central lumen (Fig. 8). An uncommon variant features microcystic dilatation of lumina within cell clusters. A clear space surrounds each tumor cell cluster, defined by intervening stroma consisting of dense fibrocollagenous tissue or a more delicate network of reticular tissue. In some instances, a lymphoid infiltrate permeates the stroma. The spongelike pattern of spaces filled by tumor cell clusters occurs in metastatic lesions as well as in the primary tumors. The spaces generally appear to be empty, but in some instances, mucinous material has been demonstrated with special stains (31). Myxoid stroma has been noted in a minority of cases (32). By electron microscopy, microvilli have been found on the cell surfaces bordering the clear spaces, suggesting that these cells are oriented as though the spaces around the tumor cell clusters were glandular lumina (31). This has been referred to as an "inside-out" growth pattern (33). In one study, immunoreactivity was detected as follows: estrogen receptor, 73%; progesterone receptor, 45%; HER2/neu, 36%; p53, 12%; and bcl-2, 70% (34). It is difficult to identify true lymphatic tumor emboli in the vicinity of the primary tumor because of the intrinsic capacity of the neoplasm to grow in a spongelike pattern. When they are present, the intravascular tumor cells are arranged in the same papillary clusters that characterize the invasive part of the tumor.

Intraductal carcinoma, which is detected in most cases, is usually micropapillary, sometimes with cribriform elements. However, solid intraductal carcinoma can be found in these tumors. Cells in the intraductal and invasive parts of the tumor often have poorly differentiated, hyperchromatic nuclei rather than the bland nuclear cytology usually associated with micropapillary intraductal carcinoma. Calcifications are sometimes found in intraductal foci and in the invasive areas.

The differential diagnosis of invasive micropapillary carcinoma includes primary mucinous carcinoma and metastatic ovarian carcinoma. Mucinous carcinoma features abundant extracellular mucin, which is absent from invasive micropapillary carcinoma. Tumor cell clusters in mucinous carcinoma usually have a smooth rather than a serrated periphery. The presence of an intraductal component serves to exclude metastatic ovarian carcinoma.

REFERENCES

Mammary Carcinoma with Osteoclast-Like Giant Cells

1. Agnantis NT, Rosen PP. Mammary carcinoma with osteoclast-like giant cells. *Am J Clin Pathol* 1979;72:383–389.

2. Holland R, Van Haelst VJGM. Mammary carcinoma with osteoclast-like giant cells. Additional observations on six cases. *Cancer* 1984;53:1963–1973.
3. Nielsen BB, Kiaer HW. Carcinoma of the breast with stromal multinucleated giant cells. *Histopathology* 1985;9:183–193.
4. Wargotz ES, Norris HJ. Metaplastic carcinomas of the breast: V. Metaplastic carcinoma with osteoclastic giant cells. *Hum Pathol* 1990;21:1142–1150.
5. Ichijima K, Kobashi Y, Ueda Y, Matsuo S. Breast cancer with reactive multinucleated giant cells: report of three cases. *Acta Pathol Jpn* 1986;36:449–457.
6. Chilose M, Bonetti F, Menestrina F, Lestani M. Breast carcinoma with stromal multinucleated giant cells [Letter to the Editor]. *J Pathol* 1987;152:55–57.
7. Phillipson J, Ostrzega N. Fine needle aspiration of invasive cribriform carcinoma with benign osteoclastlike giant cells of histiocytic origin. A case report. *Acta Cytol* 1994;38:479–482.
8. Viacava P, Naccarato AG, Nardini V, Bevilacqua G. Breast carcinoma with osteoclast-like giant cells: immunohistochemical and ultrastructural study of a case and review of the literature. *Tumori* 1995;81:135–141.

Cribriform Carcinoma

9. Page DL, Dixon JM, Anderson TJ, Lee D, Stewart HJ. Invasive cribriform carcinoma of the breast. *Histopathology* 1983;7:525–536.
10. Marzullo F, Zito FA, Marzullo A, et al. Infiltrating cribriform carcinoma of the breast. A clinico-pathologic and immunohistochemical study of 5 cases. *Eur J Gynaecol Oncol* 1996;17:228–231.
11. Stutz JA, Evans AJ, Pinder S, et al. The radiological appearances of invasive cribriform carcinoma of the breast. *Clin Radiol* 1994;49:693–695.
12. Venable JG, Schwartz AM, Silverberg SG. Infiltrating cribriform carcinoma of the breast: a distinctive clinicopathologic entity. *Hum Pathol* 1990;21:333–338.
13. Wells CA, Ferguson DJP. Ultrastructural and immunocytochemical study of a case of invasive cribriform breast carcinoma. *J Clin Pathol* 1988;41:17–20.
14. Shousha S, Schoenfeld A, Moss J, Shore I, Sinnett HD. Light and electron microscopic study of an invasive cribriform carcinoma with extensive microcalcification developing in a breast with silicone augmentation. *Ultrastruct Pathol* 1994;18:519–523.
15. Rosen PP. Adenoid cystic carcinoma of the breast: a morphologically heterogeneous neoplasm. *Pathol Annu* 1989;24(Pt 2):237–254.

Small-Cell (Oat-Cell) Carcinoma

16. Wade PM Jr, Mills SE, Read M, Cloud W, Lambert MJ III, Smith RE. Small cell neuroendocrine (oat cell) carcinoma of the breast. *Cancer* 1983;52:121–125.
17. Francois A, Chatikhine VA, Chevallier B, et al. Neuroendocrine primary small cell carcinoma of the breast. Report of a case and review of the literature. *Am J Clin Oncol* 1995;18:133–138.
18. Deeley TJ. Secondary deposits in the breast. *Br J Cancer* 1965;19:738–743.
19. Hadju SI, Urban JA. Cancers metastatic to the breast. *Cancer* 1972;29:1691–1696.

Lipid-Rich Carcinoma

20. Aboumrad MH, Horn RC, Fine G. Lipid-secreting mammary carcinoma: report of a case associated with Paget's disease of the nipple. *Cancer* 1963;16:521–525.
21. Ramos CV, Taylor HB. Lipid-rich carcinoma of the breast. A clinicopathologic analysis of 13 examples. *Cancer* 1974;33:812–819.
22. Van Bogaert L-J, Maldague P. Histologic variants of lipid-secreting carcinoma of the breast. *Virchows Arch [A]* 1977;375:345–353.
23. Mazzella FM, Sieber SC, Braza F. Ductal carcinoma of male breast with prominent lipid-rich component. *Pathology* 1995;27:280–283.

Glycogen-Rich Carcinoma

24. Fisher ER, Tavares J, Bulatao IS, Sass R, Fisher B. Glycogen-rich, clear cell breast cancer: with comments concerning other clear cell variants. *Hum Pathol* 1985;16:1085–1090.
25. Hull MT, Warfel KA. Glycogen-rich clear cell carcinomas of the breast. A clinicopathologic and ultrastructural study. *Am J Surg Pathol* 1986;10:553–559.
26. Hull MT, Priest JB, Broadie TA, Ransburg RC, McCarthy LJ. Glycogen-rich clear cell carcinoma of the breast. A light and electron microscopic study. *Cancer* 1981;48:2003–2009.
27. Sorensen FB, Paulsen SM. Glycogen-rich clear cell carcinoma of the breast: a solid variant with mucus. A light microscopic, immunohistochemical and ultrastructural study of a case. *Histopathology* 1987;11:857–869.
28. Hayes MMM, Seidman JD, Ashton MA. Glycogen-rich clear cell carcinoma of the breast: a clinicopathologic study of 21 cases. *Am J Surg Pathol* 1995;19:904–911.
29. Benisch B, Peison B, Newman R, Sobel HJ, Marquet E. Solid glycogen-rich clear cell carcinoma of the breast (a light and ultrastructural study). *Am J Clin Pathol* 1983;79:243–245.

Invasive Micropapillary Carcinoma

30. Fisher ER, Palekar AS, Redmond C, Barton B, Fisher B. Pathologic findings from the National Surgical Adjuvant Breast Project (Protocol No. 4). VI. Invasive papillary cancer. *Am J Clin Pathol* 1980;73:313–322.
31. Luna-Moré S, Gonzalez B, Acedo C, Rodrigo I, Luna C. Invasive micropapillary carcinoma of the breast. A new special type of invasive mammary carcinoma. *Path Res Pract* 1994;190:668–674.
32. Siriaunkgul S, Tavassoli FA. Invasive micropapillary carcinoma of the breast. *Mod Pathol* 1993;6:660–662.
33. Petersen JL. Breast carcinoma with an unexpected inside out growth pattern, rotation of polarisation associated with angioinvasion. *Pathol Res Pract* 1993;189:780.
34. Luna-Moré S, de los Santos F, Breton JJ, Canadas MA. Estrogen and progesterone receptors, c-erbB-2, p53, and BCL-2 in thirty-three invasive micropapillary breast carcinomas. *Pathol Res Pract* 1996;192:27–32.

CHAPTER 21

Lobular Carcinoma *In Situ* and Atypical Lobular Hyperplasia

LOBULAR CARCINOMA *IN SITU*

Lobular carcinoma *in situ* (LCIS) is a microscopic lesion that does not form a palpable tumor and is rarely detectable by mammography. In retrospective reviews, each involving several thousand breast specimens, the frequency of LCIS was 0.5% to 1.5% (1–3).

Lobular carcinoma *in situ* is typically discovered coincidentally in breast tissue removed for lesions that produce a mass or when processes that cause mammographic abnormalities lead to a biopsy. Calcifications are infrequently formed in LCIS (4). Mammography has not been an effective method for detecting LCIS and cannot be depended on to assess the multicentricity or bilaterality of the disease (5,6).

Up to 25% of LCIS patients are postmenopausal when the lobular lesion is identified (7). LCIS occurs infrequently as an isolated lesion in women younger than 35 years or older than 75 years of age. In a consecutive series of more than 1,000 patients treated for breast carcinoma, the mean age of women with LCIS (53 years) was not significantly different from the mean age of patients who had infiltrating duct carcinoma (57 years) (8). LCIS is associated with a high frequency of multicentric ipsilateral carcinoma, including occult invasive foci in 4% to 6% of women who undergo mastectomy (9,10). The contralateral breast is found to harbor LCIS in 40% of cases when a random biopsy is performed on the opposite breast in the absence of a clinical abnormality (11).

The microscopic anatomic distribution of LCIS in lobules and terminal ducts, and alterations in the morphology of these structures, influence the histopathologic appearance of LCIS in any given case. In the typical lobular form, a population of neoplastic cells replaces the normal epithelium of acini and intralobular ductules (Figs. 1,2). The abnormal cells can be sufficiently numerous to cause expansion of these structures. There may be enlargement of the entire lobule in comparison with uninvolved lobules in the adjacent breast, but lobular enlargement is not an absolute diagnostic criterion. The trend to lobular atrophy in postmenopausal women makes this an unreliable feature in that patient group (Fig. 3). If the diagnosis of LCIS is to be meaningful because it identifies a lesion associated with a substantial risk for later carcinoma, then lobular enlargement cannot be regarded as the paramount diagnostic criterion in lesions that have reached an acceptable qualitative level of cytologic abnormality.

The issue of how much lobular involvement is necessary for the diagnosis of LCIS remains unanswered and is of questionable relevance in the examination of needle core biopsy specimens, which provide limited samples. Because the number of affected lobules in a biopsy specimen has not proved to be related to the risk for subsequent carcinoma among patients not treated by mastectomy (2,12), there is presently no reason for drawing a distinction between one and two or more involved lobules as a basis for the diagnosis of LCIS (2) (Fig. 4). In some instances, the only evidence of a neoplastic lobular proliferation is one lobule in which some, but not all, of the acini are involved. At least 50% of one lobule should be involved to establish a diagnosis of LCIS (Fig. 5). Specimens with lesser lesions should be included in the category of atypical lobular hyperplasia.

Loss of cohesion is a characteristic of the neoplastic cells in LCIS, although this is not always readily apparent in acini filled and expanded by the process. When loss of cohesion is prominent and the neoplastic cells have a dissociated distribution, spaces may be created between them that can be mistaken for glandular lumina (Fig. 6). Degenerative changes may also disrupt the cellular composition of LCIS. In these situations, the neoplastic cells are not arranged in the polarized fashion that characterizes non-neoplastic cells persisting around true glandular lumina.

Typically, the neoplastic cells in LCIS have scant cytoplasm and small, round, cytologically bland nuclei that lack nucleoli. This cytologic pattern has been referred to as type A, or classic, LCIS (see Figs. 1,2,4). When greater cytologic pleomorphism is encountered, the more varied cells have been classified as type B, or pleomorphic, LCIS (Fig. 7). Type B cells have more abundant cytoplasm than cells classified as type A, and larger, more pleomorphic nuclei that sometimes have nucleoli. The cytologic features of type B cells in some instances resemble those of ductal carcinoma. When the lesion is composed entirely of type B cells, the dis-

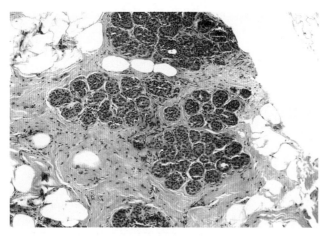

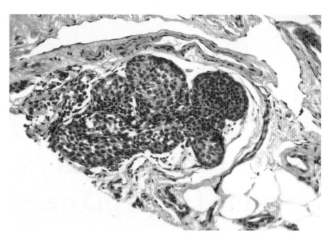

FIGURE 1. Lobular carcinoma *in situ.* The normal lobular epithelium has been replaced by neoplastic cells that fill the acinar lumina in this needle core biopsy specimen. Two contiguous lobules are affected. The biopsy was performed for mammographically detected calcifications present in lobular glands not involved by carcinoma *in situ.*

FIGURE 2. Lobular carcinoma *in situ.* A needle core biopsy specimen with a nearly completely involved lobule.

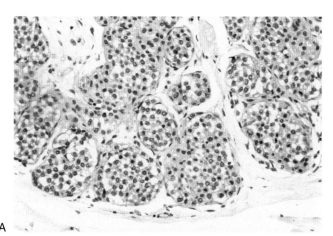

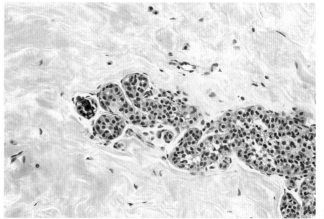

A   B

FIGURE 3. Lobular carcinoma *in situ* (LCIS). Both samples are from the same patient. **A:** LCIS as it appeared when the patient was premenopausal. The lobular glands are fully expanded. **B:** LCIS as it appeared in a biopsy specimen taken from the same breast after the menopause. This needle core biopsy was performed for mammographically detected calcifications. The lobule is markedly shrunken. One lobular gland contains a calcification.

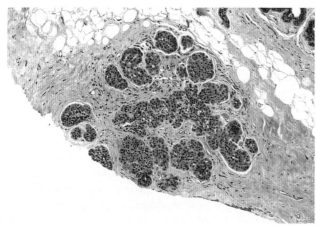

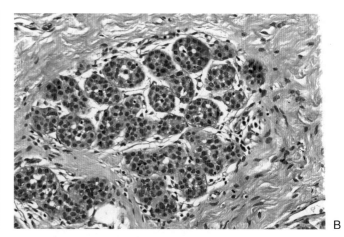

A   B

FIGURE 4. Lobular carcinoma *in situ* (LCIS). A: The only pathologic lesion in this needle core biopsy specimen was this one lobule with LCIS. **B:** This is one of several foci of LCIS found in the subsequent excisional biopsy specimen.

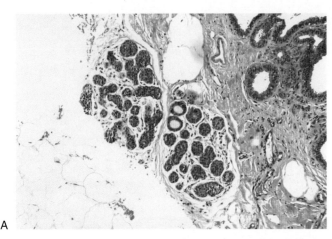
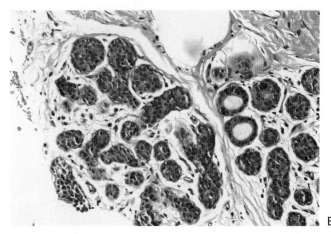

FIGURE 5. Lobular carcinoma *in situ*. A,B: A needle core biopsy specimen with minimal diagnostic evidence. Approximately 85% of the glands are involved in two lobules.

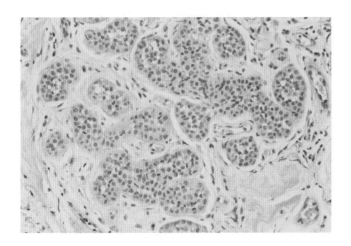

FIGURE 6. Lobular carcinoma *in situ*. Loss of cohesion and focal cellular degeneration have resulted in the formation of spaces in some lobular glands. These are not true acinar lumina.

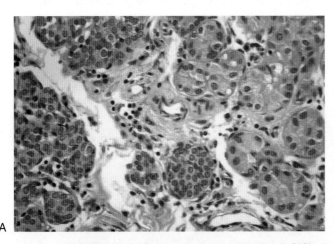
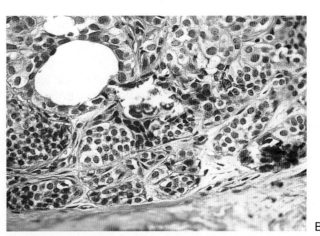

FIGURE 7. Lobular carcinoma *in situ* (LCIS). A: The carcinoma cells in acinar glands on the right have abundant cytoplasm and pleomorphic nuclei, characteristic of type B, or pleomorphic, LCIS. Type A cells are present on the left. **B:** Type A and type B cells are shown in a single lobule. Small calcifications are also present.

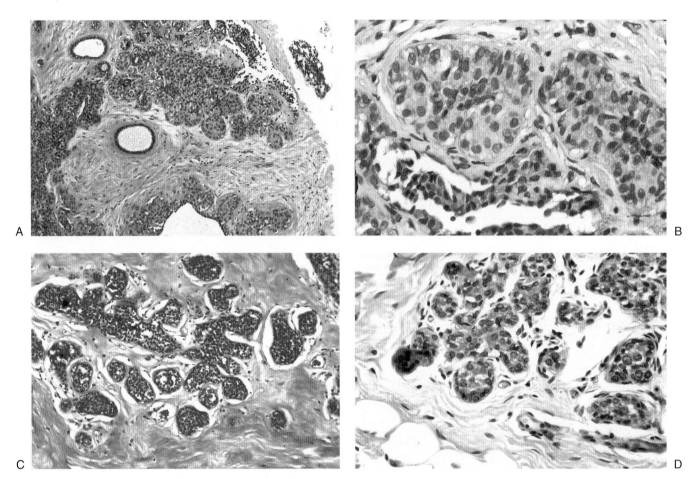

FIGURE 8. Lobular carcinoma *in situ* (LCIS). A: The lesion in this needle core biopsy specimen involves lobular glands and a duct. **B:** Intracytoplasmic mucin is stained magenta with the mucicarmine stain. **C,D:** A focus of LCIS with minimal acinar expansion. Intracytoplasmic mucin is demonstrated with the mucicarmine stain.

tinction between LCIS and intralobular extension of intraductal carcinoma may be difficult to establish. The presence of intracytoplasmic mucin secretion favors a diagnosis of LCIS. Some examples of LCIS have A and B cell types.

Intracytoplasmic vacuoles that contain mucinous secretion are usually present in some cells in LCIS, but the presence of mucin can be an inconspicuous feature that must be highlighted with a mucicarmine or alcian blue-PAS (period acid–Schiff) stain (13,14) (Fig. 8). An extreme manifestation of this phenomenon is the formation of signet-ring cells having a distended cytoplasmic vacuole that causes the nucleus to be eccentric or indented (Fig. 9). Because intracytoplasmic mucin vacuoles are uncommon in the cells of ductal carcinoma and are virtually absent in hyperplastic lesions of duct or lobular epithelium, their presence is an important but not a necessary criterion for the diagnosis of LCIS. Intracytoplasmic mucin is also present in LCIS with clear-cell change (Fig. 10).

Lobular carcinoma *in situ* in atrophic lobules and terminal ducts of postmenopausal women sometimes features cells with dark, eosinophilic-to-basophilic cytoplasm and deeply basophilic, eccentric nuclei (Fig. 11). This appearance is probably the result of cytoplasmic condensation associated

with loss of cohesion and shrinkage of cells. These cells frequently have intracytoplasmic mucin. In another variant, the cells of LCIS have a *mosaic* appearance, which results from the presence of distinct cell borders between cohesive cells

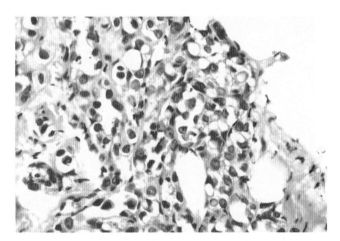

FIGURE 9. Lobular carcinoma *in situ* (LCIS) with signet-ring cells. Signet-ring cells have formed in this focus of LCIS in sclerosing adenosis at the edge of a needle core biopsy specimen.

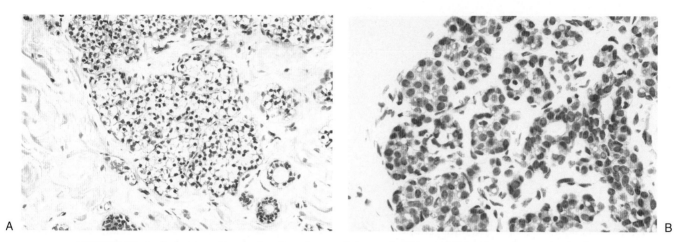

FIGURE 10. Lobular carcinoma *in situ*, clear-cell type. A: This example of carcinoma *in situ* features marked cytoplasmic clearing. **B:** Intracytoplasmic mucin is demonstrated with the mucicarmine stain. Cells in benign lobular clear-cell change do not have intracytoplasmic mucin.

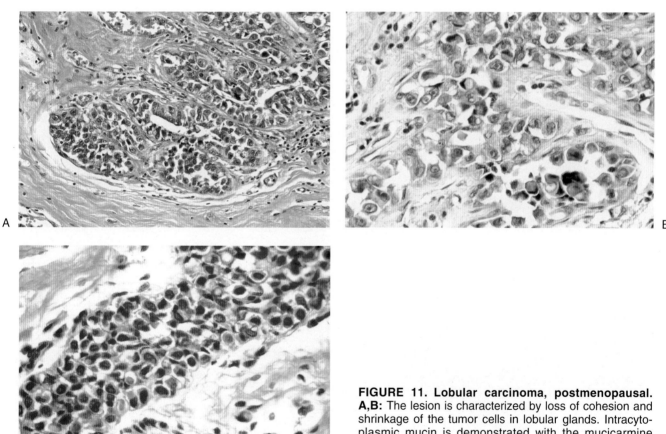

FIGURE 11. Lobular carcinoma, postmenopausal. A,B: The lesion is characterized by loss of cohesion and shrinkage of the tumor cells in lobular glands. Intracytoplasmic mucin is demonstrated with the mucicarmine stain. **C:** This example fills the lumen of a terminal duct. Some cells have intracytoplasmic vacuoles.

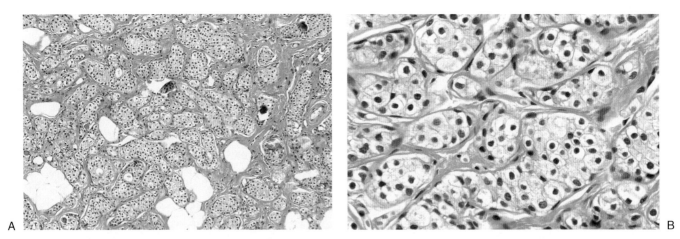

FIGURE 12. Lobular carcinoma *in situ,* mosaic pattern. A,B: The lesion involves sclerosing adenosis. Calcifications are shown in (A). The cells have distinct cytoplasmic borders, abundant pale cytoplasm, and punctate, centrally placed nuclei.

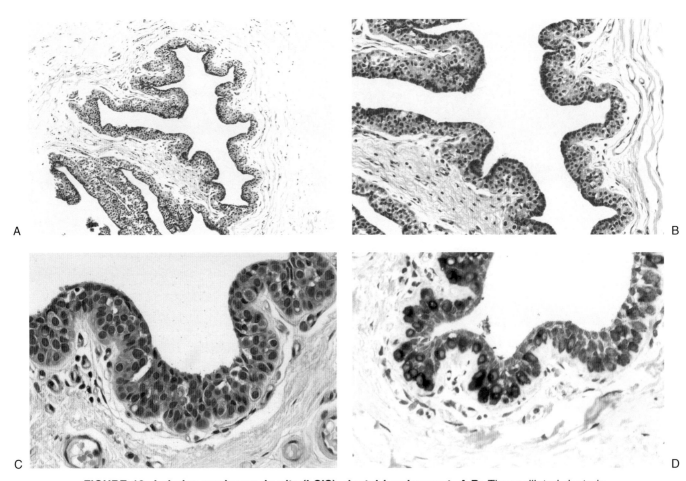

FIGURE 13. Lobular carcinoma *in situ* (LCIS), ductal involvement. A,B: These dilated ducts involved by pagetoid spread of LCIS were found in a needle core biopsy specimen. **C:** Intracytoplasmic mucin is demonstrated with the mucicarmine stain in carcinoma cells but not in the overlying residual benign ductal epithelium. **D:** The carcinoma cells are highlighted by the immunostain for epithelial membrane antigen (immunoperoxidase).

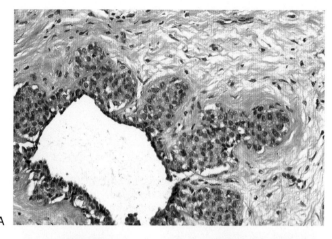

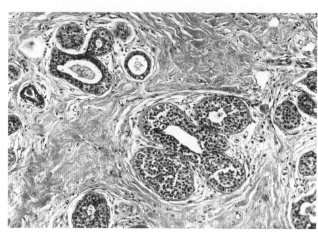

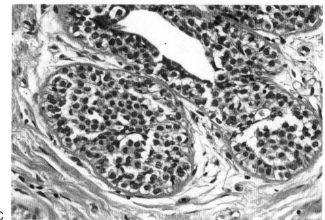

FIGURE 14. Lobular carcinoma *in situ* (LCIS), ductal origin. A: The cloverleaf pattern of ductal involvement is shown. The presence of lobulelike structures around the perimeter of the duct suggests that the neoplasm arose *de novo* at this site. A portion of this duct was illustrated at the lower border of Fig. 8A. **B,C:** This small duct exhibits florid LCIS and pagetoid spread in adjacent ductules.

and prominent, round, centrally placed nuclei surrounded by pale cytoplasm (Figs. 9,12). Intracytoplasmic mucin vacuoles can usually be found in this type of lobular carcinoma.

Lobular carcinoma *in situ* typically involves intralobular and extralobular or terminal ductules as well as acinar units within the lobule. In postmenopausal patients with atrophic lobules, duct involvement may be the only manifestation of LCIS (15). The irregular configuration of ductules affected by LCIS has been described as "sawtoothed" or as resembling a cloverleaf. LCIS cells growing beneath the non-neoplastic ductal epithelium may be distributed continuously or discontinuously along the ductal system, undermining and ultimately displacing the normal ductal epithelium (Fig. 13). The myoepithelial layer is preserved to a variable extent, and it may require an immunostain for actin to confirm that it is present. There is also evidence that the cloverleaf pattern sometimes arises *de novo* in ducts rather than by pagetoid spread (Fig. 14). Pagetoid spread of LCIS may also be encountered in papillomas or radial scar lesions. In its most florid form of ductal involvement, LCIS may proliferate to form a solid mass of tumor cells that fill and expand the duct lumen and develop central necrosis with calcification. (Fig. 15). Coexistence of LCIS and intraductal carcinoma in a single duct is a very unusual phenomenon (Fig. 16). When this occurs, the LCIS grows in a cloverleaf pattern around the perimeter of a duct lumen that contains phenotypically different intraductal carcinoma.

Lobular tissue structurally altered by various benign proliferative processes can harbor LCIS. As a consequence, LCIS has been encountered in fibroadenomas, sclerosing adenosis, papillary duct hyperplasia, collagenous spherulosis (16), and radial sclerosing lesions (Fig. 17). The diagnosis of LCIS under these circumstances rests largely on the identification of the appropriate cytologic features. The

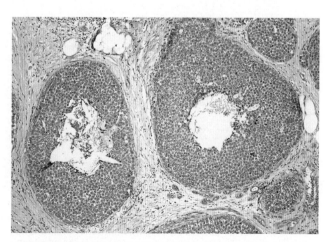

FIGURE 15. Lobular carcinoma *in situ* in a duct. The distended ducts are filled by monomorphic tumor cells with central necrosis.

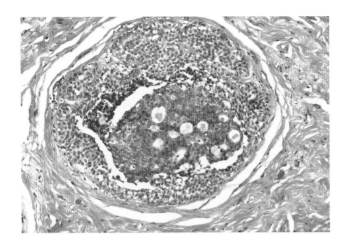

FIGURE 16. Lobular carcinoma *in situ* (LCIS) and intra-ductal carcinoma in a single duct. The lumen of the duct contains cribriform intraductal carcinoma. LCIS has a clover-leaf pattern around the perimeter of the duct.

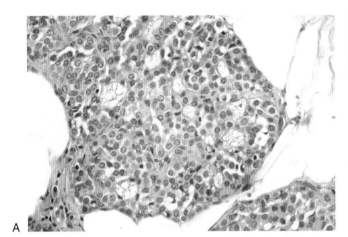

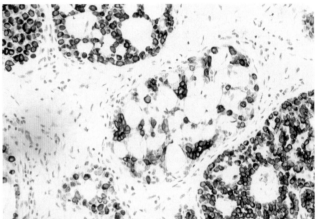

A

B

FIGURE 17. Lobular carcinoma *in situ* (LCIS) in collagenous spherulosis. A: LCIS is shown in-volving sclerosing adenosis below and collagenous spherulosis above. B: This cytokeratin stain high-lights the LCIS cells. Myoepithelial cells and strands of basement membrane material are unstained (im-munoperoxidase: CK7).

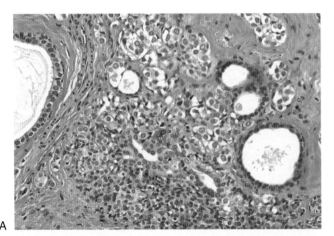

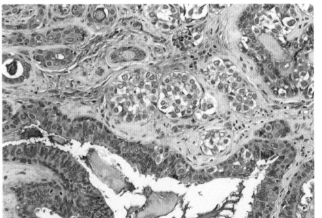

A

B

FIGURE 18. Lobular carcinoma *in situ* (LCIS) in sclerosing adenosis. A: The usual lobular struc-ture is not apparent in this area where LCIS inhabits sclerosing adenosis. B: Intracytoplasmic mucin is demonstrated as magenta spots in carcinoma cells with the mucicarmine stain. There is mucin in the lu-mina of some noncarcinomatous adenosis glands but not in the benign epithelial cells.

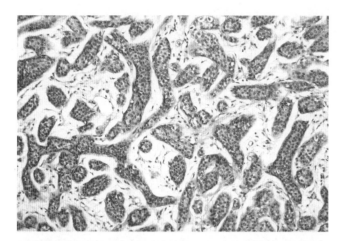

FIGURE 19. Lobular carcinoma *in situ* (LCIS) in tubular adenosis. LCIS inhabits a complex network of elongated adenosis tubules.

demonstration of intracytoplasmic mucin droplets is especially helpful for distinguishing florid adenosis from adenosis with LCIS (Fig. 18). LCIS in tubular adenosis has a striking histologic appearance (Fig. 19).

The lobular configuration is radically distorted in sclerosing lesions, and as a result it is difficult to exclude invasion when LCIS occurs in such foci (17). Careful inspection usually reveals the underlying adenosis pattern, in which glandular units are surrounded by a basement membrane, myoepithelial cells, and stroma. These elements can be highlighted with the reticulin stain and by the immunohistochemical demonstration of laminin, type IV collagen, and actin. Attenuated, spindle-shaped myoepithelial cells that proliferate in sclerosing adenosis usually persist even when the lesion is colonized by LCIS (18). Invasion is rarely detectable as long as the neoplastic cells remain confined to the configuration of sclerosing adenosis. The diagnosis of invasion is more readily made by finding carcinoma cells in the

stroma outside the sclerotic process. The appearance of such invasive foci is no different from that of invasive lobular carcinoma in the absence of a sclerosing lesion (see Chapter 22).

Most lobules are surrounded by fibrous stroma, but infrequently lobules are distributed in mammary adipose tissue. Lobules in fat are subject to the same pathologic alterations that occur in parenchymal lobules, including the development of sclerosing adenosis and LCIS. These conditions may resemble invasive carcinoma (Fig. 20). Important distinguishing features of LCIS in fat are the presence of well-defined glands containing LCIS and myoepithelial cells. The lobular glandular pattern is lost when classical infiltrating lobular carcinoma involves fat.

The risk associated with not treating LCIS by mastectomy has been estimated in several retrospective studies. The frequency of subsequent carcinoma varies from 12% to 36.4% (1–3,19–22). Studies with longer follow-up tend to report a higher frequency of subsequent carcinoma. In comparison with control populations, the relative risk of LCIS patients for subsequent development of carcinoma has been 4.0 to 12.0. In most studies, the risk for subsequent carcinoma was slightly higher in the ipsilateral than in the contralateral breast, although the difference has not been great.

Several studies prospectively assessed the follow-up of patients with LCIS after biopsy. After approximately 5 years in three studies, subsequent ipsilateral carcinoma developed in 7% to 17% of patients managed by follow-up only (12,23,24).

With few exceptions, follow-up studies of LCIS have consisted of patients who underwent biopsy for palpable clinical abnormalities in which LCIS was an incidental finding. In uncommon cases when it occurs in adenosis with calcifications or if there is marked duct distention with necrosis and calcification, LCIS rarely causes a mammographic abnormality that leads to biopsy, but it is usually discovered coin-

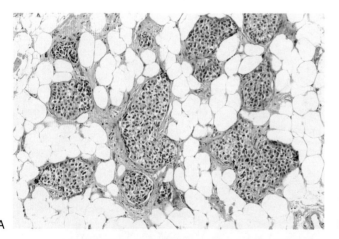

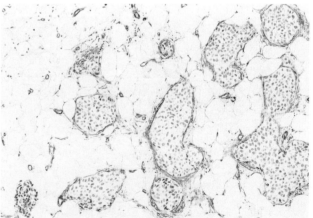

A   B

FIGURE 20. Lobular carcinoma *in situ* (LCIS) in adenosis. A: Glandular structures occupied by LCIS are shown in fat. This pattern suggests invasive carcinoma. **B:** Each glandular structure is outlined by an actin-positive border indicative of a myoepithelial cell layer, which confirms the *in situ* nature of the lesion (immunoperoxidase: smooth-muscle actin).

cidentally when a biopsy is performed for an unrelated roentgenographic finding. Zurrida et al. (25) reported the follow-up of 157 patients in whom LCIS was detected in a biopsy performed for a mammographic or palpable lesion. The ipsilateral breast was conserved in 135 cases. After a mean follow-up of 5 years, invasive carcinoma had developed in eight patients. The observed rate of carcinoma in the ipsilateral breast (4 carcinomas per 639 person-years at risk = 0.00625) was significantly (p <.05) greater than the expected rate (0.98 carcinomas per 639 person-years = 0.00152), resulting in a relative risk of 4.1 (CI, 1.1 to 10.5). The number of person-years at risk for carcinomas in either breast was 865, with an expected rate of 0.0015, an observed rate of 0.00925 (8/865), and a relative risk of 5.93 (CI, 2.6 to 11.7).

No study has thus far identified a reliable pathologic predictor of increased risk for the subsequent development of carcinoma after LCIS has been diagnosed by needle core or surgical biopsy. Lesions with marked duct distention, necrosis, and calcification are of special concern. If extensively present, treatment may be as for intraductal carcinoma. The author has found an unexpectedly high frequency of microinvasion in such cases. Three studies reported a greater risk in patients with LCIS that contained both small (type A) and large (type B) cells in comparison with patients who had LCIS with either cell type alone (2,12,19). Increased risk has also been associated with marked lobular distension (12) and the presence of 10 or more lobules with LCIS (24).

ATYPICAL LOBULAR HYPERPLASIA

There are no specific clinical features associated with the diagnosis of atypical lobular hyperplasia. The clinical indications for biopsy are the same as those leading to the detection of LCIS—a palpable lesion or a mammographic abnormality. Atypical lobular hyperplasia is usually an incidental finding not specifically associated with the abnormality that prompted the operation (Fig. 21).

The glandular proliferation in atypical lobular hyperplasia has some features of LCIS, but they are not sufficiently developed to qualify for the latter diagnosis. There are no universally accepted criteria for the precise distinction between atypical lobular hyperplasia and LCIS. Qualitative and quantitative factors must be considered. The diagnosis is rarely made solely on a quantitative basis; more often, qualitative criteria are also considered.

Quantitative criteria for the diagnosis of LCIS influence the distribution of cases classified as atypical lobular hyperplasia. Arbitrarily, the diagnosis of atypical lobular hyperplasia is made if less than 50% of the only affected lobule shows the features of LCIS (Figs. 22,23). Atypical lobular hyperplasia is characterized by the presence, within one or more lobules, of abnormal cells similar to those found in LCIS. In the least conspicuous configuration, these cells replace a portion of the normal lobular glandular epithelium, effacing some lumina. Acinar units are not enlarged at this proliferative level (Fig. 24). As the process evolves, the accumulation of a greater number of cells causes progressive acinar expansion, but the borders of individual acinar units and intralobular ductules remain indistinct (Fig. 25). Clear delineation of intralobular acinar units filled by the abnormal cell population is an important feature that distinguishes LCIS and reflects the accumulation of enough neoplastic cells to cause the individual glands to have a distinct configuration.

Similar criteria apply to the diagnosis of lobular proliferations in terminal duct structures. These alterations tend to create a cloverleaf pattern similar to that of LCIS (Figs. 25,26). The peripheral lobulelike bulges are sometimes inhabited by a mixture of normal and neoplastic cells. Atypical lobular hyperplasia of terminal ducts may also occur in a solid form that develops when the neoplastic growth is distributed in a continuous layer around the duct lumen.

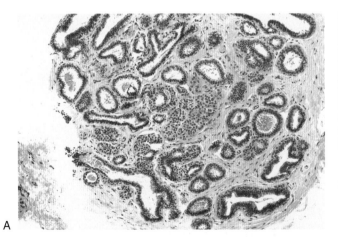
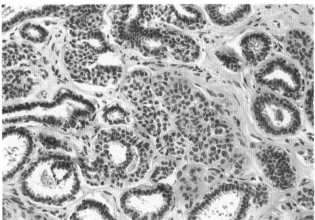

A   B

FIGURE 21. Atypical lobular hyperplasia. A,B: A needle core biopsy performed for calcifications revealed tubular carcinoma. One of the additional tissue samples had this focus of atypical lobular hyperplasia in adenosis.

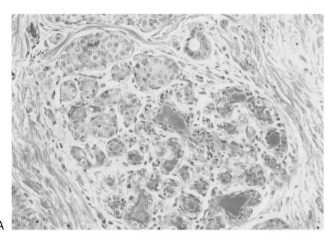
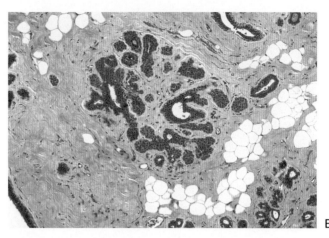

FIGURE 22. Atypical lobular hyperplasia. A,B: Examples of lobules that qualify as atypical lobular hyperplasia found in needle core biopsy specimens.

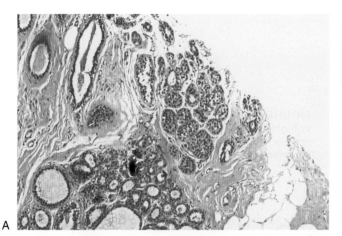
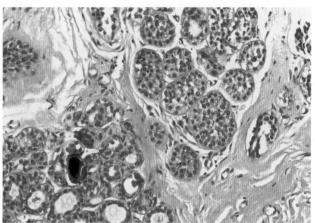

FIGURE 23. Atypical lobular hyperplasia. A,B: One partially involved lobule is present at the edge of this needle core biopsy specimen. The procedure was performed for calcifications that were present in sclerosing adenosis next to the atypical lobular hyperplasia in a premenopausal patient.

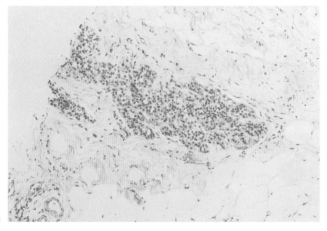
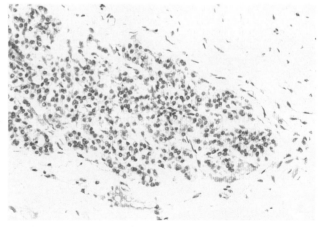

FIGURE 24. Atypical lobular hyperplasia. A,B: Atypical lobular hyperplasia in this needle core biopsy specimen involves a terminal duct-lobular unit from a postmenopausal woman.

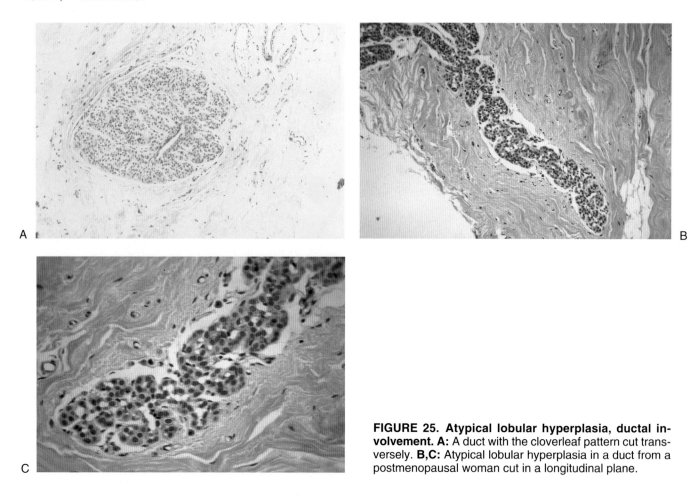

FIGURE 25. Atypical lobular hyperplasia, ductal involvement. A: A duct with the cloverleaf pattern cut transversely. B,C: Atypical lobular hyperplasia in a duct from a postmenopausal woman cut in a longitudinal plane.

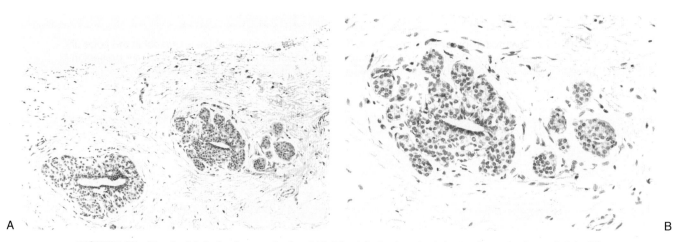

FIGURE 26. Atypical lobular hyperplasia. A,B: The lobular-terminal duct unit on the lower left in (A) shows moderate atypical hyperplasia with a cloverleaf pattern. The unit on the right has a developed lobular pattern that approaches lobular carcinoma *in situ.*

Estimates of the risk for subsequent carcinoma in women with atypical lobular hyperplasia are clouded by the absence of a uniform definition for this lesion. Some investigators who did not distinguish between atypical lobular hyperplasia and LCIS have reported relative risk estimates for both lesions under the heading of lobular neoplasia (19,20). The relative risk of patients for subsequent development of carcinoma is about four times that of age-matched controls (21). The risk is higher in women with a family history of breast carcinoma and when ducts are involved by the atypical lobular proliferation (26).

REFERENCES

1. Andersen J. Lobular carcinoma *in situ*: a long-term follow-up in 52 cases. *Acta Pathol Microbiol Scand A* 1974;82:519–533.
2. Rosen PP, Lieberman PH, Braun DW Jr, Kosloff C, Adair F. Lobular carcinoma *in situ* of the breast. Detailed analysis of 99 patients with average follow-up of 24 years. *Am J Surg Pathol* 1978;2:225–251.
3. Page DL, Kidd TE Jr, Dupont WD, Simpson JF, Rogers LW. Lobular neoplasia of the breast: higher risk for subsequent invasive cancer predicted by more extensive disease. *Hum Pathol* 1991;22:1232–1239.
4. Hutter RVP, Snyder RE, Lucas J, Foote FW Jr, Farrow JH. Clinical and pathologic correlation with mammographic findings in lobular carcinoma *in situ*. *Cancer* 1969;23:826–839.
5. Mackarem G, Yacoub LK, Lee AKC, Barbarisi LJ, Cuttino JT Jr, Hughes KS. Effects of screening on detection of lobular carcinoma *in situ* of the breast: nonspecificity of mammography and physical examination. *Breast Dis* 1994;7:339–345.
6. Morris DM, Walker AP, Cocker DC. Lack of efficacy of xeromammography in preoperatively detecting lobular carcinoma *in situ* of the breast. *Breast Cancer Res Treat* 1982;1:365–368.
7. Rosen PP, Senie R, Ashikari R, Schottenfeld D. Age, menstrual status, and exogenous hormone usage in patients with lobular carcinoma *in situ* (LCIS). *Surgery* 1979;85:219–224.
8. Rosen PP, Lesser ML, Senie RT, Duthie KJ. Epidemiology of breast carcinoma IV: age and histologic tumor type. *J Surg Oncol* 1982;19:44–47.
9. Shah JP, Rosen PP, Robbins GF. Pitfalls of local excision in the treatment of carcinoma of the breast. *Surg Gynecol Obstet* 1973;136:721–725.
10. Carter D, Smith AL. Carcinoma *in situ* of the breast. *Cancer* 1977;40:1189–1193.
11. Urban JA. Biopsy of the "normal" breast in treating breast cancer. *Surg Clin North Am* 1969;49:291–301.
12. Fisher ER, Costantino J, Fisher B, et al., for the National Surgical Adjuvant Breast and Bowel Project Collaborating Investigators. Pathologic findings from the National Surgical Adjuvant Breast Project (NSABP) Protocol B-17. Five-year observations concerning lobular carcinoma *in situ*. *Cancer* 1996;78:1403–1416.
13. Andersen JA, Vendelhoe ML. Cytoplasmic mucous globules in lobular carcinoma *in situ*. Diagnosis and prognosis. *Am J Surg Pathol* 1981;5:251–255.
14. Gad A, Azzopardi JG. Lobular carcinoma of the breast: a special variant of mucin-secreting carcinoma. *J Clin Pathol* 1975;28:711–716.
15. Haagensen CD, Lane N, Lattes R. Neoplastic proliferation of the epithelium of the mammary lobules: adenosis, lobular neoplasia and small cell carcinoma. *Surg Clin North Am* 1972;52:497–524.
16. Sgroi D, Koerner FC. Involvement of collagenous spherulosis by lobular carcinoma *in situ*. Potential confusion with cribriform ductal carcinoma *in situ*. *Am J Surg Pathol* 1995;19:1366–1370.
17. Fechner RE. Lobular carcinoma *in situ* in sclerosing adenosis. A potential source of confusion with invasive carcinoma. *Am J Surg Pathol* 1981;5:233–239.
18. Oberman HA, Markey BA. Noninvasive carcinoma of the breast presenting in adenosis. *Mod Pathol* 1991;4:31–35.
19. Haagensen CD, Lane N, Lattes R, Bodian C. Lobular neoplasia (so-called lobular carcinoma *in situ*) of the breast. *Cancer* 1978;42:737–769.
20. Bodian CA, Perzin KH, Lattes R, Huffman P, Abernathy TG. Prognostic significance of benign proliferative breast disease. *Cancer* 1993;71:3896–3907.
21. Page DL, Dupont WD, Rogers LW, Rados MS. Atypical hyperplastic lesions of the female breast. A long-term follow-up study. *Cancer* 1985;55:2698–2708.
22. Bodian CA, Perzin KH, Lattes R. Lobular neoplasia. Long-term risk of breast cancer and relation to other factors. *Cancer* 1996;78:1024–1034.
23. Ciatto S, Cataliotti C, Cardona G, Bianchi S. Risk of infiltrating breast cancer subsequent to lobular carcinoma *in situ*. *Tumori* 1992;78:244–246.
24. Ottesen GL, Graversen HP, Blichert-Toft M, Zedeler K, Andersen JA. Lobular carcinoma *in situ* of the female breast. Short-term results of a prospective nationwide study. *Am J Surg Pathol* 1993;17:14–21.
25. Zurrida S, Bartoli C, Galimberti V, Raselli R, Barletta L. Interpretation of the risk associated with the unexpected finding of lobular carcinoma *in situ*. *Ann Surg Oncol* 1996;3:57–61.
26. Page DL, Dupont WD, Rogers LW. Ductal involvement by cells of atypical lobular hyperplasia in the breast: a long-term follow-up study of cancer risk. *Hum Pathol* 1988;19:201–207.

CHAPTER 22

Invasive Lobular Carcinoma

When the diagnosis is restricted to tumors with the so-called classic histologic appearance, 3% to 4% of carcinomas qualify for a diagnosis of invasive lobular carcinoma (1–3). If the classification is broadened to include variant forms, the frequency of invasive lobular carcinoma has reportedly been as high as 10% to 14% of invasive carcinomas (4–6). Invasive lobular carcinoma occurs throughout virtually the entire age range of breast carcinoma in adult women (28 to 86 years). Most studies have placed the median age at diagnosis between 45 and 56 years (2,3,5–7). Invasive lobular carcinoma is relatively more common among women older than 75 years (11%) than in women 35 years or younger.

The presenting symptom in almost all cases is a mass, often with ill-defined margins. In some cases, the only evidence of the neoplasm is vague thickening or fine, diffuse nodularity of the breast. Invasive lobular carcinoma is not prone to form calcifications, but calcifications may be present coincidentally in benign proliferative lesions such as sclerosing adenosis (8). A lower frequency of calcifications detected by mammography has been reported in invasive lobular carcinomas than in duct carcinomas (9–11). The mammographic estimate of tumor size tends to be less than the grossly measured size in a significant proportion of cases (12). Rodenko et al. (13) found that magnetic resonance (MR) imaging was more effective than mammography in a significant proportion of cases for determining the extent of the primary invasive lobular carcinoma, but the presence of metastatic carcinoma in axillary lymph nodes was not detected in four cases examined.

A comparison between mammograms of invasive lobular and other types of carcinoma revealed that lobular carcinomas were more often spiculated and associated with retraction of the nipple or skin. Carcinomas with mixed lobular and duct features tended to have mammographic features between those of the two groups. The most common mammographic manifestations of invasive lobular carcinoma are asymmetric, ill-defined or irregular, spiculated masses (8,9,11,14). In one study, the findings of 46% of mammograms from patients who ultimately proved to have invasive lobular carcinoma were initially reported to be negative (10). The absence of well-defined margins and, in some cases, a tendency to form multiple small nodules throughout the breast are features that may hinder the radiologic detection of invasive lobular carcinoma and lead to a false-negative diagnosis. Patients with a spiculated mass are less likely to have residual carcinoma when excision is repeated than are those with ill-defined or asymmetric lesions (14).

Patients with invasive lobular carcinoma are reported to have a relatively high frequency of bilateral carcinoma when compared with women who have other types of carcinoma (15). Prior and concurrent contralateral carcinomas have been described in 6% to 28% of cases (5,7,16,17). The reported incidence of subsequent contralateral carcinoma ranges from 1.0 (16,18) to 2.38 (19) per 100 women per year. There is some evidence that the frequency of bilaterality is higher in patients with classic invasive lobular carcinoma than in patients with variant subtypes (19). A lobular component has been found in the majority of synchronous or metachronous contralateral carcinomas, and at least 50% of these have been invasive (7,16–18). In one series, random concurrent contralateral biopsies in 108 patients revealed intraductal carcinoma in 6% and invasive carcinoma in 10% (20). Biopsies performed for clinical indications in an additional 22 cases yielded intraductal carcinoma in 5% and invasive carcinoma in 32%. The probability of detecting contralateral invasive carcinoma was significantly greater in women who had multicentric invasive carcinoma in the ipsilateral breast or who had ipsilateral lymph node metastases.

Several growth patterns may be encountered in lesions classified as classic, or pure, invasive lobular carcinoma. The common denominator is the virtual absence of solid, alveolar, papillary, and gland-forming aggregates of cells. In the two-dimensional plane of a histologic section, the slender strands of cells are arranged in a linear fashion not more than one or two cells across (Fig. 1). If the tumor cells are arranged around ducts and lobules in a concentric fashion, the distribution is described as having a targetoid appearance (Fig. 2). In a minority of cases, the linear, strand-forming pattern is not conspicuous, and the tumor cells tend to grow mainly in dispersed, disorderly foci (Fig. 3). The small tumor cells in such foci may be mistaken for lymphocytes or plasma cells in areas of fibrosis or fat when sections are examined at low magnification (Figs. 4,5). Invasive lobular carcinoma is only rarely accompanied by a notable lymphocytic reaction (Fig. 6).

Tumors with the cytologic features of invasive lobular

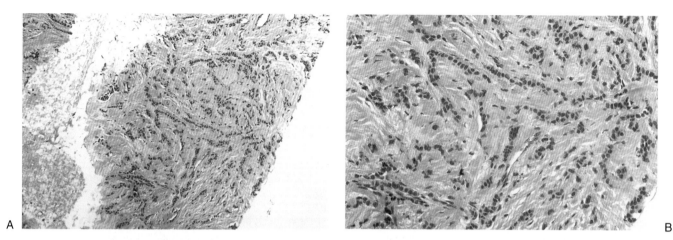

FIGURE 1. Invasive lobular carcinoma, classic type. A,B: The small cells with scant cytoplasm and dark, homogeneous nuclei are arranged in a linear pattern in this needle core biopsy specimen.

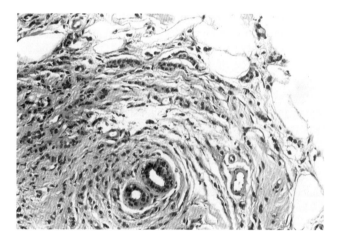

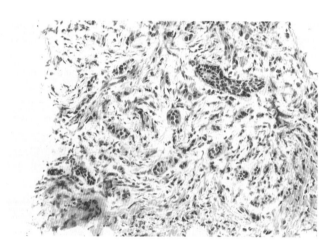

FIGURE 2. Invasive lobular carcinoma, classic type with targetoid growth. The linear cellular infiltrate is arranged in circumferential rings around a duct.

FIGURE 3. Invasive lobular carcinoma, classic type. The linear growth pattern is obscured by stromal reaction around a terminal duct and lobular glands in this needle core biopsy specimen.

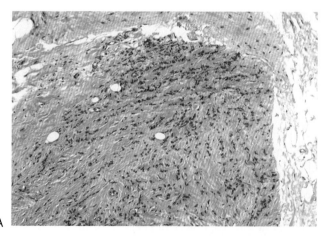

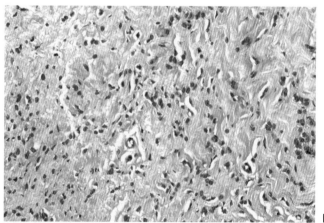

FIGURE 4. Invasive lobular carcinoma obscured by fibrosis. A,B: The small invasive carcinoma cells in this needle core biopsy specimen are obscured by dense fibrosis and a subtle form of pseudoangiomatous stromal hyperplasia. The specimen was obtained from an area of increased density found by mammography at the site of prior breast conservation therapy for infiltrating duct carcinoma.

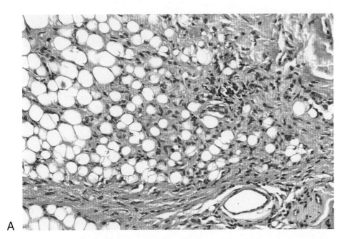

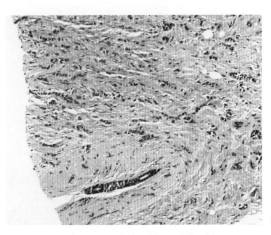

A

B

FIGURE 5. Invasive lobular carcinoma obscured by fat. A: Carcinoma cells infiltrating fat in this needle core biopsy specimen create an appearance that superficially resembles fat necrosis. **B:** Another portion of the specimen contained classic invasive lobular carcinoma.

carcinoma and substantial elements of nonlinear growth have been referred to as "variant" forms of invasive lobular carcinoma (2,5,6). Areas of classic invasive lobular carcinoma with a linear pattern are found in most variant forms, but they will not necessarily be present in a needle core biopsy specimen. These carcinomas are composed of cells typically found in classic invasive lobular carcinoma (6). Solid, tubular, trabecular, and alveolar variants have been described, extending the diagnosis of invasive lobular carcinoma to a larger group of tumors. The solid type consists of compact nests of tumor cells (Fig. 7). Trabecular lobular carcinoma refers to tumors with prominent bands two or more cells broad (Fig. 8). Usually, the trabecular pattern is found in association with other variants, and the tumors are classified as mixed. The alveolar pattern is defined by rounded ag-

gregates or clumps of cells, a configuration that overlaps somewhat with the solid pattern (Fig. 9). Lobular carcinoma *in situ* is associated with about 85% of the tumors. The observation that many examples of classic invasive lobular carcinoma have minor components of alveolar, tubular, trabecular, or solid growth is further evidence for classifying neoplasms that express these features prominently as variants of invasive lobular carcinoma.

Occasionally, the sample obtained by needle core biopsy contains minimal, inconspicuous evidence of invasive lobular carcinoma that can easily be overlooked or mistaken for an inflammatory cell infiltrate (Figs. 10,11). When lobular carcinoma *in situ* is identified in a needle core biopsy specimen, all tissue should be carefully inspected for occult invasion.

All the cytologic appearances found in lobular carcinoma *in situ* may also be present in invasive lobular carcinoma. Classic invasive lobular carcinoma consists of small, uniform cells with round nuclei and inconspicuous nucleoli. A variable proportion of cells have intracytoplasmic lumina (Fig. 12). Mucin is demonstrable in these vacuoles with the mucicarmine and alcian blue stains (21,22). When the secretion is prominent, the cells have a signet-ring configuration. The majority of so-called signet-ring cell carcinomas are forms of invasive lobular carcinoma (5,21–23).

Some invasive lobular carcinomas consist entirely or in part of cells with relatively abundant cytoplasm and enlarged, hyperchromatic nuclei (Fig. 13). These cells have been referred to as histiocytoid (24) and pleomorphic lobular carcinoma (25). Eusebi et al. (25) emphasized the presence of apocrine differentiation in pleomorphic invasive lobular carcinoma and concluded that these patients have an especially aggressive clinical course because recurrences developed in 9 of 10 patients in their series (Fig. 14).

Perineural invasion is uncommon in invasive lobular carcinoma but may occur when the lesion is very extensive.

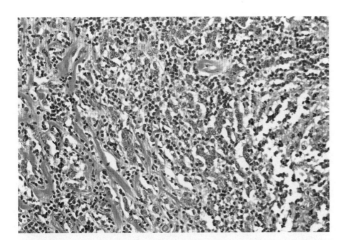

FIGURE 6. Invasive lobular carcinoma with lymphocyte reaction. The carcinoma cells have a linear growth pattern that is difficult to appreciate in the midst of the lymphocytic reaction.

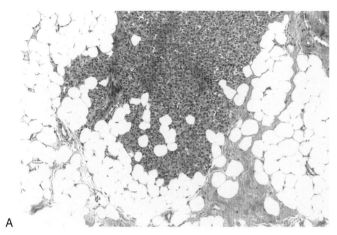
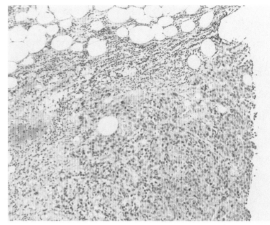

A
B

FIGURE 7. Invasive lobular carcinoma, solid variant. A: The tumor cells form a solid mass with uneven borders infiltrating fat (hematoxylin-phloxine-saffranin). **B:** A needle core biopsy specimen in which the border of solid invasive lobular carcinoma is defined by a lymphocytic reaction.

Lymphatic tumor emboli are also rarely found in this type of carcinoma, and in some situations, shrinkage artifacts may simulate carcinoma in lymphatic spaces. When lymphatic tumor emboli are present, the tumor cells tend to form cohesive aggregates rather than being individually dispersed.

The majority of invasive lobular carcinomas exhibit nuclear immunoreactivity for estrogen receptor, and usually for progesterone receptor as well (Fig. 15). Histiocytoid or pleomorphic invasive lobular carcinoma is positive for gross cystic disease fluid protein-15 (GCDFP-15) (25). The HER2/neu gene product is only rarely detected immunohistochemically in *in situ* or invasive lobular carcinoma (26). When compared with infiltrating duct carcinoma, invasive lobular carcinoma is more often positive for cathepsin D, but it is typically negative for p53 protein and vimentin (27).

Metastatic deposits of lobular carcinoma tend to duplicate the cytologic features of the primary tumor. Axillary lymph node metastases derived from invasive lobular carcinoma of the classic type may be distributed largely in sinusoids, sparing lymphoid areas. If lymph node involvement is sparse, the distinction between tumor cells and histiocytes may be difficult. Isolated tumor cells in the bone marrow may resemble hematopoietic elements (28). When compared with ductal carcinoma, lobular carcinoma is associated with a statistically significantly greater frequency of metastases in the peritoneum and retroperitoneum, leptomeninges, gastrointestinal tract, and gynecologic organs, and a lower frequency of pulmonary or pleural metastases (29). In the uterus, the carcinoma cells blend with normal endometrial stromal cells and may be overlooked in endometrial curettings (30). Metastases involving the stomach can produce clinical and pathologic findings indistinguishable from those of a pri-

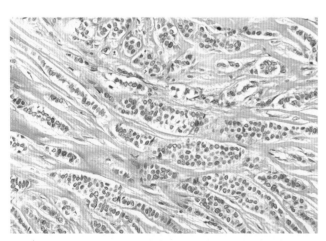

FIGURE 8. Invasive lobular carcinoma, trabecular variant. This tumor has a linear growth pattern formed by bands of cells arrayed two to four across.

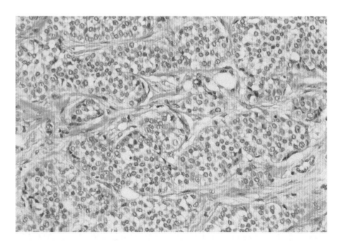

FIGURE 9. Invasive lobular carcinoma, alveolar type. The tumor cells form rounded masses that duplicate the appearance of lobular carcinoma *in situ*.

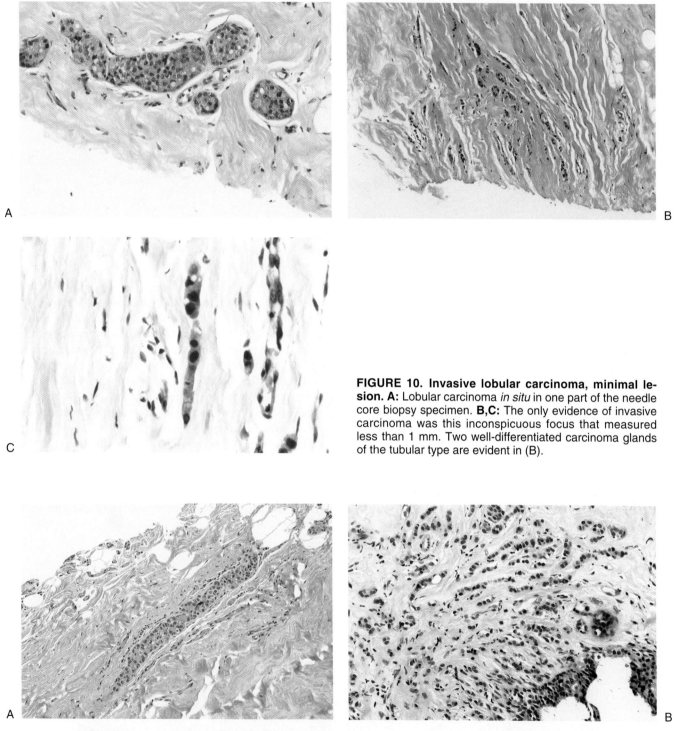

FIGURE 10. Invasive lobular carcinoma, minimal lesion. A: Lobular carcinoma *in situ* in one part of the needle core biopsy specimen. **B,C:** The only evidence of invasive carcinoma was this inconspicuous focus that measured less than 1 mm. Two well-differentiated carcinoma glands of the tubular type are evident in (B).

FIGURE 11. Invasive lobular carcinoma, minimal lesion. A: *In situ* lobular carcinoma involving a terminal duct was present in the needle core biopsy specimen. **B:** This 1-mm focus of invasive lobular carcinoma was initially diagnosed incorrectly as a periductal lymphocytic reaction. No other evidence of carcinoma was found in the specimen, which consisted of several tissue cores.

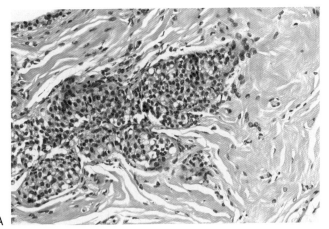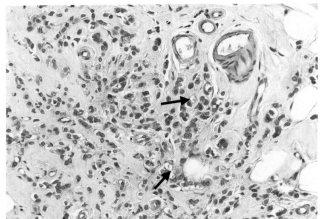

A   B

FIGURE 12. Invasive lobular carcinoma with signet-ring cells. A,B: Signet-ring cells (*arrows*) in *in situ* and invasive lobular carcinoma were found in this needle core biopsy specimen.

mary gastric carcinoma (31). Estrogen receptors have been detected in gastric adenocarcinomas by immunohistochemical procedures, but diffuse, strong staining would favor metastatic lobular carcinoma (32,33). No significant differences have been found in the distribution of metastases between patients with the classic and variant patterns of invasive lobular carcinoma (5).

Studies of prognosis in patients with invasive lobular carcinoma have not shown a consistent difference between them and patients with invasive duct carcinoma treated by mastectomy when stage at diagnosis is taken into consideration (2,5,19,34). Patients with classic invasive lobular carcinoma have a slightly better prognosis than those with variant forms as a group, but the differences have not been statistically significant. No reproducible differences in prognosis

have been demonstrated among patients with different variant lesions, and it is evident that very large numbers of cases would be needed to document significant differences if they exist. Consequently, no distinction should be made between classic and variant forms of invasive carcinoma with regard to therapy. The most important determinants of prognosis and treatment are primary tumor size and nodal status.

Several reports of successful treatment by breast conservation with radiotherapy have appeared (14,35–38). These studies indicate that survival for patients with invasive lobular carcinoma treated by breast conservation is similar to the result obtained for duct carcinoma at 5 years of follow-up. Patients with multifocal invasive lobular carcinoma have a greater frequency of breast recurrence than those with unifocal tumors (39).

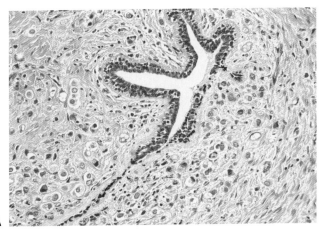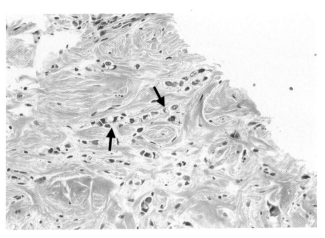

A   B

FIGURE 13. Invasive lobular carcinoma, pleomorphic and histiocytoid types. A linear growth pattern is present in these two different needle core biopsy specimens. **A:** Invasive lobular carcinoma with histiocytoid features is shown surrounding a duct. The carcinoma cells have relatively abundant cytoplasm. Signet-ring cell forms are present. **B:** Some of the carcinoma cells in this needle core biopsy specimen have cytoplasmic vacuoles and a signet-ring cell appearance (*arrows*) despite the pleomorphic nuclei.

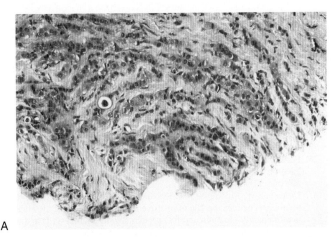

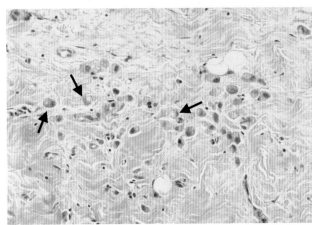

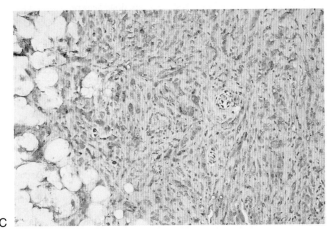

FIGURE 14. Invasive lobular carcinoma, pleomorphic type with apocrine differentiation. A: The carcinoma cells have relatively abundant cytoplasm and pleomorphic hyperchromatic nuclei. **B:** This example features cells with a prominent histiocytoid appearance and intracytoplasmic vacuoles (*arrows*). **C:** Intracytoplasmic mucin appears magenta in this mucicarmine stain.

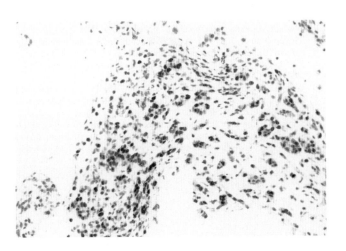

FIGURE 15. Invasive lobular carcinoma, estrogen receptors. This immunoperoxidase-stained section of a needle core biopsy specimen displays diffuse, strong nuclear immunoreactivity for estrogen receptor.

REFERENCES

1. Henson D, Tarone R. A study of lobular carcinoma of the breast based on the Third National Cancer Survey in the United States of America. *Tumori* 1979;65:133–142.
2. Dixon JM, Anderson TJ, Page DL, Lee D, Duffy W. Infiltrating lobular carcinoma of the breast. *Histopathology* 1982;6:149–161.
3. Ashikari R, Huvos AG, Urban JA, Robbins GF. Infiltrating lobular carcinoma of the breast. *Cancer* 1973;31:110–116.
4. Martinez V, Azzopardi JG. Invasive lobular carcinoma of the breast: incidence and variants. *Histopathology* 1979;3:467–488.
5. DiCostanzo D, Rosen PP, Gareen I, Franklin S, Lesser M. Prognosis in infiltrating lobular carcinoma: an analysis of "classical" and variant tumors. *Am J Surg Pathol* 1990;14:12–23.
6. Fechner RE. Histologic variants of infiltrating lobular carcinoma of the breast. *Hum Pathol* 1975;6:373–378.
7. Fechner RE. Infiltrating lobular carcinoma without lobular carcinoma in situ. *Cancer* 1972;29:1539–1545.
8. Mendelson EB, Harris KM, Doshi N, Tobon H. Infiltrating lobular carcinoma: mammographic patterns with pathologic correlation. *AJR Am J Roentgenol* 1989;153:265–271.
9. Helvie MA, Paramagul C, Oberman HA, Adler DD. Invasive lobular carcinoma: imaging features and clinical detection. *Invest Radiol* 1993; 28:202–207.
10. Krecke KN, Gisvold JJ. Invasive lobular carcinoma of the breast: mammographic findings and extent of disease at diagnosis in 184 patients. *AJR Am J Roentgenol* 1993;161:957–960.
11. Le Gal M, Ollivier L, Asselain B, et al. Mammographic features of 455 invasive lobular carcinomas. *Radiology* 1992;185:705–708.
12. Yeatman TJ, Cantor AB, Smith TJ, et al. Tumor biology of infiltrating lobular carcinoma. Implications for management. *Ann Surg* 1995;222: 549–561.
13. Rodenko GN, Harms SE, Pruneda JM, et al. MR imaging in the management before surgery of lobular carcinoma of the breast: correlation with pathology. *AJR Am J Radiol* 1996;167:1415–1419.
14. White JR, Gustafson GS, Wimbish K, et al. Conservative surgery and radiation therapy for infiltrating lobular carcinoma of the breast. The role of preoperative mammograms in guiding treatment. *Cancer* 1994; 74:640–647.
15. Broët P, de la Rochefordiére A, Scholl SM, et al. Contralateral breast cancer: annual incidence and risk parameters. *J Clin Oncol* 1995;13: 1578–1583.
16. Dixon JM, Anderson TJ, Page DL, Lee D, Duffy SW, Stewart HJ. Infiltrating lobular carcinoma of the breast: an evaluation of the incidence and consequence of bilateral disease. *Br J Surg* 1983;70:513–516.
17. Lesser ML, Rosen PP, Kinne DW. Multicentricity and bilaterality in invasive breast carcinoma. *Surgery* 1982;1:234–240.
18. Hislop TG, Ng V, McBride ML, Coldman AJ, Worth AJ. Incidence and risk factors for second breast primaries in women with lobular breast carcinoma. *Breast Dis* 1990;3:95–105.
19. du Toit RS, Locker AP, Ellis IO, Elston CW, Nicholson RI, Blamey RW. Invasive lobular carcinomas of the breast—the prognosis of histopathological subtypes. *Br J Cancer* 1989;60:605–609.
20. Simkovich AH, Sclafani LM, Masri M, Kinne DW. Role of contralateral breast biopsy in infiltrating lobular cancer. *Surgery* 1993;114: 555–557.
21. Breslow A, Brancaccio ME. Intracellular mucin production by lobular breast carcinoma cells. *Arch Pathol Lab Med* 1976;100:620–621.
22. Gad A, Azzopardi JG. Lobular carcinoma of the breast: a special variant of mucin-secreting carcinoma. *J Clin Pathol* 1975;28:711–716.
23. Steinbrecher JS, Silverberg SG. Signet ring cell carcinoma of the breast. The mucinous variant of infiltrating lobular carcinoma. *Cancer* 1976;37:828–840.
24. Allenby PL, Chowdhury LN. Histiocytic appearance of metastatic lobular breast carcinoma. *Arch Pathol Lab Med* 1986;110:759–760.
25. Eusebi V, Magalhaes F, Azzopardi JG. Pleomorphic lobular carcinoma of the breast: an aggressive tumor showing apocrine differentiation. *Hum Pathol* 1992;23:655–662.
26. Porter PL, Garcia R, Moe R, Corwin DJ, Gown AM. C-erbB-2 oncogene protein in in situ and invasive lobular breast neoplasia. *Cancer* 1991;68:331–334.
27. Domagala W, Markiewski M, Kubiak R, Bartowiak J, Osborn M. Immunohistochemical profile of invasive lobular carcinoma of the breast: predominantly vimentin and p53 protein negative cathepsin D and oestrogen receptor positive. *Virchows Arch A* 1993;423:497–502.
28. Bitter MA, Fiorito D, Corkell ME, et al. Bone marrow involvement by lobular carcinoma of the breast cannot be identified reliably by routine histological examination alone. *Hum Pathol* 1994;25:781–788.
29. Harris M, Howell A, Chrissohou M, Swindell RIC, Hudson M, Sellwood RA. A comparison of the metastatic pattern of infiltrating lobular carcinoma and infiltrating duct carcinoma of the breast. *Br J Cancer* 1984;50:23–30.
30. Kumar NB, Hart WR. Metastases to the uterine corpus from extragenital cancers. A clinicopathologic study of 63 cases. *Cancer* 1982;50: 2163–2169.
31. Cormier WJ, Gaffey TA, Welch JM, Welch JS, Edmonson JH. Linitis plastica caused by metastatic carcinoma of the breast. *Mayo Clin Proc* 1980;55:747–753.
32. Harrison JD, Morris DL, Ellis IO, Jones JA, Jackson I. The effect of tamoxifen and estrogen receptor status on survival in gastric carcinoma. *Cancer* 1989;64:1007–1010.
33. Yokozaki H, Takemura N, Takanashi A, Tabuchi J, Haruta R, Tahara E. Estrogen receptors in gastric adenocarcinoma: a retrospective immunohistochemical analysis. *Virchows Arch A* 1988;413:297–302.
34. Frost AR, Terahata S, Siegel RS, Overmoyer B, Silverberg SG. An analysis of prognostic features in infiltrating lobular carcinoma of the breast. *Mod Pathol* 1995;8:830–836.
35. Kurtz JM, Jacquemier J, Torhorst J, et al. Conservation therapy for breast cancers other than infiltrating ductal carcinoma. *Cancer* 1989; 63:1630–1635.
36. Poen JC, Tran L, Juillard G, et al. Conservation therapy for invasive lobular carcinoma of the breast. *Cancer* 1992;69:2789–2795.
37. Sastre-Garau X, Jouve M, Asselain B, et al. Infiltrating lobular carcinoma of the breast. Clinicopathologic analysis of 975 cases with reference to data on conservative therapy and metastatic patterns. *Cancer* 1996;77:113–120.
38. Warneke J, Berger R, Johnson C, Stea D, Villar H. Lumpectomy and radiation treatment for invasive lobular carcinoma of the breast. *Am J Surg* 1996;172:496–500.
39. Schnitt SJ, Connolly JL, Recht A, Silver B, Harris JR. Influence of lobular histology on local tumor control in breast cancer patients treated with conservative surgery and radiotherapy. *Cancer* 1989;64:448–454.

CHAPTER 23

Mesenchymal Tumors

BENIGN MESENCHYMAL TUMORS

Fibromatosis is an infiltrating, histologically low-grade spindle-cell neoplasm composed of fibroblastic cells with variable amounts of collagen.

Patients with mammary fibromatosis range in age from 13 to 80 years at diagnosis, averaging 37 to 49 years in three reported series (1–3). They usually present with a palpable, firm, painless mass that may suggest carcinoma on clinical examination. Bilateral fibromatosis is very uncommon. Mammography reveals a stellate tumor that may be indistinguishable from carcinoma (1,3–6). Calcifications are rarely formed in mammary fibromatosis, but they may be present in a benign proliferative lesion, such as sclerosing adenosis, that has been engulfed by the tumor. Rarely, the tumor may be nonpalpable and initially detected by mammography (7). Antecedent injury or surgery has been reported at the site of fibromatosis in some patients, and an association with breast augmentation implants has been reported in several cases. Tumor size averages 2.5 to 3.0 cm (2,3).

A single lesion may have varied growth patterns, a feature that complicates the diagnosis of fibromatosis by needle core biopsy. The microscopic components of the tumor are spindle cells and collagen. Areas in which the collagenous element is accentuated have a keloidal appearance (Fig. 1). More commonly, the lesion is composed of a moderately cellular spindle-cell proliferation in which there is modest collagen deposition. Mitotic figures are very infrequent or undetectable. In most tumors, the cells have small, pale, oval or spindly nuclei with little pleomorphism (Fig. 2). The tumor cells are usually distributed in broad sheets, sometimes in a storiform configuration or in the form of interlacing bundles. Actin-positive myofibroblasts are usually inconspicuous. In addition to varied amounts of collagenization, the stroma sometimes has focal myxoid areas. Focal lymphocytic infiltrates are found in nearly half of the tumors, especially at the periphery (Fig. 3). Regardless of how well demarcated the lesions seem to be grossly, all have at least some stellate extensions into the surrounding fat and glandular parenchyma. It is usually possible to find ducts and lobules engulfed by these extensions at the periphery of the tumor (Fig. 4). The differential diagnosis of mammary fibromatosis includes scarring from trauma or prior surgery, metaplastic spindle-cell carcinoma, and other spindle-cell mesenchymal tumors, including cystosarcoma.

Recommended treatment is wide local excision. The frequency of local recurrence ranges from 21% to 27% (1–3). Histologic features such as cellularity, mitotic activity, and cellular pleomorphism are not helpful for predicting recurrence. Although the risk for recurrence is higher in patients with documented positive margins, recurrences have been observed in cases with apparently negative margins (3).

Fibrous tumor (focal fibrous disease) is a discrete breast tumor composed of collagenized mammary stroma (8). Fibrous tumor is a disease of premenopausal women. Mammography reveals an area of density with borders varying from irregular to smooth. Calcifications are not a feature of fibrous tumor. This benign stromal proliferation is treated by local excision.

Histologically, examination reveals normal-appearing collagenous stroma in which ductal and lobular elements are markedly decreased or absent (8,9). The findings in a needle core biopsy specimen are nonspecific and are usually reported as "fibrosis" (Fig. 5). Capillaries, other vascular structures, and nerves are very sparse; perivascular and perilobular inflammatory infiltrates are absent. Cysts, apocrine metaplasia, sclerosing adenosis, and duct hyperplasia are not features of fibrous tumor. Pseudoangiomatous stromal hyperplasia is not a feature of fibrous tumor.

Pseudoangiomatous stromal hyperplasia (PASH) can be mistaken for angiosarcoma. The term pseudoangiomatous was proposed to emphasize the fact that the histologic pattern mimics but does not actually constitute a vasoformative proliferation. PASH is a tumor formed by myofibroblasts with variable expression of myoid and fibroblastic features. Glandular hyperplasia is sometimes also present.

With one exception, reported examples of tumor-forming PASH have been in women. It is a frequent incidental microscopic component of gynecomastia, having been found in 44 of 93 consecutive male breast biopsy specimens (47.4%); 43 of the 44 male specimens with PASH were from patients with gynecomastia (10). Age at diagnosis in female patients ranges from the teens to the middle fifties, with a median age in the middle to late thirties (11–13). Almost all patients have been premenopausal, but PASH can occur in postmenopausal women on estrogen. Most women have a palpable, painless, unilateral mass that is firm or rubbery. Palpable tumors average 5 cm in diameter. Skin necrosis has been

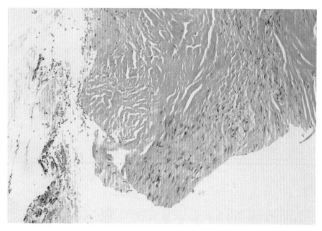

FIGURE 1. Fibromatosis, keloidal. This needle core biopsy specimen shows an area of dense collagenous tissue adjacent to a more cellular component of the lesion. The slit-shaped spaces in the keloidal tissue create a resemblance to pseudoangiomatous stromal hyperplasia.

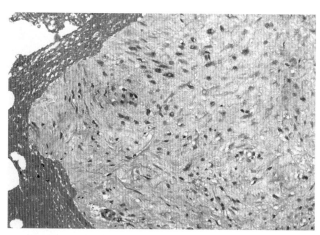

FIGURE 2. Fibromatosis. A needle core biopsy specimen showing average cellularity and slight stromal edema. The tumor cells have uniform, round-to-oval nuclei.

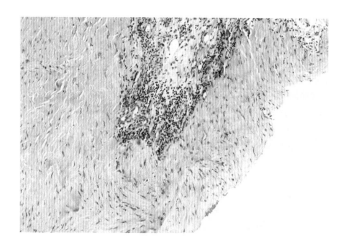

FIGURE 3. Fibromatosis. A perivascular lymphocytic infiltrate is apparent in this needle core biopsy specimen.

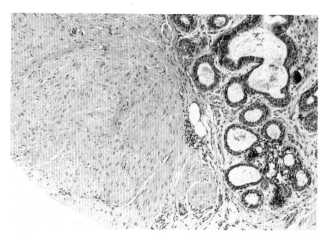

FIGURE 4. Fibromatosis. The tumor invades up to a lobule in this part of a needle core biopsy specimen.

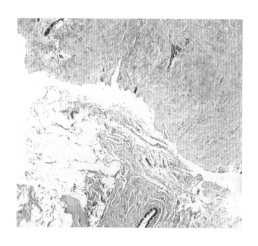

FIGURE 5. Fibrous tumor. The upper sample in this needle core biopsy specimen shows collagenous tissue from the tumor. In the lower sample, a duct is surrounded by normal fibrofatty tissue.

observed in patients who have massive breast enlargement caused by PASH during pregnancy.

Pseudoangiomatous stromal hyperplasia has been detected by mammography in patients who were asymptomatic (14,15). The lesions present as masses without calcification. The borders are usually smooth, but a minority of the tumors are spiculated or have ill-defined margins sometimes obscured by surrounding tissue. Ultrasound reveals a well-defined hypoechoic mass (15). Clinically asymptomatic PASH detected by mammography may occur in postmenopausal patients, whereas palpable lesions are almost always found in premenopausal women or in postmenopausal women who have been treated with hormone replacement therapy.

The tumors are composed of intermixed stromal and epithelial elements. The lobular and duct structures of the breast parenchyma are usually separated by an increased amount of stroma. Collagenization of intralobular stroma and duct attenuation producing fibroadenoma-like features are common. Nonspecific proliferative epithelial changes include mild hyperplasia of duct and lobular epithelium, often with some accentuation of myoepithelial cells, and apocrine metaplasia with or without cyst formation.

The most striking histologic finding is a complex pattern of anastomosing, slit-shaped spaces in the intralobular as well as interlobular stroma (Fig. 6). Myofibroblasts present singly and intermittently at the margins of the spaces resemble endothelial cells. The nuclei of most of the myofibroblasts are attenuated, lack atypia, and rarely show mitotic activity. Rarely, some of these cells are enlarged and have noticeably hyperchromatic nuclei. Also present in the stroma are round or oval blood-containing true capillaries lined by endothelial cells (Figs. 6,7).

The myofibroblasts may accumulate in distinct bundles or fascicles in a background of more conventional PASH (Figs. 8,9). The most pronounced examples of this cellular form of PASH have a growth pattern reminiscent of a myofibroblastoma. This is especially the case when the myofibroblasts have abundant cytoplasm and PASH occurs as a localized tumor rather than as a diffuse process. Myofibroblastoma and PASH are related conditions, possibly representing the extremes of a spectrum of lesions that share a common histogenesis in the myofibroblasts. An atypical form of PASH is composed of pleomorphic nuclei and mitotic figures (Fig. 10).

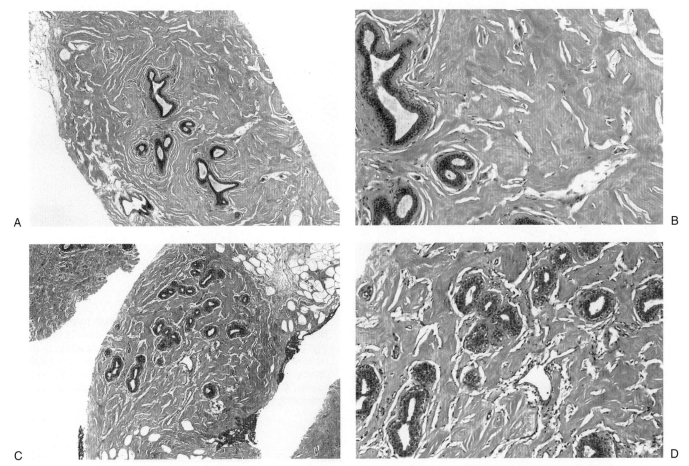

FIGURE 6. Pseudoangiomatous stromal hyperplasia. Needle core biopsy specimens from two patients. **A,B:** In this instance, myofibroblasts are inconspicuous, and the slit-shaped spaces are largely unconnected. Collagen fibrils extend across some of the spaces. **C,D:** This very pronounced pseudoangiomatous proliferation involves a lobule and the surrounding stroma.

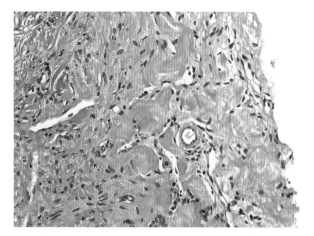

FIGURE 7. Pseudoangiomatous stromal hyperplasia.
Small blood vessels are distributed among the pseudoangiomatous spaces in this needle core biopsy specimen.

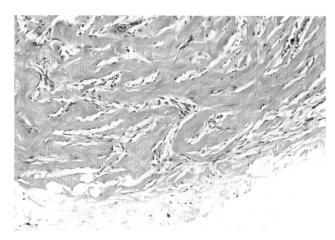

FIGURE 8. Pseudoangiomatous stromal hyperplasia.
The lesion in this needle core biopsy specimen has a circumscribed border. The presence of myofibroblastic nuclei in
some of the spaces is an early phase in the development of
the fascicular pattern.

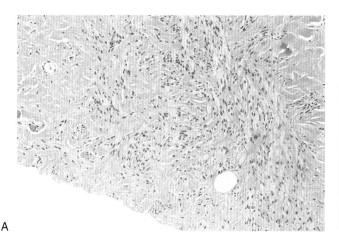

A

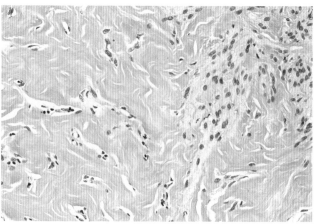

B

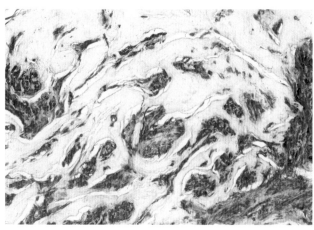

C

**FIGURE 9. Pseudoangiomatous stromal hyperplasia,
fascicular. A:** Myofibroblasts have formed distinct bundles
that are distributed in the pseudoangiomatous pattern in this
needle core biopsy specimen. **B:** Another portion of the
specimen showing pseudoangiomatous and fascicular elements. **C:** The myofibroblasts are immunoreactive for actin
(immunoperoxidase).

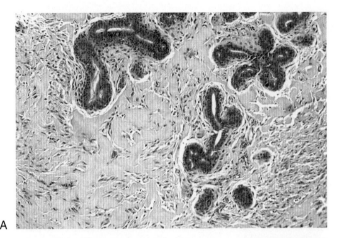

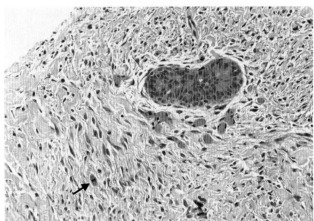

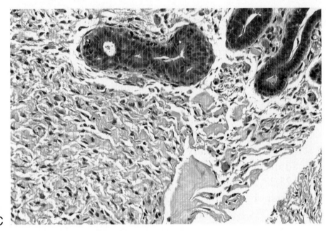

FIGURE 10. Atypical pseudoangiomatous stromal hyperplasia, fascicular. A–C: This needle core biopsy specimen was obtained from a 12-cm tumor in a 29-year-old woman. The stroma has occasional mitotic figures (*arrow*) and is focally very cellular. The pseudoangiomatous pattern is maintained in cellular foci. Ductal hyperplasia is also evident.

Basement membrane material is not demonstrable around the slitlike spaces. Myofibroblasts defining the pseudo-angiomatous spaces exhibit strong immunoreactivity for vimentin and variable reactivity for actin. They show no immunoreactivity for vascular markers. The nuclei of myofibroblasts in PASH are sometimes immunoreactive for progesterone receptor (11,16). Estrogen receptor is absent or only weakly present when the tissues are examined by immunohistochemistry (16,17). CD34 reactivity can be demonstrated in the majority of lesions (16).

Pseudoangiomatous stromal hyperplasia that forms a clinically palpable tumorous mass appears to be an exaggerated manifestation of physiologic changes commonly encountered microscopically. Ibrahim et al. (12) found microscopic foci of PASH in 23% of 200 consecutive breast specimens obtained for benign or malignant conditions. Eighty-nine percent of the patients were younger than 50 years. The majority of these specimens also exhibited epithelial hyperplasia, sometimes including secretory changes in lobules. Most patients have remained well after excisional biopsy, but ipsilateral recurrences have developed in some cases. Bilateral involvement, an infrequent occurrence, may be simultaneous or metachronous.

Myofibroblastoma is a benign tumorous proliferation of myofibroblasts. These spindle-shaped or fusiform mesenchymal cells have cytoplasmic actinlike microfilaments measuring 5 to 7 nm in diameter with focal dense bodies and pinocytotic vesicles. In contrast to myoepithelial cells, they lack prekeratin tonofilaments and are not immunoreactive for cytokeratin. Desmosomes are absent or poorly formed between myofibroblasts. Depending on their phenotypic state, the cells may be reactive with antiactin antibodies.

The patient typically presents with a solitary unilateral mass in the breast. The median age is about 65 years. The majority of patients reported to have myofibroblastoma have been men, but the lesion also occurs in women (18). Radiographically, the tumors are homogeneous, lobulated, and well circumscribed, and they lack microcalcifications (19,20). The average diameter of the tumor is about 2 cm, with most smaller than 4 cm. Extremes of size include one lesion that measured 0.9 cm (18) and one 10-cm tumor (21). Excisional biopsy is adequate treatment in most cases, and local recurrence is infrequent.

The classic type of myofibroblastoma is composed of bundles of slender, bipolar, uniform, spindle-shaped cells, typically arranged in clusters separated by broad bands of hyalinized collagen distributed throughout the tumor (22) (Fig. 11). Multinucleated giant cells are uncommon, and mitotic figures are sparse or undetectable. Fat cells, ducts, and lobules are present in a minority of lesions. Some lesions have foci of leiomyomatous differentiation. A perivascular lymphoplasmacytic infiltrate is sometimes identified. The

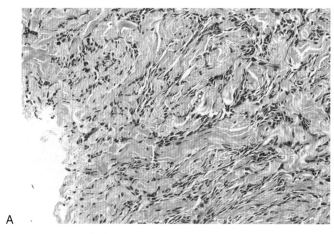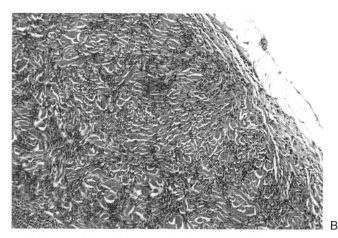

A   B

FIGURE 11. Myofibroblastoma. A: This needle core biopsy specimen shows the characteristic fascicles of myofibroblasts and intervening bands of collagen. **B:** The excised tumor had a circumscribed bor-

border of the tumor is usually circumscribed microscopically, but in a minority of cases the tumor has an invasive margin. The majority of myofibroblastomas are immunoreactive for desmin, vimentin, actin, and CD34. The tumors are not immunoreactive for cytokeratin or factor VIII and only rarely weakly reactive for S-100 protein.

Variant forms of myofibroblastoma have received little attention. In a *collagenized* myofibroblastoma, the spindle cells are distributed in diffusely collagenized stroma (Fig. 12). Irregular, slitlike spaces formed between tumor cells and the stroma are reminiscent of PASH. The *epithelioid* variant features polygonal or epithelioid cells arranged in alveolar groups (Fig. 13) mixed with classic myofibroblastoma elements. A *cellular, infiltrating* type of myofibroblastoma is formed by dense proliferation of spindle-shaped neoplastic myofibroblasts with cytologic atypia. Collagenous bands may be absent in some parts of the lesion. These tumors tend to have infiltrative borders microscopically (Fig. 14).

Granular-cell neoplasms are derived from the Schwann cells of peripheral nerves. They occur throughout the body,

with about 5% of them originating in the breast (23). The patient usually presents with a solitary firm or hard painless mass, most often located in the upper and medial breast quadrants. On mammography, granular-cell tumor of the breast (GCTB) is difficult to distinguish from carcinoma (24,25), and coexistence of the two lesions has been described (26). It typically forms a stellate mass lacking calcifications, but circumscribed lesions have been reported (24,25,27,28). Ultrasound usually reveals a solid mass with posterior shadowing, suggestive of carcinoma (27,28). Benign GCTB is treated by wide excision. Local recurrence may develop after incomplete excision. Fewer than 1% of all granular-cell tumors, including mammary lesions, are malignant.

Granular-cell tumor of the breast is composed of compact nests or sheets of cells that contain eosinophilic cytoplasmic granules (Fig. 15). In some lesions, there is a tendency to cytoplasmic vacuolization and clearing. The cytoplasmic granules are positive for periodic acid–Schiff (PAS) and diastase-resistant. Cell borders are typically well defined, and the cells vary from polygonal to spindle-shaped. Variable amounts of collagenous stroma are present. Nuclei are round to slightly oval with an open chromatin pattern. Nucleoli tend to be prominent. A modest amount of nuclear pleomorphism, occasional multinucleated cells, and rare mitoses may be found, but these features should not be interpreted as evidence of a malignant neoplasm. Small nerve bundles are sometimes seen in the tumor or in close association with the peripheral invasive border. Ducts and lobules are typically surrounded by the invasive tumor cells and incorporated into the lesion.

The differential diagnosis of GCTB includes apocrine carcinoma and histiocytic or granulomatous lesions. The presence of intraductal carcinoma, often of the comedo type, as well as marked cytologic pleomorphism usually serve to identify apocrine carcinoma, but these features may be absent from a needle core biopsy specimen. The lesions can be distinguished with confidence by histochemical studies. GCTB is not reactive for epithelial markers and does not

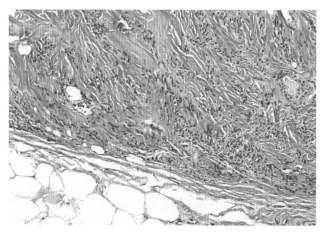

FIGURE 12. Myofibroblastoma, collagenized. Inconspicuous bundles of myofibroblasts are distributed between prominent bands of collagen. The tumor has a circumscribed border.

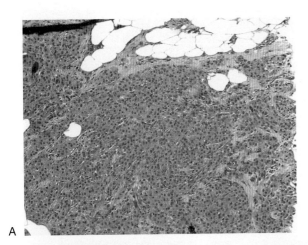

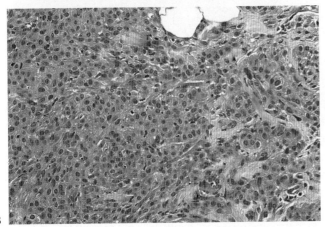

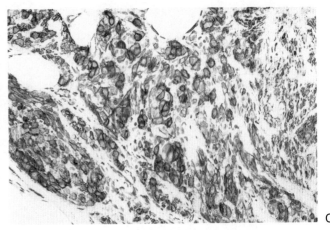

FIGURE 13. Myofibroblastoma, epithelioid. A,B: Epithelioid myofibroblasts form alveolar clusters and small bundles in this very cellular needle core biopsy specimen. This appearance could be mistaken for invasive carcinoma. **C:** The cells are strongly immunoreactive for smooth-muscle actin (immunoperoxidase).

contain mucin. The strong, diffuse immunoreactivity for S-100 protein and carcinoembryonic antigen (CEA) that characterizes granular-cell tumors does not by itself distinguish these lesions from mammary carcinoma (25,29–31). A high proportion of granular-cell tumors are reactive for vimentin, and they are negative for estrogen and progesterone receptors. GCTB is immunohistochemically negative for histio-

cyte-associated antigens such as alpha$_1$-antitrypsin and muramidase (25,29).

Tumors of nerve and nerve sheath origin of the breast have usually been diagnosed as "neurilemomas" (32–34) or as schwannomas. The age range at diagnosis is 15 to 78 years, with most patients in their thirties and forties. The lesion presents as a painless, well-defined mass. One schwan-

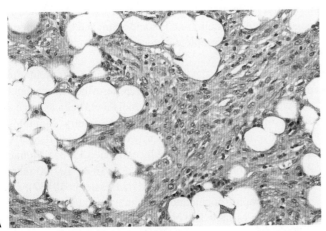

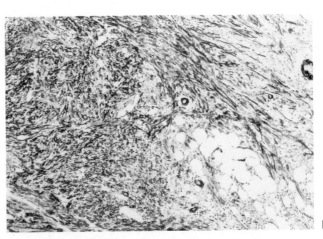

FIGURE 14. Myofibroblastoma, infiltrating. A: Tumor cells in fat might be mistaken for infiltrating carcinoma in this needle core biopsy specimen. **B:** The tumor cells are strongly immunoreactive for smooth-muscle actin (immunoperoxidase).

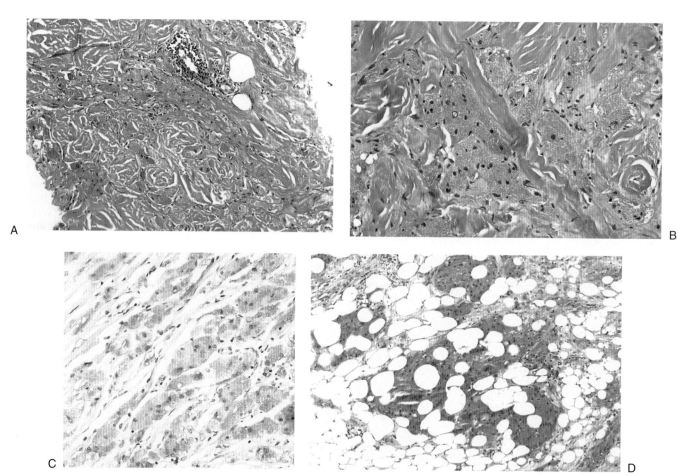

FIGURE 15. Granular-cell tumor. A,B: Bundles of elongated and polygonal tumor cells are present in the collagenous breast stroma in this needle core biopsy specimen. This appearance could be mistaken for infiltrating apocrine carcinoma. **C:** The tumor cells are strongly immunoreactive for S-100 protein (immunoperoxidase). **D:** Another lesion, in which a granular-cell tumor infiltrates fat and resembles infiltrating apocrine carcinoma.

noma was an asymptomatic 7-mm lesion detected by mammography (34). Microscopic examination reveals the typical histologic features of a benign nerve sheath tumor, consisting of spindle cells in bundles, sometimes with nuclei arranged in a palisading pattern (Antoni type A) (Fig. 16). Less

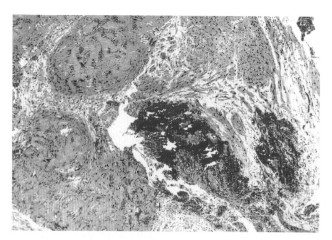

FIGURE 16. Schwannoma. The lesion has the Antoni type A pattern. Hemorrhage is at the site of a prior needle core biopsy.

cellular areas with thick-walled blood vessels, the Antoni B pattern, may be present as well. Vascular thrombi, hyalinized blood vessels, cells with atypical nuclei, and xanthomatous areas are found in sclerotic schwannomas. The diagnosis of a benign peripheral nerve sheath tumor is supported by a positive immunohistochemical stain for S-100 protein, a negative immunostain for CEA and actin, and the absence of mitotic activity. Complete excision provides adequate therapy.

Hamartoma of the breast occurs most often in premenopausal women, but it has been described in teenagers and women in their sixties. The tumors have been as large as 17 cm, often resulting in substantial asymmetry. Mammography reveals a well-circumscribed, dense, round or oval mass surrounded by a narrow lucent zone (35–37). Hamartomas of the breast were diagnosed in 16 of 10,000 mammography examinations reviewed by Hessler et al. (37). The ultrasonographic appearance of mammary hamartoma is reported to be variable and not specific (38).

There are two common histologic variants of mammary hamartoma. Radiologic examination of an ***adenolipoma*** demonstrates a sharply defined round or oval tumor that appears to be encapsulated and surrounded by a radiolucent

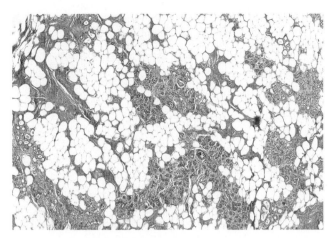

FIGURE 17. Adenolipoma. Normal lobules are distributed in lipomatous adipose tissue.

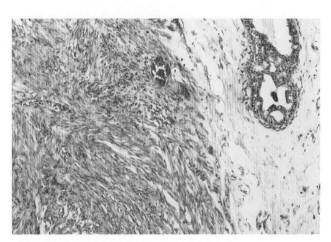

FIGURE 19. Leiomyoma. There is a suggestion of palisading in the arrangement of the smooth-muscle cells in this circumscribed tumor. There is micropapillary hyperplasia in an adjacent duct.

ring. Appearance in the mammogram varies with the composition of the tumor. Predominantly fatty tumors may have the lucent appearance of lipomas, whereas those with abundant glandular tissue appear dense (39,40). Ultrasonography reveals a mixed pattern of echogenic and sonolucent regions (41). Microscopically, the tissue consists of mature fat and mammary parenchyma mixed in varying proportions, delimited by a pseudocapsule of compressed breast tissue (Fig. 17). Lobules and ducts present in the lesion appear structurally normal with little or no proliferative change, the most significant abnormality being the unusual tissue distribution. *Chondrolipomas* are composed of mature adipose tissue and hyaline cartilage (42,43). Mammography reveals a well-circumscribed mass without calcification resembling a fibroadenoma (43). Histologically, the tumor consists of islands of hyaline cartilage distributed in mature fat and fibrofatty glandular mammary parenchyma (Fig. 18).

Leiomyomas of the breast arise most often from smooth muscle in the nipple and areola (44). Parenchymal leiomyomas probably arise as a result of smooth-muscle metaplasia of myoepithelial and myofibroblastic cells or from blood vessels. Radiologic examination reveals a circumscribed tu-

mor without calcification (45,46). Complete excision is recommended. Local recurrence is very uncommon.

Microscopically, the growth pattern features interlacing fascicles of spindle cells with eosinophilic cytoplasm (Fig. 19). Cytologic atypia, mitoses, and necrosis, which characterize leiomyosarcoma, are absent. The tumor cells are immunoreactive for desmin and actin but not for S-100 protein.

The so-called *leiomyomatous ("myoid") hamartoma* is a tumorous form of sclerosing adenosis with leiomyomatous myoid metaplasia of the myoepithelial cell component (47). Mammography reveals a well-demarcated tumor of variable density (48–50). The histologic composition of myoid hamartomas depends on the relative proportions of glandular, cystic, myomatous, and fibrous elements. In most lesions, interlacing bundles of smooth muscle constitute a focal leiomyoma, but in a minority of tumors, the myoid component mingles more diffusely with adipose and fibrous tissue (Fig. 20). Epithelioid differentiation of myoepithelial cells can result in a pattern resembling infiltrating lobular carcinoma, especially in the limited sample obtained by needle core biopsy (51). Adequate sampling reveals foci of sclerosing adenosis in virtually all examples of myoid hamartoma, and at these sites origin of the myoid element can be traced to myoepithelial cells. Associated "fibrocystic changes" include cystic apocrine metaplasia and duct hyperplasia (48,49).

Lipomas of the breast are usually solitary tumors, but multiple lipomas may be encountered. The tumors are circumscribed, well-defined masses of mature adipose tissue. In some instances, a clinically palpable lesion proves to be mature fat without the characteristic circumscription of lipoma. *Hibernomas* are composed of brown fat found in the axillary tail of the breast or in the axilla (Fig. 21). A *fibrolipoma* consists of mature adipose tissue and collagenous stroma that contains slightly prominent fibroblasts. Occasional ducts and lobular glands can be found in the substance of the tumor.

The *perilobular hemangioma* is a benign microscopic vascular lesion detected in sections of breast tissue taken to

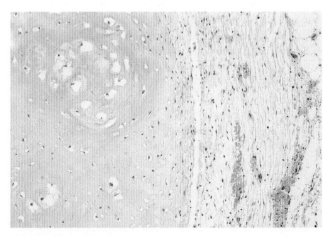

FIGURE 18. Chondrolipoma. Mature hyaline cartilage in a chondrolipoma.

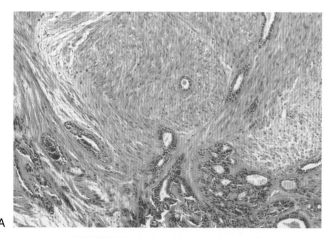
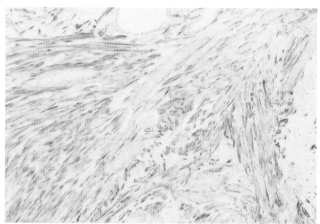

A   B

FIGURE 20. Leiomyoma ("myoid hamartoma"). A: Myomatous proliferation of myoepithelial cells is present in this nodular focus of adenosis. **B:** There is immunoreactivity for smooth-muscle actin in the myomatous areas. Adenosis glands are also apparent.

evaluate various unrelated benign and malignant lesions (52). A few have reportedly measured between 2 and 4 mm on a histologic section, but none was grossly or mammographically apparent (53,54). They have been found in 1.3% of specimens from mastectomies for carcinoma, 4.5% of specimens from biopsies for benign breast lesions, and in 11.0% of women whose breast tissue was sampled in forensic autopsies (52,53). Multiple perilobular hemangiomas may be found in one breast, and a number of patients have had these lesions in both breasts. There is no evidence that angiosarcomas arise from these lesions, although the existence of cytologically atypical variants leaves this issue open to speculation.

Microscopically, perilobular hemangiomas are not limited to a perilobular distribution. Many are partially or completely within the lobular stroma, whereas others are located in extralobular stroma, sometimes in proximity to ducts or apparently in no particular relationship to a duct or lobule. The lesion is typically a localized collection of distinct, capillary-size vascular channels arranged in a meshwork fashion (Fig. 22). Anastomosing channels may be seen. The thin, delicate vessels consist of endothelial cells encased in incon-

spicuous stroma. Some perilobular hemangiomas have endothelial cells that appear cytologically atypical because they have prominent, hyperchromatic nuclei (52).

Hemangiomas are benign vascular tumors large enough to be clinically palpable or detected by mammography (52). A substantial number of hemangiomas are currently detected by mammography in the absence of a clinically palpable tumor. Hemangiomas range in size from 0.4 to 2.0 cm, with a mean diameter of 0.9 cm. The majority of patients have been women 19 to 82 years of age (mean, 60 years). The mammographic appearance is usually that of a well-defined lobulated mass that may have fine or coarse calcifications (55,56). Almost all palpable vascular tumors of the male breast have been hemangiomas.

Cavernous hemangiomas are the most common form of mammary hemangioma. Microscopic examination reveals dilated vessels congested with red blood cells (Fig. 23). Small vessels of capillary dimension may be seen in portions of a cavernous hemangioma. The individual channels appear to be independent, there being few if any anastomosing vessels. Endothelial nuclei are inconspicuous and flat. Calcification may occur in the stroma. Thrombosis within cavernous channels sometimes elicits a lymphocytic reaction, and endothelial proliferation may be seen within the organizing clot. These alterations can result in papillary endothelial hyperplasia, which should not be mistaken for angiosarcoma. There is considerable variability in the degree of circumscription seen microscopically. In many cavernous hemangiomas, vascular channels drift into the fatty parenchyma, becoming smaller at the periphery (Fig. 24). This pattern duplicates the histologic appearance of peripheral parts of well-differentiated angiosarcoma.

Capillary hemangiomas tend to be cellular, with an average size of 1 cm. Many of these lesions have been detected by mammography. Fibrous septa frequently divide capillary hemangiomas into segments, resulting in a lobulated structure (Fig. 25). Some of the tumors have prominent anastomosing vascular channels. Papillary endothelial hyperplasia may be present at sites of organizing thrombosis. The small vascular

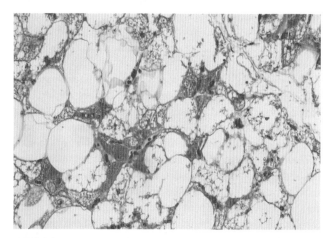

FIGURE 21. Hibernoma. Brown fat in a tumor from the axillary tail of the breast.

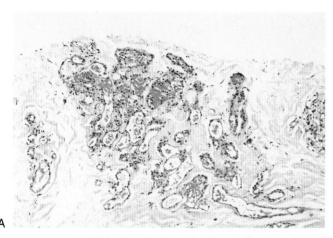

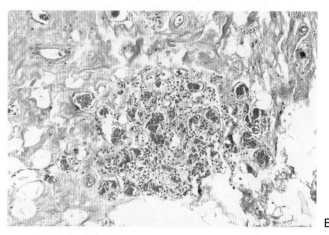

FIGURE 22. Perilobular hemangioma. A: This vascular lesion was an incidental finding in the specimen from a needle core biopsy performed to sample a nearby focus of nonpalpable calcifications in sclerosing adenosis. The hemangioma is located in interlobular stroma. **B:** An intralobular hemangioma in another needle core biopsy specimen. Several atrophic lobular glands are present in the lesion.

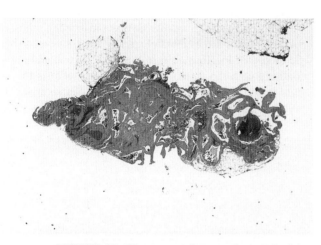

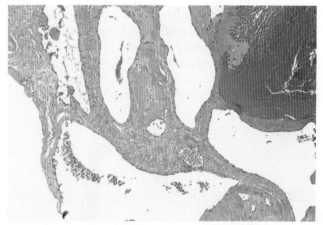

FIGURE 23. Cavernous hemangioma. A: A low-magnification view of the entire needle core biopsy specimen. Dilated vascular spaces are evident, some congested with red blood cells. **B:** The cavernous vascular channels are separated by slender fibrous bands and have a flat, inconspicuous lining of endothelial cells.

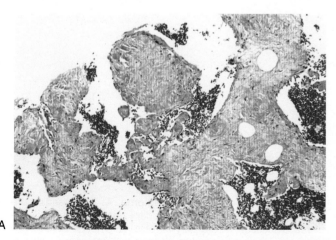

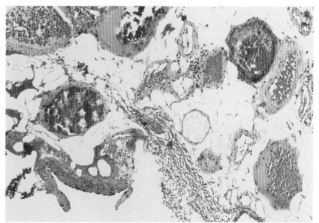

FIGURE 24. Cavernous hemangioma. A: A needle core biopsy specimen showing a portion of the lesion composed of dense fibrous stroma with a vaguely papillary structure. **B:** Another part of the tumor, with vascular structures extending into fat. *Figure continues*

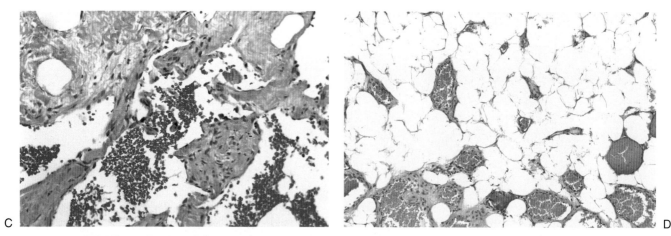

C

D

FIGURE 24. *Continued.* **C:** A papillary area in the excised hemangioma. The endothelium is flat and inconspicuous. **D:** Dilated vascular channels congested with red blood cells are growing into fat at the periphery of the excised tumor.

channels are lined by endothelial cells that may have hyperchromatic nuclei (Fig. 26). Muscular blood vessels may be found within and at the periphery of the tumor, apparently constituting the vessel that gave origin to the lesion.

Complex hemangiomas, consisting of dilated vascular channels of varying size as well as compact, dense aggregates of capillary structures, may also be detected by mammography. These lesions have an average size of 0.7 cm.

Some complex hemangiomas have conspicuous anastomosing vascular channels (Fig. 27).

Hemorrhage and infarction can occur in hemangiomas, especially lesions detected radiologically and subjected to needle biopsy or localization (see Fig. 23). This should not be confused with the pattern of hemorrhagic necrosis that results in the formation of "blood lakes," characteristically found in angiosarcomas. Calcification may occur in orga-

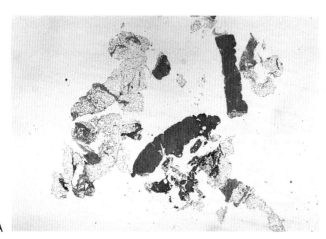

A

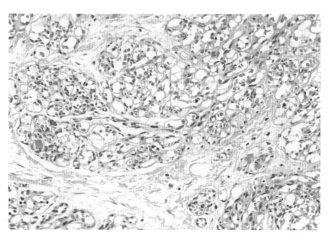

B

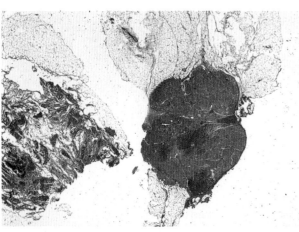

C

FIGURE 25. Capillary hemangioma. A: This needle core biopsy specimen contains two dark red cylinders of dense vascular tissue. **B:** Capillary vessels in the needle core biopsy specimen are arranged in clusters with intervening fibrous septa. **C:** The excised tumor has a lobular configuration.

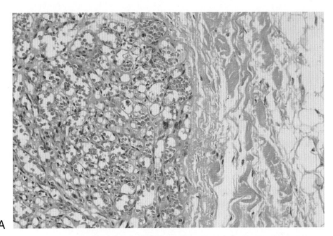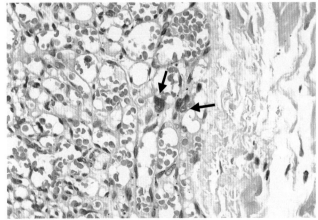

FIGURE 26. Capillary hemangioma. A,B: This needle core biopsy specimen shows the circumscribed border of the tumor. Some endothelial cells have prominent hyperchromatic nuclei (*arrows*).

nized thrombi, sometimes associated with endothelial hyperplasia, or in fibrous septa between vascular spaces. Marked septal fibrosis is sometimes found in hemangiomas.

Because of their dimensions, atypical cytologic features with mitoses in some instances, and concern that they might be precursors of angiosarcoma, some vascular lesions have been characterized as *"atypical" hemangiomas* (52) (Figs. 28,29). Additional follow-up has demonstrated that so-called atypical angiomas are not borderline or low-grade variants of angiosarcoma and provides no evidence that they predispose to the development of angiosarcoma (57).

Complete excision is necessary for accurate diagnosis. The material obtained with a needle core biopsy is not always sufficient for this purpose. Peripheral portions of a cavernous hemangioma may be indistinguishable from low-grade angiosarcoma in a small sample. Until recently, it has been possible to rely on the observation that hemangiomas rarely exceed 2.0 cm in diameter, whereas few angiosarcomas are smaller than 3.0 cm. This conclusion has been based primarily on data obtained from clinically palpable tumors. Currently, the availability of needle core biopsy samples

from small, nonpalpable vascular tumors has created a situation in which lesions smaller than 3 cm with the histologic appearance of angiosarcoma can be encountered.

Angiomatosis is a diffuse benign vascular lesion that produces a mass. The tumors have measured 9 to 11 cm and are grossly cystic. Microscopically, they are composed of anastomosing, large vascular channels extending diffusely in the breast parenchyma. They surround ducts and lobules but do not invade the lobular stroma. The vessels are lined by flat, inconspicuous endothelium with sparse supporting mural tissue that is virtually devoid of smooth muscle (Fig. 30). The lesions consist predominantly of hemangiomatous erythrocyte-containing channels or lymphangiomatous empty channels accompanied by lymphoid aggregates, or a mixture of the two. Angiomatosis may occur in breast tissue involved by other conditions, such as fibroadenoma.

The microscopic distinction between low-grade angiosarcoma and angiomatosis may be difficult, especially in a small biopsy sample, because anastomosing channels that are "empty" or contain erythrocytes occur in both lesions. In angiosarcomas, the vascular channels grow into lobules that

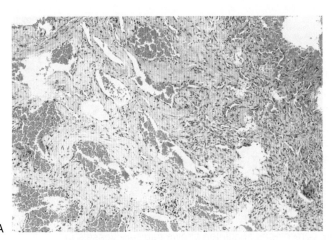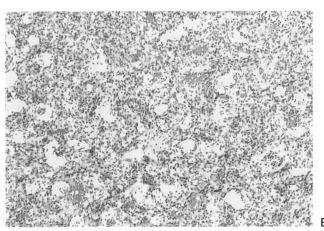

FIGURE 27. Complex hemangiomas. A: Vessels on the left have a cavernous appearance, whereas on the right there is a more cellular capillary network. **B:** Another hemangioma, in which cellular fibrous stroma is distributed between capillary vessels.

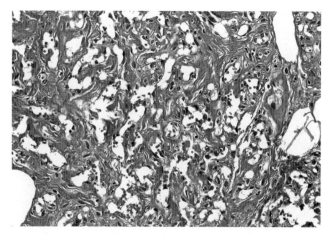

FIGURE 28. Atypical hemangioma. Endothelial cells in this needle core biopsy specimen have large, hyperchromatic nuclei.

are consequently destroyed, whereas lobules are spared in angiomatosis as the vascular proliferation surrounds but does not invade them.

Venous hemangiomas usually present as palpable tumors in patients averaging 40 years of age, but the lesion may be small enough to be detected only by mammography. The tumors have measured from 1.0 to 5.3 cm in greatest diameter (average, 3.2 cm). All have open venous channels with smooth-muscle walls of varying structural completeness (Fig. 31). Red blood cells are present in the lumina of some vascular spaces. Others are empty or contain lymph. Thick-walled arterial channels and capillaries are usually not conspicuous. Lobules and ducts can be found distributed in the mammary stroma between the vascular channels, and focal, perivascular lymphocytic infiltrates are usually present in the stroma.

Nonparenchymal mammary hemangiomas occur in the mammary region (58). Some lesions occur in the inframammary region, whereas others are distributed in various quadrants. The presenting symptom is a mass in most cases, but nonpalpable lesions have been detected by mammography. Tumor size ranges from 0.8 to 3.2 cm, averaging 1.8 cm. Breast parenchyma may be included in the biopsy specimen. The lesion is classified as nonparenchymal if the neoplastic vessels do not mingle with the glandular tissue. Several types of hemangiomas have been identified: angiolipoma, cavernous hemangioma, papillary endothelial hyperplasia, and capillary hemangiomas (Figs. 32,33). The histologic appear-

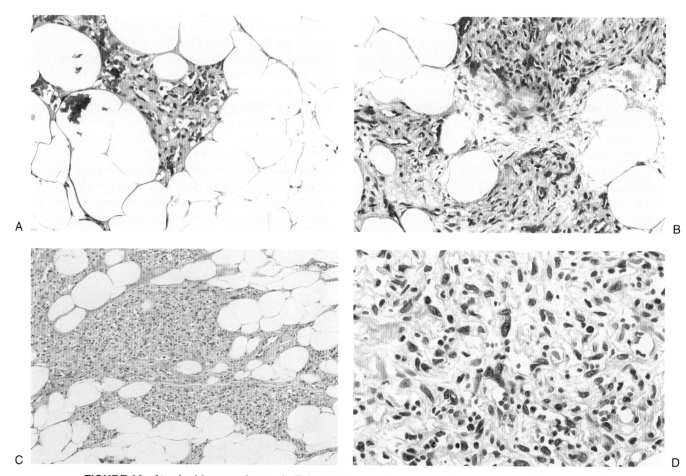

FIGURE 29. Atypical hemangioma. A: This needle core biopsy specimen shows capillary vessels in fat. **B:** A more compact portion of the same specimen. **C,D:** The excised tumor has an invasive growth pattern. Endothelial cell nuclei in the anastomosing capillary channels are pleomorphic and hyperchromatic. No mitotic figures were identified.

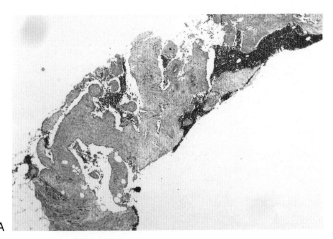
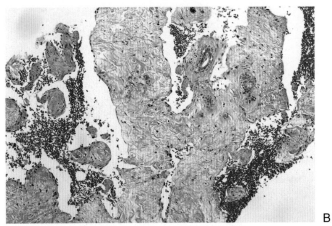

A

B

FIGURE 30. Angiomatosis. A,B: This needle core biopsy specimen reveals anastomosing dilated vascular spaces in fibrous breast stroma that contains several ducts.

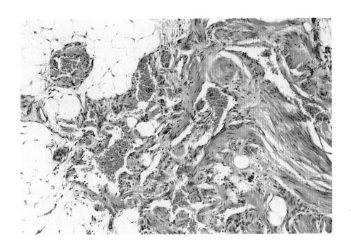

FIGURE 31. Venous hemangioma. The lesion in this needle core biopsy specimen is composed of vascular structures of various sizes with mural smooth muscle.

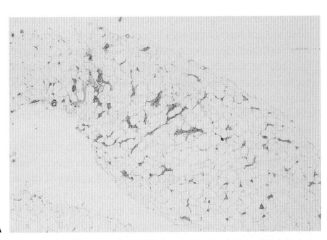
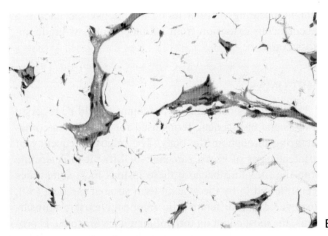

A

B

FIGURE 32. Nonparenchymal angiolipoma. A,B: Capillaries are dispersed in fat in this needle core biopsy specimen. A specimen such as this should be interpreted with caution because areas with a very similar histologic appearance can be found at the periphery of an angiosarcoma.

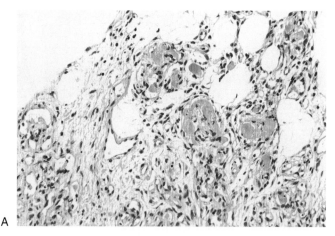

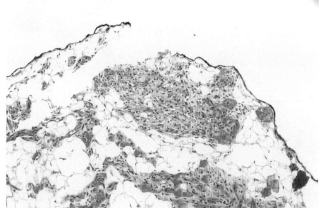

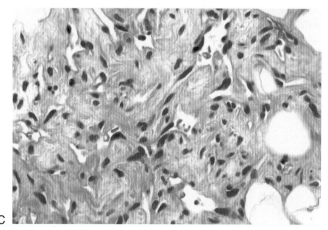

FIGURE 33. Nonparenchymal angiolipoma with atypia.
A: This needle core biopsy specimen displays a compact area of capillary proliferation. Some cells have hyperchromatic nuclei. Microthrombi, which characterize angiolipomas, are present. **B:** The excised tumor extended to an inked margin. **C:** This part of the excised tumor resembles the needle core biopsy specimen. Prominent hyperchromatic endothelial nuclei are shown.

ances of various types of hemangiomas in the mammary subcutaneous tissue does not differ from those of comparable lesions in other subcutaneous locations. Some hemangiomas found in mammary subcutaneous tissue feature interconnected vascular channels. Areas in which the septa are disrupted have a pseudopapillary pattern. Encapsulation, which characterizes many hemangiomas, cannot always be reliably assessed in a core biopsy sample. Complete removal of the tumor may be necessary to exclude the possibility that the benign-appearing vascular lesion in a biopsy specimen is a subcutaneous extension from an underlying low-grade angiosarcoma.

SARCOMAS

The diagnosis of mammary sarcomas should be reported in the same histogenetic terms used for soft-part sarcomas occurring throughout the body. The relative frequency of different types of breast sarcomas is difficult to determine from the literature because these lesions have sometimes been referred to by the general term stromal sarcoma (59). However, some differences in frequency exist. Angiosarcoma, the most common form of mammary sarcoma, is proportionately less frequent among somatic sarcomas. Other distinct mammary sarcomas include liposarcoma, fibrosarcoma, leiomyosarcoma, sarcomas with bone and cartilage, and malignant fibrous histiocytoma. A review of the re-

ported incidence of local recurrence in relation to primary treatment suggests that total mastectomy should be recommended for most sarcomas of the breast. When total mastectomy or a more extensive operation was the initial treatment, 8% had local failures, whereas recurrence in the breast was reported in 53% of patients treated by excisional surgery. Axillary lymph node metastases are exceedingly uncommon at the time of primary therapy, and therefore routine axillary dissection is not indicated (60,61).

A diagnosis of mammary sarcoma can be established only after metaplastic carcinoma has been excluded. Perhaps the most difficult distinction lies between fibrosarcoma and a metaplastic spindle-cell squamous carcinoma. Immunohistochemical studies for epithelial markers may be useful for detecting inconspicuous foci of epithelial expression in a carcinoma that has undergone virtually complete conversion into a spindle-cell neoplasm.

Angiosarcoma arises in the breast more often than in any other organ. With rare exceptions, the initial clinical finding is a painless mass. Blue or purple discoloration of the skin accompanies large or superficial tumors, but in some cases there are no external features to suggest angiosarcoma. Mammographic examination reveals an ill-defined, lobulated tumor with areas of high and low echogenicity on sonography (62,63). Rarely, nonpalpable angiosarcomas measuring less than 3 cm have been detected by mammography.

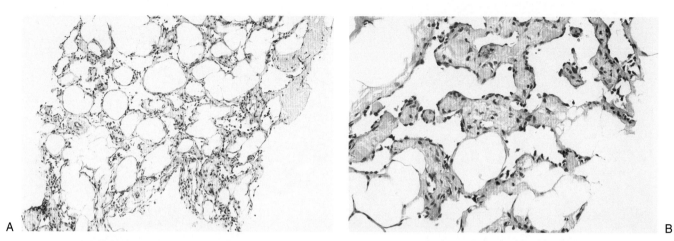

FIGURE 34. Angiosarcoma, low-grade. A,B: Open, empty, irregularly shaped vascular channels are distributed diffusely in this needle core biopsy specimen. The endothelial layer is flat, with slightly prominent nuclei.

Age at diagnosis ranges from the teens to older than 80 years, with a mean age at diagnosis of about 35 years. A statistically significant correlation between age at diagnosis and tumor grade was reported in one study (64). The median ages of patients with low-, intermediate-, and high-grade tumors were 43, 34, and 29 years, respectively. Because of the relative youth of patients with mammary angiosarcoma, it is not unexpected that a number of the patients were also pregnant (64,65).

A substantial number of angiosarcomas have been described in the breast after breast-conserving surgery and irradiation for carcinoma (66–68). The interval between radiation and the diagnosis of angiosarcoma ranged from 3 to 12 years, with the majority occurring within 6 years after radiotherapy (67). Almost all of these women were more than 50 years of age when treated for mammary carcinoma (67). Cutaneous presentation of angiosarcoma of the breast is more frequent after therapeutic irradiation for mammary carcinoma than is parenchymal angiosarcoma in the conserved breast. Many patients who present with angiosarcoma in the

skin also have parenchymal involvement (69–72). The estimated risk of cutaneous or parenchymal angiosarcoma of the breast after breast conservation and radiation for carcinoma is about 0.4% (69). Rarely, angiosarcoma has been found in a breast affected by mammary carcinoma without a history of radiotherapy (73).

The tumors average about 5 cm, with very few angiosarcomas smaller than 2 cm. There is no significant difference in the average size of high- and low-grade lesions.

Studies in the past decade have shown mammary angiosarcoma to be a morphologically heterogeneous group of neoplasms in which grade is prognostically significant (64,74,75). Three histologic patterns of growth in the primary tumor have been described. Low-grade (type 1) tumors are composed of open, anastomosing vascular channels that have proliferated diffusely in mammary glandular tissue and fat (Fig. 34). Infiltration into lobules is characterized by spread of the vascular channels within the intralobular stroma, a process that leads to separation and atrophy of the lobular glandular units (Fig. 35). Endothelial cells are dis-

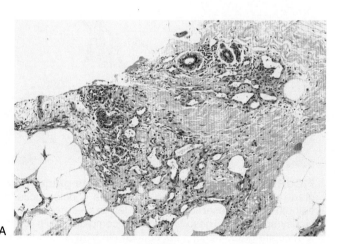
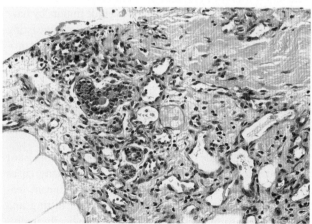

FIGURE 35. Angiosarcoma, low-grade. A,B: Neoplastic vascular channels invade around and into lobules in this needle core biopsy specimen.

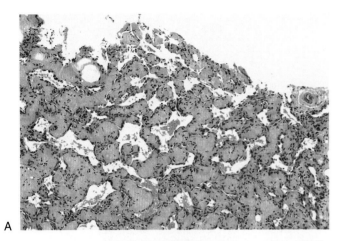

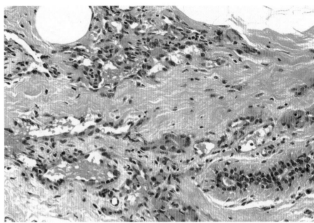

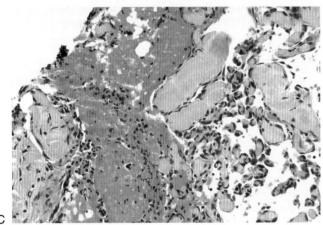

FIGURE 36. Angiosarcoma, intermediate-grade. A: This needle core biopsy sample shows a low-grade area with fibrous stroma between anastomosing vascular channels. **B:** The endothelial cells have enlarged, hyperchromatic nuclei. **C:** This region in the specimen shows focal intermediate-grade angiosarcoma with papillary endothelial growth and thrombosis.

tributed in a flat, single-cell layer around the vascular spaces, with papillary formations absent or at most very infrequent. Some prominent, hyperchromatic endothelial nuclei may be found, but the endothelial cells often have inconspicuous nuclei. Mitotic figures are rarely seen in the neoplastic endothelial cells. The vascular lumina are usually open and interanastomosing. Red blood cells are typically present in small numbers, but occasional lesions are congested.

Low-grade components can be found in high-grade lesions, sometimes comprising the bulk of the tumor. This is particularly true for intermediate-grade (type 2) angiosarcomas, which are distinguished from low-grade tumors by having scattered focal areas of cellular proliferation consisting of small buds or papillary fronds of endothelial cells that project into the vascular lumina (Fig. 36). Less often, the focally cellular areas feature polygonal and spindle cells, or there are foci that combine spindle-cell and papillary elements (Fig. 37). Mitoses may be found in papillary or spindle-cell cellular areas. Some spindle-cell foci resemble lesions encountered in Kaposi sarcoma.

Part of a high-grade (type 3) angiosarcoma may consist of low- and intermediate-grade elements, but in many cases more than half of the tumor has high-grade malignant features. These consist of prominent endothelial tufting and solid papillary formations that contain cytologically malignant endothelial cells, or conspicuous solid and spindle-cell

areas virtually devoid of vascular elements (Fig. 38). Mitoses are usually present. Necrosis is found only in high-grade angiosarcomas. Some high-grade angiosarcomas, especially those that arise after radiotherapy, are composed of cells with epithelioid cytology and vesicular nuclei with

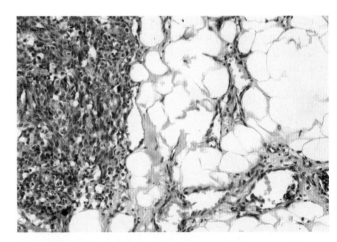

FIGURE 37. Angiosarcoma, intermediate-grade. Low-grade growth is shown on the right and a nodular focus of spindle-cell angiosarcoma on the left in this needle core biopsy specimen. These findings are compatible with an intermediate-grade tumor if the nodular element is found to be limited to isolated foci in the excised tumor.

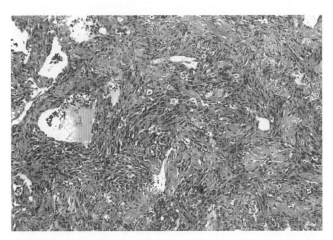

FIGURE 38. Angiosarcoma, high-grade. A relatively solid spindle-cell area is shown.

prominent nucleoli. The epithelioid appearance of these tumors may be mistaken for carcinoma (Fig. 39).

With few exceptions, angiosarcomas have infiltrative borders composed of well-formed or low-grade vascular channels. In some cases, the peripheral vascular component is so orderly that the neoplastic vascular channels are structurally indistinguishable from existing capillaries in the normal parenchyma. The tendency for peripheral portions to have a low-grade structure is likely to be misleading when a superficial biopsy specimen has been obtained from an intermediate- or high-grade tumor (76). If the initial sample does not indicate a high-grade lesion, thorough histologic evaluation of the entire tumor is required before the differentiation or grade of the tumor can be determined.

Two studies of mammary angiosarcomas reported more intense staining for factor VIII in well-differentiated than in poorly differentiated portions of the tumor (75,77). Angiosarcomas also exhibit reactivity for CD34, the hematopoietic progenitor cell antigen, and for CD31.

Tumor grade is the most important prognostic factor (64,74). The majority of patients with orderly or low-grade

lesions remain disease-free, whereas virtually all women with high-grade tumors have died of recurrent sarcoma within 5 years. Analysis of survival curves for patients stratified on the basis of tumor grade revealed the following estimated probabilities of disease-free survival 5 to 10 years after treatment: low grade, 76%; intermediate grade, 70%; and high grade, 15%. The median duration of disease-free survival was also correlated with tumor grade (low, >15 years; intermediate, >12 years; high, 15 months). The prognosis of angiosarcoma arising in the breast after radiotherapy is also determined by the degree of differentiation of the tumor, and when patients are stratified according to tumor grade, the prognosis does not appear to differ substantially from that of parenchymal angiosarcoma. Total mastectomy is the recommended primary surgical therapy. Axillary dissection is not indicated, as metastases rarely involve these lymph nodes.

Leiomyosarcoma of the breast usually originates from blood vessels or the smooth muscle of the nipple-areolar complex. A predisposition of smooth muscle in the nipple to give rise to neoplasms is evidenced by reports of leiomyomas and leiomyosarcomas at this site (78–81). The presenting symptom is a mass averaging about 4 cm. Mammography reveals a dense, noninvasive lesion. Approximately 25% of patients with mammary leiomyosarcoma with reported follow-up have died of metastatic sarcoma (81,82). Microscopically, the neoplasm consists of interlacing bundles of fusiform cells, characteristic of a smooth-muscle tumor, with typical blunt-ended nuclei (Fig. 40). Cells with an epithelioid phenotype are variably present. Malignant cytologic features are nuclear hyperchromasia, pleomorphism (sometimes with multinucleated giant cells), and readily identified mitoses. Focal areas of necrosis or hyalinized stromal fibrosis may be encountered. Immunohistochemical stains are positive for desmin and actin.

Liposarcoma of the breast occurs in patients 26 to 76 years of age at the time of diagnosis, with an average age of 49 years (83). The average size of mammary liposarcomas is 8 cm.

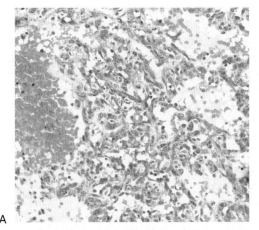
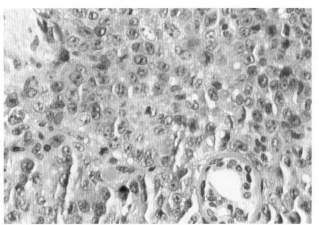

FIGURE 39. Angiosarcoma, high-grade epithelioid. A: This angiosarcoma arose in the breast 4 years after conservative surgery and radiotherapy. **B:** High-grade postradiation angiosarcoma with an epithelioid appearance. The tumor cells have characteristic vesicular nuclei and prominent nucleoli.

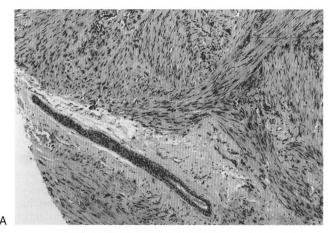
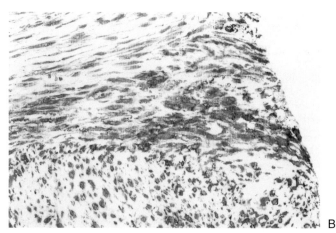

A   B

FIGURE 40. Leiomyosarcoma. A: A needle core biopsy specimen showing the sarcoma infiltrating around a duct. Note the cylindrical and pleomorphic tumor cell nuclei. **B:** The sarcoma is immunoreactive for smooth-muscle actin (immunoperoxidase).

The histologic features of liposarcoma in the breast are identical to those of liposarcoma arising in the extremities or trunk. Among 25 mammary tumors classified in these terms, 12 (48%) were myxoid, 6 (24%) were well differentiated, 4 (16%) were pleomorphic, and 3 (12%) were poorly differentiated (83–85) (Fig. 41).

Osteogenic sarcoma and chondrosarcoma of the mammary stroma are very uncommon. The precise frequency of these neoplasms is difficult to determine because some case reports do not clearly exclude metaplastic carcinoma or cystosarcoma. Mammography reveals a dense mass that may exhibit calcifications (86). One tumor was positive in a technetium diphosphonate Tc 99 scan (87). Age at diagnosis averages 55 years (88,89).

The tumors have had an average size of 10 cm. Histologic examination reveals osteogenic sarcoma and chondrosarcoma associated with a prominent component of high-grade spindle-cell sarcoma that has a variable mitotic rate. Chondrosarcomas are less frequent than sarcomas with osseous differentiation (Fig. 42). Multinucleated osteoclastic giant

cells are usually present in areas of bone formation. Rarely, giant cells constitute a conspicuous element, and they may be associated with hemorrhagic cysts with a telangiectatic appearance. Special stains, including immunohistochemistry for cytokeratin, are helpful in ruling out an epithelial component. Areas with cartilaginous differentiation can be immunoreactive for epithelial membrane antigen, and staining for S-100 protein is sometimes found in spindle-cell portions of the lesion (89).

Malignant fibrous histiocytoma presents as a mass averaging 7 cm in diameter (90,91). Necrosis and calcification are infrequent. The microscopic hallmark of malignant fibrous histiocytoma is a storiform growth pattern in which the spindle cells are arranged in a pinwheel pattern (Fig. 43). Capillaries or small blood vessels may be found at the center of the storiform complex. Giant cells, usually with multiple nuclei, myxoid change, and a chronic inflammatory cell infiltrate are variably present. High-grade lesions are characterized by easily identified mitoses, marked cellular pleomorphism, and necrosis. Low-grade tumors have little mitotic activity and minimal pleomorphism or necrosis.

Fibrosarcoma is a tumor in which the dominant growth pattern is formed by elongated spindle cells arranged in broad, interdigitating sheets, bands, or fascicles (so-called herringbone pattern) (90). Some fibrosarcomas lacking the classic herringbone pattern have a loosely structured fibroblastic proliferation. In one study, tumors with the fibrosarcomatous herringbone pattern tended to be low-grade histologically and to have a better prognosis than sarcomas with the malignant fibrous histiocytoma pattern, which were more often of a high grade (90).

Hemangiopericytoma of the breast is an uncommon neoplasm derived from the pericytes of blood vessels (92–94). Mammography in one case revealed a well-circumscribed, dense mass that was hypoechogenic with posterior enhancement on sonography (94). Reported follow-up in 15 cases varies from less than a year to 276 months, averaging 5 years. Approximately equal numbers of patients have been

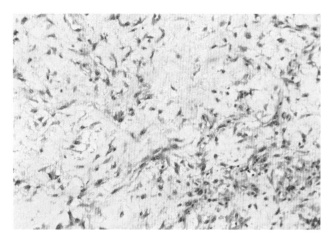

FIGURE 41. Liposarcoma. Myxoid liposarcoma with a characteristic network of capillary proliferation.

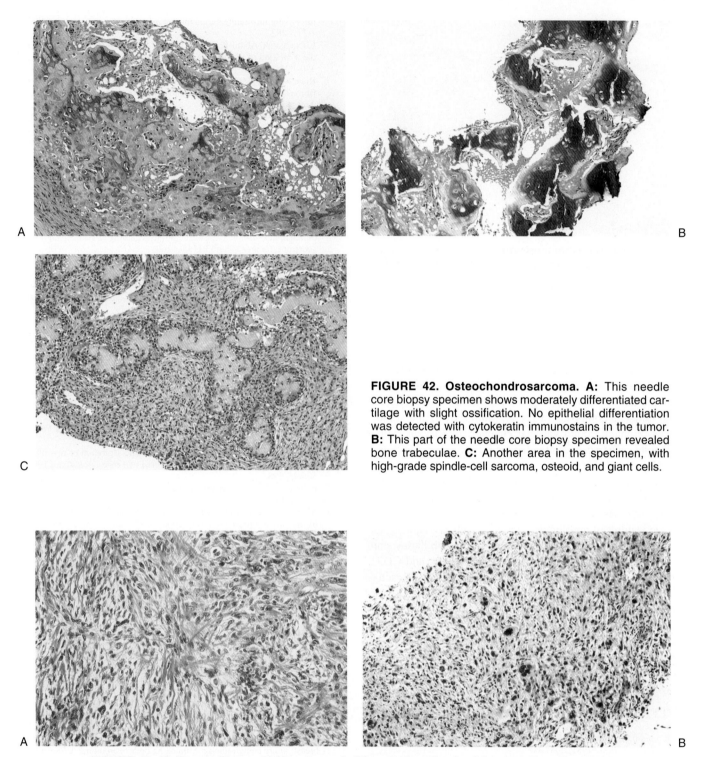

FIGURE 42. Osteochondrosarcoma. A: This needle core biopsy specimen shows moderately differentiated cartilage with slight ossification. No epithelial differentiation was detected with cytokeratin immunostains in the tumor. **B:** This part of the needle core biopsy specimen revealed bone trabeculae. **C:** Another area in the specimen, with high-grade spindle-cell sarcoma, osteoid, and giant cells.

FIGURE 43. Malignant fibrous histiocytoma. A: The spindle-cell tumor has a typical storiform structure. No epithelial differentiation was detected in the tumor. **B:** This needle core biopsy specimen from another tumor shows giant cells.

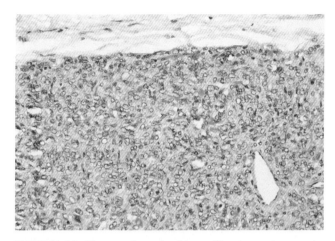

FIGURE 44. Hemangiopericytoma. The tumor has a circumscribed border. Numerous capillaries are highlighted by red blood cells. The dilated, empty vascular space in the lower right corner is a characteristic element.

treated by mastectomy and local excision. Local recurrence or systemic metastases have developed in none of the patients, whether treated by local excision or mastectomy. As a consequence, mammary hemangiopericytomas that lack high-grade features such as necrosis or numerous mitoses should be considered low-grade neoplasms. Histologically, the tumor is composed of round, plump, oval, and spindle cells oriented around vascular channels of varying caliber (Fig. 44). The vessels often have a branching or "staghorn" configuration. More compact zones have a spongiform appearance. The endothelium is supported by a delicate reticulin stroma without appreciable collagen or smooth-muscle cells. Mitoses are infrequent, and the cells lack other cytologic features of high-grade sarcomas, such as anaplasia and pleomorphic cells. Endothelial cells of the capillaries stain for *Ulex europaeus I* lectin, factor VIII, CD34, and CD31, but no reactivity has been found in the tumor cells. Reactivity for vimentin and variable staining for actin have been reported (92,93).

Other sarcomas described in the breast include ***malignant myofibroblastoma*** (95), ***angioblastic sarcoma, malignant peripheral nerve sheath tumors*** (96), and ***rhabdomyosarcoma*** (97,98).

REFERENCES

1. Gump FE, Sternschein MJ, Wolff, M. Fibromatosis of the breast. *Surg Gynecol Obstet* 1981;15:57–60.
2. Rosen PP, Ernsberger D. Mammary fibromatosis. A benign spindle cell tumor with significant risk for local recurrence. *Cancer* 1989;63:1363–1369.
3. Wargotz ES, Norris HJ, Austin RM, Enzinger FM. Fibromatosis of the breast. A clinical and pathological study of 28 cases. *Am J Surg Pathol* 1987;11:38–45.
4. Cederlund CG, Gustavsson S, Linell F, Moquist-Olsson I, Andersson I. Fibromatosis of the breast mimicking carcinoma at mammography. *Br J Radiol* 1984;57:98–101.
5. Kalisher L, Long JA, Peyster RG. Extra-abdominal desmoid of the axillary tail mimicking breast carcinoma. *Am J Roentgenol* 1976;126:903–906.
6. Leal SM, Poppiti RJ, Surujon I, Matallana R. Fibromatosis of the breast mimicking infiltrating carcinoma on mammography. *Breast Dis* 1989;1:277–282.
7. El-Naggar A, Abdul-Karim FW, Marshalleck JJ, Sorensen K. Fine needle aspiration of fibromatosis of the breast. *Diagn Cytopathol* 1987;3:320–322.
8. Rivera-Pomar JM, Vilanova JR, Burgos-Bretones JJ, Arocena G. Focal fibrous disease of breast. A common entity in young women. *Virchows Arch A* 1980;386:59–64.
9. Puente JL, Potel J. Fibrous tumor of the breast. *Arch Surg* 1974;109:391–394.
10. Badve S, Sloane JP. Pseudoangiomatous hyperplasia of male breast. *Histopathology* 1995;26:463–466.
11. Anderson C, Ricci A Jr, Pedersen CA, Cartun RW. Immunocytochemical analysis of estrogen and progesterone receptors in benign stromal lesions of the breast. Evidence for hormonal etiology in pseudoangiomatous hyperplasia of mammary stroma. *Am J Surg Pathol* 1991;15:145–149.
12. Ibrahim RE, Sciotto CG, Weidner N. Pseudoangiomatous hyperplasia of mammary stroma. Some observations regarding its clinicopathologic spectrum. *Cancer* 1989;63:1154–1160.
13. Vuitch MF, Rosen PP, Erlandson RA. Pseudoangiomatous hyperplasia of mammary stroma. *Hum Pathol* 1986;17:185–191.
14. Polger MR, Denison CM, Lester S, Meyer JE. Pseudoangiomatous stromal hyperplasia: mammographic and sonographic appearances. *AJR Am J Roentgenol* 1996;166:349–352.
15. Cohen MA, Morris EA, Rosen PP, Dershaw DD, Liberman L, Abramson AF. Pseudoangiomatous stromal hyperplasia: mammographic, sonographic and clinical patterns. *Radiology* 1996;198:117–120.
16. Powell CM, Cranor ML, Rosen PP. Pseudoangiomatous stromal hyperplasia (PASH): a mammary stromal tumor with myofibroblastic differentiation. *Am J Surg Pathol* 1995;19:270–277.
17. Fisher CJ, Hanby AM, Robinson L, Millis RR. Mammary hamartoma—a review of 35 cases. *Histopathology* 1992;20:99–106.
18. Hamele-Bena D, Cranor ML, Sciotto C, Erlandson R, Rosen PP. Uncommon presentation of mammary myofibroblastoma. *Hum Pathol* 1996;9:786–790.
19. Ordi J, Riverola A, Solé M, et al. Fine needle aspiration of myofibroblastoma of the breast in a man: a report of two cases. *Acta Cytol* 1992;36:194–198.
20. Rebner M, Raju U. Myofibroblastoma of the male breast. *Breast Dis* 1993;6:157–160.
21. Ali S, Teichberg S, Derisi DC, Urmacher C. Giant myofibroblastoma of the male breast. A case report. *Am J Surg Pathol* 1994;18:1170–1176.
22. Wargotz ES, Weiss SW, Norris HJ. Myofibroblastoma of the breast. Sixteen cases of a distinctive benign mesenchymal tumor. *Am J Surg Pathol* 1987;11:493–502.
23. Turnbull AD, Huvos AG, Ashikari R, Strong EW. Granular-cell myoblastoma of the breast. *N Y State J Med* 1971;71:436–438.
24. Bassett LW, Cove HC. Myoblastoma of the breast. *AJR Am J Roentgenol* 1979;132:122–123.
25. Willen R, Willen H, Balldin G, Albrechtsson V. Granular cell tumor of the mammary gland simulating malignancy. *Virchows Arch A* 1984;403:391–400.
26. Tai G, Costa H, Lee D, Watkins RM, Jones P. Case report: coincident granular cell tumour of the breast with invasive ductal carcinoma. *Br J Radiol* 1995;68:1034–1036.
27. Vos LD, Tham RTOTA, Vroegindweij D, Vrints LWMA. Granular cell tumor of the breast: mammographic and histologic correlation. *Eur J Radiol* 1994;19:56–59.
28. Green DH, Clark AH. Case report: granular cell myoblastoma of the breast: a rare benign tumour mimicking breast carcinoma. *Clin Radiol* 1995;50:799.
29. Buley ID, Gatter KC, Kelly PMA, Heryet A, Millard PR. Granular cell tumours revisited. An immunohistochemical and ultrastructural study. *Histopathology* 1988;12:263–274.
30. Hahn HJ, Iglesias J, Flenker H, Kreuzer G. Granular cell tumor in differential diagnosis of tumors of the breast. *Pathol Res Pract* 1992;188:1091–1094.
31. Ingram DL, Mossler JA, Snowhite J, Leight GS, McCarty KS Jr. Granular cell tumors of the breast. Steroid receptor analysis and localization of carcinoembryonic antigen, myoglobin and S-100 protein. *Arch Pathol Lab Med* 1984;108:897–901.
32. Majmudar B. Neurilemoma presenting as a lump in the breast. *South Med J* 1976;69:463–464.

33. van der Walt JD, Reid HA, Shaw JHF. Neurilemoma appearing as a lump in the breast. *Arch Pathol Lab Med* 1982;106:539–540.
34. Gultekin SH, Cody HS III, Hoda SA. Schwannoma of the breast. *South Med J* 1996;89:238–239.
35. Linell F, Ostberg G, Soderstrom J, Andersson I, Hildell J, Ljungqvist U. Breast hamartomas. An important entity in mammary pathology. *Virchows Arch A* 1979;383:253–264.
36. Evers K, Yeh I-T, Troupin RH, Patterson EA, Friedman AK. Mammary hamartomas. The importance of radiologic-pathologic correlation. *Breast Dis* 1992;5:35–43.
37. Hessler C, Schnyder P, Ozzello L. Hamartoma of the breast: Diagnostic observation of 16 cases. *Radiology* 1978;126:95–98.
38. Adler DD, Jeffries DO, Helvie MA. Sonographic features of breast hamartomas. *J Ultrasound Med* 1990;9:85–90.
39. Crothers JG, Butler NF, Fortt RW, Gravelle IH. Fibroadenolipoma of the breast. *Br J Radiol* 1985;58:191–202.
40. Jackson FI, Lalani Z, Swallow J. Adenolipoma of the breast. *J Can Assn Radiol* 1988;39:288–289.
41. Yasuda S, Kubota M, Noto T, et al. Two cases of adenolipoma of the breast. *Tokai J Exp Clin Med* 1992;17:139–144.
42. Lugo M, Reyes JM, Putony PB. Benign chondrolipomatous tumor of the human female breast. *Arch Pathol Lab Med* 1982;106:691–692.
43. Marsh WL Jr, Lucas JG, Olsen J. Chondrolipoma of the breast. *Arch Pathol Lab Med* 1989;113:369–371.
44. Nascimiento AG, Rosen PP, Karas M. Leiomyoma of the nipple. *Am J Surg Pathol* 1979;3:151–154.
45. Diaz-Arias AA, Hurt MA, Loy TS, Seeger RM, Bickel JT. Leiomyoma of the breast. *Hum Pathol* 1989;20:396–399.
46. Velasco M, Ubeda B, Autonel F, Serra C. Leiomyoma of the male areola infiltrating the breast tissue. *AJR Am J Roentgenol* 1995;164:511–512.
47. Eusebi V, Cunsolo A, Fedeli F, Severi B, Scarani P. Benign smooth muscle cell metaplasia in breast. *Tumori* 1980;66:643–653.
48. Huntrakoon M, Lin F. Muscular hamartoma of the breast. *Virchows Arch A* 1984;403:307–312.
49. Shepstone BJ, Wells CA, Berry AR, Ferguson JDP. Mammographic appearance and histopathological description of a muscular hamartoma of the breast. *Br J Radiol* 1985;58:459–461.
50. Fiirgaard B, Kristensen. Muscular hamartomas of the breast. A case report. *Acta Radiol* 1992;33:115–116.
51. Garfein CF, Aulicino MR, Leytin A, Drossman S, Hermann G, Bleiweiss IJ. Epithelioid cells in myoid hamartoma of the breast. *Arch Pathol Lab Med* 1996;120:676–680.
52. Jozefczyk MA, Rosen PP. Vascular tumors of the breast II. Perilobular hemangiomas and hemangiomas. *Am J Surg Pathol* 1985;9:491–503.
53. Lesueur GC, Brown RW, Bhathal PS. Incidence of perilobular hemangioma in the female breast. *Arch Pathol Lab Med* 1983;107:308–310.
54. Rosen PP, Ridolfi RL. The perilobular hemangioma. A benign vascular lesion of the breast. *Am J Clin Pathol* 1977;68:21–23.
55. Webb LA, Young JR. Case report: haemangioma of the breast—appearances on mammography and ultrasound. *Clin Radiol* 1996;51:523–524.
56. Tabar L, Dean PB. *Teaching atlas of mammography*, 2nd ed. New York: Thieme Medical Publishers, 1985:45,209.
57. Hoda SA, Cranor ML, Rosen, PP. Hemangiomas of the breast with atypical histological features. Further analysis of histological subtypes confirming their benign character. *Am J Surg Pathol* 1992;16:553–560.
58. Rosen PP. Vascular tumors of the breast V. Non-parenchymal hemangiomas of mammary subcutaneous tissue. *Am J Surg Pathol* 1985;9:723–729.
59. Berg JW, DeCrosse JJ, Fracchia AA, Farrow J. Stromal sarcomas of the breast: a unified approach to connective tissue sarcomas other than cystosarcoma phyllodes. *Cancer* 1962;13:419–424.
60. Gutman H, Pollock RE, Ross MI, et al. Sarcoma of the breast: implications for extent of therapy. The MD Anderson experience. *Surgery* 1994;116:505–509.
61. McGregor GI, Knowling MA, Este FA. Sarcoma and cystosarcoma phyllodes tumors of the breast—a retrospective review of 58 cases. *Am J Surg* 1994;167:477–480.
62. Grant EG, Holt RW, Chung B, Richardson JD, Orson LW, Cigtay OS. Angiosarcoma of the breast: sonographic, xeromammographic and pathologic appearance. *AJR Am J Roentgenol* 1983;141:691–692.
63. Liberman L, Dershaw DD, Kaufman RJ, Rosen PP. Angiosarcoma of the breast. *Radiology* 1992;183:649–654.
64. Rosen PP, Kimmel M, Ernsberger D. Mammary angiosarcoma. The prognostic significance of tumor differentiation. *Cancer* 1988;62:2145–2151.
65. Chen KTK, Kirkeguard DD, Bocian JJ. Angiosarcoma of the breast. *Cancer* 1980;46:368–371.
66. Del Mastro L, Garrone O, Guenzi M, et al. Angiosarcoma of the residual breast after conservative surgery and radiotherapy for primary carcinoma. *Ann Oncol* 1994;5:163–165.
67. Cafiero F, Gipponi M, Peressini A, et al. Radiation-associated angiosarcoma. Diagnostic and therapeutic implications—two case reports and a review of the literature. *Cancer* 1996;77:2496–2502.
68. Pendlebury SC, Bilous M, Langlands AO. Sarcomas following radiation therapy for breast cancer: a report of three cases and a review of the literature. *Int J Radiat Oncol Biol Phys* 1994;31:405–410.
69. Wijnmaalen A, van Ooijen B, van Geel BN, Henzen-Logmans SC, Treurniet-Donker A. Angiosarcoma of the breast following lumpectomy, axillary lymph node dissection, and radiotherapy for primary breast cancer: three case reports and a review of the literature. *Int J Radiat Oncol Biol Phys* 1993;26:135–139.
70. Fineberg S, Rosen PP. Angiosarcoma and atypical cutaneous vascular lesions after radiation therapy for breast carcinoma. *Am J Clin Pathol* 1994;102:757–763.
71. Timmer SJ, Osuch JR, Colony LH, Edminster RR, Gayar H, Igram R. Angiosarcoma of the breast following lumpectomy and radiation therapy for breast carcinoma: case report and review of the literature. *Breast J* 1997;3:40–47.
72. Bolin DJ, Lukas GM. Low-grade dermal angiosarcoma of the breast following radiotherapy. *Am Surg* 1996;62:668–672.
73. Benda JA, Al-Jurf AS, Benson AJB III. Angiosarcoma of the breast following segmental mastectomy complicated by lymphedema. *Am J Clin Pathol* 1987;87:651–655.
74. Donnell RM, Rosen PP, Lieberman PH, et al. Angiosarcoma and other vascular tumors of the breast. Pathologic analysis as a guide to prognosis. *Am J Surg Pathol* 1981;5:629–642.
75. Merino MJ, Berman M, Carter D. Angiosarcoma of the breast. *Am J Surg Pathol* 1983;7:53–60.
76. Britt LD, Lambert P, Sharma R, Ladaga LE. Angiosarcoma of the breast. Initial misdiagnosis is still common. *Arch Surg* 1995;130:221–223.
77. Guarda LA, Ordonez NG, Smith JL Jr, Hanssen G. Immunoperoxidase localization of factor VIII in angiosarcomas. *Arch Pathol Lab Med* 1982;106:515–516.
78. Cameron HM, Stamperl H, Warambo W. Leiomyosarcoma of the breast originating from myothelium (myoepithelium). *J Pathol* 1974;114:89–92.
79. Pardo-Mindan J, Garcia-Julian G, Altuna ME. Leiomyosarcoma of the breast. *Am J Clin Pathol* 1974;62:477–480.
80. Hernandez FJ. Leiomyosarcoma of the male breast originating in the nipple. *Am J Surg Pathol* 1978;2:299–304.
81. Parham DM, Robertson AJ, Hussein KA, Davidson AIG. Leiomyosarcoma of the breast: cytological and histological features, with a review of the literature. *Cytopathology* 1992;3:245–252.
82. Callery CD, Rosen PP, Kinne DW. Sarcoma of the breast. A study of 32 patients with reappraisal of classification and therapy. *Ann Surg* 1985;201:527–532.
83. Odom JW, Mikhailova B, Pryce E, Sabatini MT, Oropeza R. Liposarcoma of the breast. Report of a case and review of the literature. *Breast Dis* 1991;4:293–298.
84. Austin RM, Dupree WB. Liposarcoma of the breast: a clinicopathologic study of 20 cases. *Hum Pathol* 1986;17:906–913.
85. Pollard SG, Marks PV, Temple LN, Thompson HH. Breast sarcoma. A clinicopathologic review of 25 cases. *Cancer* 1990;66:941–944.
86. Remadi S, Doussis-Anagnostopoulu I, Mac Gee W. Primary osteosarcoma of the breast. *Pathol Res Pract* 1995;191:471–474.
87. Savage AP, Sagor GR, Dovey P. Osteosarcoma of the breast: a case report with an unusual diagnostic feature. *Clin Oncol* 1984;10:295–298.
88. Going JJ, Lumsden AB, Anderson JJ. A classical osteogenic sarcoma of the breast: histology, immunohistochemistry and ultrastructure. *Histopathology* 1986;10:631–641.
89. Muller AGS, Van Zyl JA. Primary osteosarcoma of the breast. *J Surg Oncol* 1993;52:135–136.
90. Jones MW, Norris HJ, Wargotz ES, Weiss SW. Fibrosarcoma-malignant fibrous histiocytoma of the breast. A clinicopathologic study of 32 cases. *Am J Surg Pathol* 1992;16:667–674.
91. Rossen K, Stamp I, Sorensen IM. Primary malignant fibrous histiocytoma of the breast. A report of four cases and review of the literature. *APMIS* 1991;99:696–702.

92. Arias-Stella J, Rosen PP. Hemangiopericytoma of the breast. *Mod Pathol* 1988;1:98–103.

93. Mittal KR, Gerald W, True LD. Hemangiopericytoma of breast: report of a case with ultrastructural and immunohistochemical findings. *Hum Pathol* 1986;17:1181–1183.

94. van Kints MJ, Tjon A Tham RTO, Klinkhamer PJJM, van den Bosch HCH. Hemangiopericytoma of the breast: mammographic and sonographic findings. *AJR Am J Roentgenol* 1994;163:61–63.

95. Taccagni G, Rovere E, Masullo M, Christensen L, Eyden B. Myofi-broblastoma of the breast. Review of the literature on myofibroblastic tumors and criteria for defining myofibroblastic differentiation. *Am J Surg Pathol* 1997;21:489–496.

96. Catania S, Pacifico E, Zurrida S, Cusumano. Malignant schwannoma of the breast. *Eur J Surg Oncol* 1992;18:80–81.

97. Barnes L, Pietruszka M. Sarcomas of the breast. A clinicopathologic analysis of 10 cases. *Cancer* 1977;40:1577–1585.

98. Howarth GB, Caces JN, Pratt CB. Breast metastases in children with rhabdomyosarcoma. *Cancer* 1980;46:2520–2524.

CHAPTER 24

Lymphoid and Hematopoietic Tumors

NON-HODGKIN'S LYMPHOMA

The diagnosis of primary mammary lymphoma is limited to patients without evidence of systemic lymphoma or leukemia at the time that the breast lesion is detected (1). Clinically, the disease should involve only the breast or the breast and ipsilateral lymph nodes. Fewer than 0.5% of all malignant lymphomas and about 2% of extranodal lymphomas involve the breast (2). The occurrence of synchronous and metachronous lymphoma and breast carcinoma has been described (3). Mammary involvement by lymphoma occurs in some but not all of these patients.

With rare exceptions, patients described in the literature have been women ranging in age from 13 to 90 years at diagnosis, averaging about 55 years. Bilateral disease is present in about 10% of patients at the time of diagnosis.

The presenting symptom in virtually all cases is a mass, located most often in the upper outer quadrant. A history of recent onset and rapid growth is not unusual. The tumor is often solitary, but patients with multiple lesions and diffuse infiltration have been described. Enlarged axillary lymph nodes have been found clinically in 30% to 50% of patients (4–6). Mammographically, the tumor may be well-defined and circumscribed or irregular and thus difficult to distinguish from other lesions (7,8). It has been suggested that diffuse infiltration and multiple ill-defined lesions are radiologic clues to the diagnosis of lymphoma. There is no association between specific subtypes of lymphoma and radiologic findings on mammography (9,10). Mammary lymphomas may be hypoechoic when studied by ultrasonography (10). The tumors have measured 1 to 12 cm, averaging about 3 cm. Histologic examination often reveals that the lymphomatous infiltrate extends into the breast parenchyma beyond the grossly evident mass.

The largest subgroup of primary mammary lymphomas has been described as diffuse histiocytic when classified by the Rappaport system (1,4,5,7) or as diffuse large-cell (11) (Fig. 1). Poorly differentiated lymphocytic lymphomas, the majority of which are diffuse, and mixed lymphomas, equally nodular and diffuse, are the second and third most common types, respectively (5) (Fig. 2). Well-differentiated lymphocytic, lymphoblastic, undifferentiated, and Burkitt's lymphomas account for 5% to 10% of mammary lymphomas in most series. Immunoblastic lymphoma and lymphoplas-macytic immunocytoma are uncommon in the breast (Fig. 3). Diffuse large cleaved, diffuse small cleaved, and diffuse or follicular mixed-cell lymphomas are the three most common cell types according to the Working Formulation (5). The majority of female mammary lymphomas are of the B-cell type, with infrequent examples of T-cell and histiocytic lymphoma described (11–14).

Lymphoma in the breast typically consists of a dense population of tumor cells that diffusely infiltrate the mammary parenchyma. Ducts and lobules in the central portion of the lesion are usually obliterated, and in some cases, a dense sclerotic reaction develops in the stroma that tends to be associated with blood vessels (Fig. 4). Ducts and lobules are better preserved away from the center of the lesion, where there is a tendency for the lymphomatous infiltrate to concentrate in and around these structures (Fig. 5). A reactive lymphoid infiltrate composed of small lymphocytes is very commonly present at the periphery of the tumor, often localized around epithelial elements and blood vessels. Germinal centers may be formed in these reactive infiltrates (Fig. 6). Calcifications are not usually an intrinsic feature of mammary lymphoma, but they may occur coincidentally in epithelial lesions or in fat necrosis.

Extension of lymphoma cells into the glandular epithelium may mimic *in situ* carcinoma or pagetoid spread of carcinoma. In some instances, the linear pattern assumed by lymphoma cells in the stroma closely resembles invasive lobular carcinoma (11). Signet-ring cell lymphoma bears a striking resemblance to signet-ring cell lobular carcinoma, and it may require immunostains for lymphoid and epithelial markers to distinguish between these entities. The appearance of lymphoma involving mammary stroma that is altered by pseudoangiomatous stromal hyperplasia may also be mistaken for invasive carcinoma (Fig. 7). Distinguishing large-cell lymphoma from poorly differentiated carcinoma is sometimes difficult, especially when the tumor lacks a classic intraductal component. Large-cell lymphoma may assume solid, diffuse, and sometimes alveolar growth patterns that resemble carcinoma. The limited samples of needle core biopsies provide a setting in which there is a risk of mistaking lymphoma for carcinoma.

The term pseudolymphoma has been applied to tumor-forming lymphoid lesions that are thought to be benign reac-

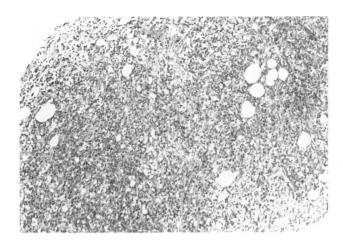

FIGURE 1. Malignant lymphoma. This patient presented with an ill-defined breast mass and ipsilateral axillary lymph node enlargement. This needle core biopsy specimen of the breast tumor revealed diffuse large-cell lymphoma.

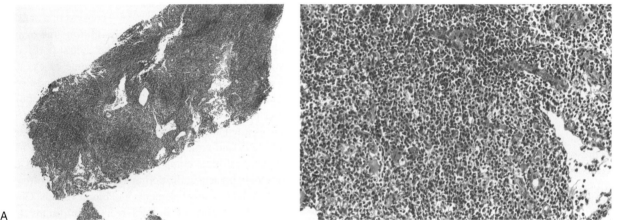

A   B

FIGURE 2. Malignant lymphoma. A,B: Diffuse poorly differentiated lymphocytic lymphoma in a needle core biopsy specimen of the breast.

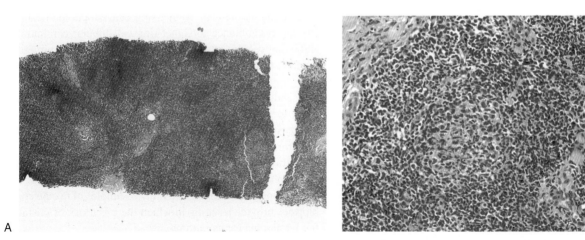

A   B

FIGURE 3. Malignant lymphoma. A,B: This lymphoplasmacytic lymphoma in the breast has nodular and diffuse areas. Focal perivascular fibrosis is evident.

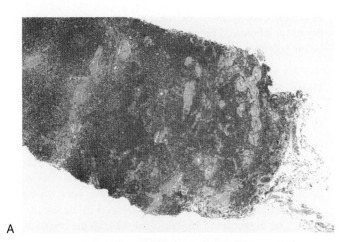
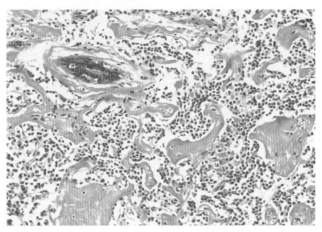

A

B

FIGURE 4. Malignant lymphoma. A,B: Diffuse lymphocytic lymphoma with perivascular sclerosis. A residual mammary duct is shown in (B).

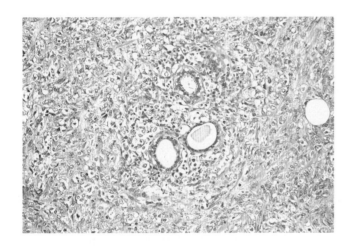

FIGURE 5. Malignant lymphoma. Diffuse large-cell lymphoma has infiltrated and partially destroyed this lobular gland, creating an appearance that could be mistaken for perilobular infiltrating carcinoma.

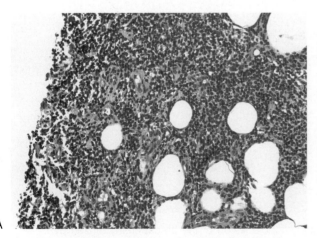
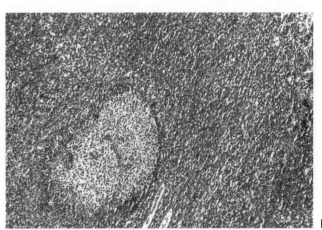

A

B

FIGURE 6. Malignant lymphoma. A,B: This needle core biopsy specimen contained small lymphocytes and germinal center formation in an atypical lymphoid infiltrate suggestive of lymphoma.

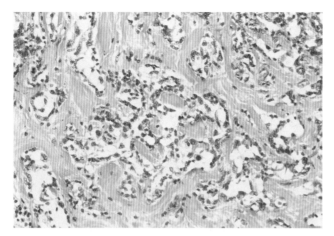

FIGURE 7. Malignant lymphoma. Malignant lymphoma shown here growing in mammary stroma altered by pseudoangiomatous hyperplasia can be mistaken for a vascular lesion or invasive lobular carcinoma.

tive conditions. Fewer than 20 cases have been reported in the breast (15,16). The number of unreported patients initially given a diagnosis of mammary pseudolymphoma in whom malignant lymphoma later developed is not known. Tumors described as pseudolymphomas have been characterized by an infiltrate composed largely of mature lymphocytes. Germinal centers are often present, especially at the periphery, and they are sometimes numerous (Fig. 8). The infiltrate tends to concentrate in the stroma, on occasion accompanied by fat necrosis and fibrosis. The epithelium of ducts and lobules is largely spared, although these structures can be surrounded by the infiltrative process. Analysis of the tissue for cell markers reveals a polyclonal cellular infiltrate. The sample obtained in a needle core biopsy is not a reliable basis for a diagnosis of mammary pseudolymphoma. Comparable foci

of lymphocytic reaction are often encountered at the periphery of lymphomas. Fragments of lymph node tissue may also be mistaken for a pseudolymphomatous lesion histologically.

HODGKIN'S DISEASE

Hodgkin's disease very rarely involves the breast. Mammary infiltration is usually the result of direct extension from axillary or mediastinal lymph nodes, part of regional disease with discontinuous axillary nodal involvement, or a manifestation of systemic disease (17). Most of the patients with primary mammary Hodgkin's disease have been women, and systemic disease ultimately developed in almost all of them. The diagnosis of Hodgkin's disease in the breast may be suspected in a needle core biopsy specimen. Reed-Sternberg cells are the diagnostic feature. The identification of Reed-Sternberg cells can be confirmed by immunohistochemical staining for Leu-M1.

PLASMACYTIC TUMORS

Extramedullary plasmacytoma localized to the breast has been described in very few patients. In one case, mammography revealed a circumscribed mass that was hypoechoic and solid on ultrasound (18). Solitary plasmacytomas of the breast have generally measured between 2 and 4 cm in diameter. In patients with multiple myeloma, the tumors have been composed of "abnormal" or "immature" plasma cells, whereas solitary plasmacytomas contain a mixture of mature and immature plasma cells. Mitoses, nuclear pleomorphism, and multinucleated plasma cells may be seen in solitary plasmacytomas. Mammary glandular structures are largely effaced in the region where the plasma cell infiltrate is most concentrated. Mammary plasmacytoma should be distinguished from plasma cell mastitis, amyloid tumor, and plasma cell granuloma (19). If appropriate samples are avail-

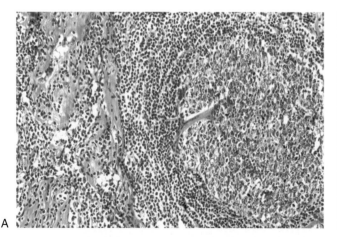

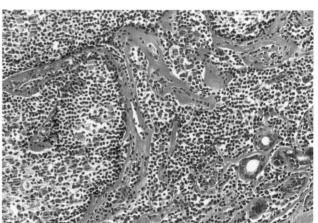

FIGURE 8. "Pseudolymphoma." A,B: This atypical lymphoid lesion of the breast characterized by stromal fibrosis and prominent germinal centers proved to be composed of a polyclonal infiltrate.

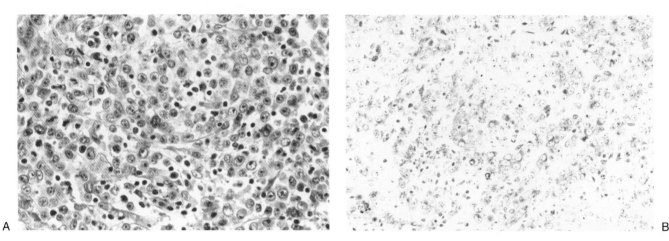

FIGURE 9. Granulocytic leukemia. A: The infiltrate consists of largely undifferentiated granulocytic cells. A few cells have cytoplasmic granules. **B:** Granulocytic differentiation is manifested by this immunostain for muramidase (immunoperoxidase).

able, immunohistochemical studies for immunoglobulins may be performed on the tissue to determine if the infiltrate has the monoclonal character of a neoplastic process or if it is a reactive polyclonal lesion. Amyloid is absent from mammary plasmacytoma, and the plasma cells associated with amyloid tumor are mature.

LEUKEMIC INFILTRATION

Leukemic infiltration of the breast occurs not uncommonly at an advanced stage but only rarely as the initial manifestation of the disease or as the site of localized recurrence (20). Tumor involvement of the breast by *granulocytic leukemia* is referred to as granulocytic sarcoma (21). The term *chloroma* has been used to describe extramedullary tumor-forming granulocytic leukemic infiltrates, in which a green color develops as a result of the enzymatic action of myeloperoxidase (verdoperoxidase) contained in the neoplastic cells. Mammary infiltrates have also been described

as a secondary manifestation in patients with established leukemia (22). Microscopically, the growth pattern may simulate invasive lobular carcinoma or malignant lymphoma (22). The neoplastic cells, which form broad sheets or cords, surround and invade normal mammary parenchymal structures (Fig. 9). Intraepithelial extension of the leukemic infiltrate simulates *in situ* carcinoma. The diagnosis of granulocytic sarcoma may be suggested by cytoplasmic granules in maturing myeloid cells or by the presence of relatively numerous mature myeloid cells scattered throughout the lesion. The myeloid granules in immature cells are reactive histochemically with the naphthol-ASD-chloroacetate esterase stain and immunohistochemically for lysozyme (muramidase). The differential diagnosis includes tumorous myeloid metaplasia in the breast, which is distinguished by the presence of abundant mature and maturing cells of all stem lines (23,24).

Mammary infiltration has been described in patients with lymphocytic leukemia (25,26) (Fig. 10). The lesions tend to be bilateral. Coincidental bone marrow and hematogenous involvement are usually present.

INTRAMAMMARY LYMPH NODES

The differential diagnosis of lymphoid tissue noted in a needle core biopsy specimen includes intramammary lymph nodes, which may be single or multiple (Fig. 11). Mammographic examination usually reveals a well-circumscribed mass that may have a lucent center and a peripheral "hilar" notch (27). Lymph nodes measuring 3 to 15 mm have been described (28). Enlargement of intramammary lymph nodes may be caused by lymphoid hyperplasia, sinus histiocytosis, involvement by or reaction to inflammatory conditions, and neoplasms such as metastatic tumor or lymphoma (29,30) (Figs. 12–14). The distinction between medullary carcinoma and metastatic carcinoma in an intramammary lymph node is sometimes difficult.

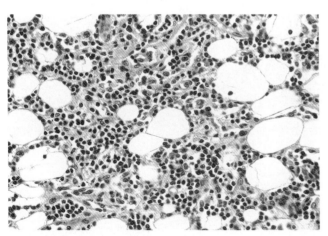

FIGURE 10. Lymphocytic leukemia. Well-differentiated lymphocytic leukemia is shown.

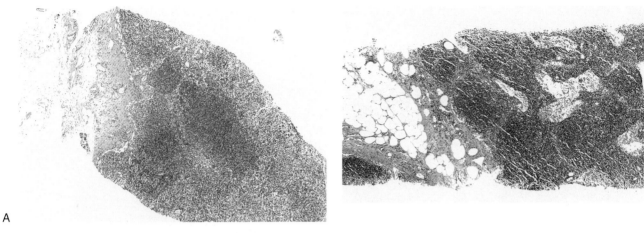

A

B

FIGURE 11. Intramammary lymph node. A: This needle core biopsy specimen demonstrates the lymph node capsule and subcapsular sinus partly obscured by lymphoid hyperplasia. **B:** The lymph node capsule is not conspicuous in this intramammary lymph node with sinusoidal dilatation.

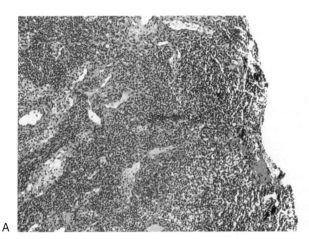

A

FIGURE 12. Intramammary lymph node. A,B: This needle core biopsy specimen of an intramammary lymph node reveals some cells that contain pigment (*arrows*). **C:** The pigment stained black with the Fontana-Masson stain, indicative of melanin. The patient was an African-American woman with a history of chronic periductal mastitis and a cutaneous sinus. The intramammary lymph node was interpreted as showing dermatopathic lymphadenitis.

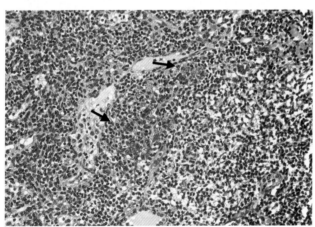

B

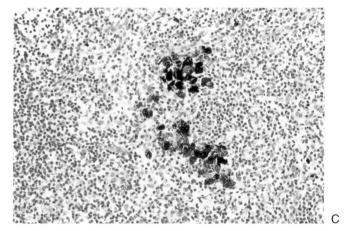

C

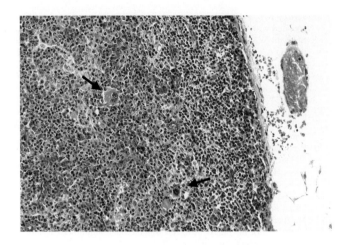

FIGURE 13. Intramammary lymph node. Extramedullary hematopoiesis was present in this intramammary lymph node from a patient with myelofibrosis. Several megakaryocytes are evident (*arrows*).

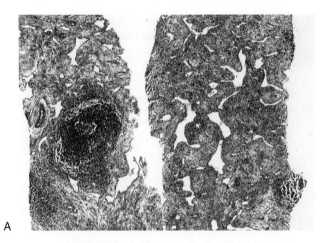

A

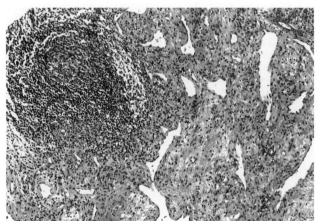

B

FIGURE 14. Intramammary lymph node. A,B: The patient had breast conservation treatment, including radiotherapy for invasive mammary carcinoma. A follow-up mammogram disclosed a nonpalpable, well-circumscribed nodule in the treated breast. The needle core biopsy specimen shown here revealed a lymph node with lymphoid depletion secondary to radiotherapy.

REFERENCES

1. Wiseman C, Liao KT. Primary lymphoma of the breast. *Cancer* 1972; 29:1705–1712.
2. Giardini R, Piccolo C, Rilke F. Primary non-Hodgkin's lymphomas of the female breast. *Cancer* 1992;69:725–735.
3. Sanford DB, Yeomans-Kinney A, McLaughlin PW, Hortobagyi GN, Dhingra K. Ninety-one cases of breast cancer and chronic lymphoproliferative neoplasm: a retrospective review of a population at high risk for multiple malignancies. *Breast J* 1996;2:312–319.
4. Liu F-F, Clark RM. Primary lymphoma of the breast. *Clin Radiol* 1986; 37:567–570.
5. Brustein S, Filippa DA, Kimmel M, Lieberman PH, Rosen PP. Malignant lymphoma of the breast: a study of 53 patients. *Ann Surg* 1987; 205:144–150.
6. Lamovec J, Jancar J. Primary malignant lymphoma of the breast. Lymphoma of the mucosa-associated lymphoid tissue. *Cancer* 1987;60: 3033–3041.
7. Dixon JM, Lumsden AB, Krajewski A, Elton RA, Anderson TJ. Primary lymphoma of the breast. *Br J Surg* 1987;74:214–217.
8. Meyer JE, Kopans DB, Long JC. Mammographic appearance of malignant lymphoma of the breast. *Radiology* 1980;135:623–626.
9. Liberman L, Giess CS, Dershaw DD, Louis DC, Deutch BM. Non-Hodgkin lymphoma of the breast: imaging characteristics and correlation with histopathologic findings. *Radiology* 1994;192:157–160.
10. DiPiro PJ, Lester S, Meyer JE, Denison CM, Takvorian T. Non-Hodgkin lymphoma of the breast: clinical and radiologic presentations. *Breast J* 1996;2:380–384.
11. Lin Y, Govindan R, Hess JL. Malignant hematopoietic breast tumors. *Am J Clin Pathol* 1997;107:177–186.
12. Aozasa K, Ohsawa M, Saeki K, Horiuchi K, Kawano K, Taguchi T. Malignant lymphoma of the breast. Immunologic type and association with lymphocytic mastopathy. *Am J Clin Pathol* 1992;97:699–704.
13. Kosaka M, Tsuchihashi N, Takishita M, et al. Primary adult T-cell lymphoma of the breast. *Acta Haematol* 1992;87:202–205.
14. Bobrow LG, Richards MA, Happerfield LC, Isaacson PG, Lammie GA, Millis RR. Breast lymphomas: a clinicopathologic review. *Hum Pathol* 1993;24:274–278.
15. Lin JJ, Farha GJ, Taylor RJ. Pseudolymphoma of the breast I. In a study of 8,654 consecutive tylectomies and mastectomies. *Cancer* 1980;45: 973–978.
16. Jeffrey KM, Pantazis CG, Wei JP. Pseudolymphoma of the breast associated with Graves' thyrotoxicosis. *Breast Dis* 1994;7:169–173.
17. Shehata WM, Pauke TW, Schleuter JA. Hodgkin's disease of the breast. A case report and review of the literature. *Breast* 1985;11: 19–21.
18. Kim EE, Sawwaf ZW, Sneige N. Multiple myeloma of the breast: magnetic resonance and ultrasound imaging findings. *Breast Dis* 1996;9: 229–233.
19. Pettinato G, Manivel JC, Insabato L, DeChiara A, Petrella G. Plasma cell granuloma (inflammatory pseudo-tumor) of the breast. *Am J Clin Pathol* 1988;90:627–632.
20. Weinblatt ME, Kochen J. Breast nodules as the initial site of relapse in childhood leukemia. *Med Pediatr Oncol* 1990;18:510–512.
21. Sears HF, Reid J. Granulocytic sarcoma. Local presentation of a systemic disease. *Cancer* 1976;37:1808–1813.
22. Pascoe RH. Tumors composed of immature granulocytes occurring in breast in chronic granulocytic leukemia. *Cancer* 1970;25:697–704.
23. Martinelli G, Santini D, Bazzocchi F, Pileri S, Casanova S. Myeloid metaplasia of the breast. A lesion which clinically mimics carcinoma. *Virchows Arch A* 1983;401:203–207.
24. Zonderland HM, Michiels JJ, Tenkate FJW. Mammographic and sonographic demonstration of extramedullary hematopoiesis of the breast. *Clin Radiol* 1991;44:64–65.
25. Gogoi PK, Stewart ID, Keane PF, Scott R, Dunn GD, Catovsky D. Chronic lymphocytic leukemia presenting with bilateral breast involvement. *Clin Lab Haematol* 1989;11:57–60.
26. Seale DL, Riddervoid HO, Tears CD, Stone DD. Roentgenographic appearance of chronic lymphatic leukemia involving the female breast. *AJR Am J Roentgenol* 1972;115:808–810.
27. Kopans DB, Meyer JE, Murphy GF. Benign lymph nodes associated with dermatitis presenting as breast masses. *Radiology* 1980;137: 15–19.
28. McSweeney MB, Egan RL. Prognosis of breast cancer related to intramammary lymph nodes. *Recent Results Cancer Res* 1984;90:166–172.
29. Arnaout AH, Shousha S, Metaxas N, Husain OAN. Intramammary tuberculous lymphadenitis. *Histopathology* 1990;17:91–93.
30. Lindfors KK, Kopans DB, McCarthy KA, Koerner FC, Meyer JE. Breast cancer metastasis to intramammary lymph nodes. *AJR Am J Roentgenol* 1986;146:133–136.

CHAPTER 25

Metastases in the Breast from Nonmammary Malignant Neoplasms

It is important to consider metastatic tumor in the differential diagnosis when faced with a breast lesion that has unusual clinical, radiologic, gross, or microscopic features. The nonmammary primary lesion may be a new, occult neoplasm not evident to the patient's physicians. The preoperative clinical workup of an apparently healthy patient with a breast mass is often perfunctory and unlikely to exclude an occult malignant extramammary primary tumor.

A lesion in the breast is the initial manifestation of a nonmammary malignant neoplasm in a minority of patients who have metastatic tumor in the breast. The occult primary tumor is usually a carcinoma, and one of the most common sites is the lung (1–3). A surprising number of the occult lung lesions have been oat-cell carcinomas (2,4). Other sites of occult, clinically inapparent neoplasms that have presented with metastases in the breast include the kidney, stomach, and ovary (5,6), and breast metastasis has been reported as a manifestation of intestinal carcinoid tumors (7,8). Previously diagnosed tumors that have given rise to metastases in the breast, sometimes rather late in the clinical course, include malignant melanoma (4,9), sarcomas (4), carcinoma of the lung (9,10), and transitional-cell carcinoma of the urinary bladder (11). Several types of malignant lymphoma have sometimes been included under the heading of metastases in the breast. However, these neoplasms in the breast are best regarded as primary tumors or as part of a systemic disease affecting the lymphoid system.

Adenocarcinomas of the gastrointestinal tract, especially the colon and rectum, are rarely the source of metastatic carcinoma in the breast despite their relative frequency in the population at large (12). On the other hand, carcinoid tumors of the small bowel are a surprisingly frequent source of breast metastases (13). Without knowledge of an extramammary primary, metastatic carcinoid tumor in the breast can be mistaken for a primary mammary carcinoma with endocrine differentiation.

Mammary metastases from medulloblastoma (14), rhabdomyosarcoma (15,16), and neuroblastoma have been reported in children and adults. Metastatic melanoma presenting clinically as a breast tumor may be difficult to recognize if the primary lesion is occult or if the pathologist is not in-

formed that the patient received prior treatment for such a lesion. When a breast mass is discovered in a man known to have prostatic carcinoma, histochemical studies for mucin and immunohistochemical studies for prostate-specific antigen and prostatic acid phosphatase should be performed (17,18). Examining the tissue for estrogen receptor is not likely to be helpful, because this protein can be found in mammary and prostatic carcinomas.

Radiographically, metastatic lesions tend to be discrete, round shadows without spiculation (4). They are usually not distinguishable from circumscribed primary papillary, medullary, or colloid breast carcinomas. Microcalcifications are very uncommon but have been described in metastatic ovarian carcinoma (19). Metastatic foci in the breast are usually solitary initially, but they may become multiple and bilateral with progression of the patient's clinical course (4).

Some clinical features are helpful in recognizing that a neoplasm in the breast is a metastatic tumor. The average interval to the development of a mammary metastasis is approximately 2 years for patients with previously treated cancer. Usually, there have already been metastases at other sites, or they are detected coincidentally. Isolated metastases initially limited to the breast are uncommon. Metastases have been described in ipsilateral axillary lymph nodes in a substantial proportion of patients.

An unusual histologic pattern and clinical information about a prior neoplasm are the best clues for identifying a metastatic tumor in the breast. It is important to be sensitive to morphologic patterns that are not typical for breast carcinoma, but some histologic appearances present especially difficult problems because similar tumors arise in the breast and other organs. Included in this group are pulmonary large-cell carcinoma (Fig. 1); mucinous (colloid), mucoepidermoid, and clear-cell carcinomas (Fig. 2); and malignant melanoma (Fig. 3). Metastatic ovarian carcinomas have generally been serous rather than mucinous, and in the absence of a known ovarian primary, they may be mistaken for papillary mammary carcinoma (5) (Fig. 4). Metastatic endometrial carcinoma with a solid growth pattern may mimic poorly differentiated or solid papillary mammary carcinoma (Fig. 5). Among sarcomas metastatic to the breast, heman-

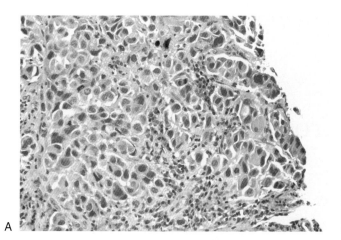

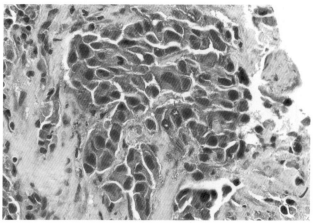

FIGURE 1. Metastatic lung carcinoma. A: Large-cell adenocarcinoma in a needle core biopsy specimen of the breast. Without a history of pulmonary carcinoma, this tumor could be interpreted as mammary carcinoma. **B:** Intracytoplasmic mucin appears magenta with the mucicarmine stain. The patient had a histologically identical large-cell carcinoma of the lung treated previously.

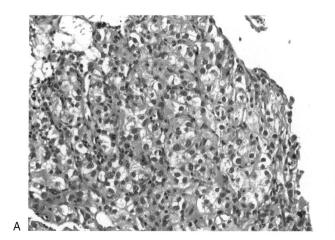

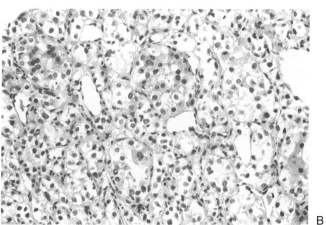

FIGURE 2. Metastatic renal carcinoma. A: A needle core biopsy specimen of the breast showing metastatic tumor with an alveolar structure and cytoplasmic clearing. **B:** The cells in this metastatic lesion from the kidney resemble apocrine carcinoma with clear-cell change.

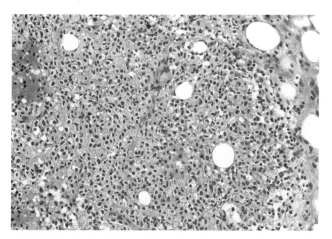

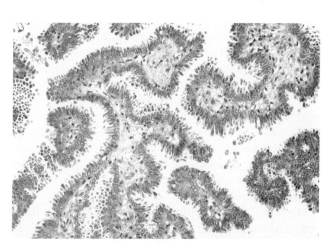

FIGURE 3. Metastatic malignant melanoma. Diffusely infiltrating tumor cells with an epithelioid appearance.

FIGURE 4. Metastatic ovarian carcinoma. Part of a needle core biopsy specimen of the breast that demonstrates metastatic papillary serous ovarian carcinoma.

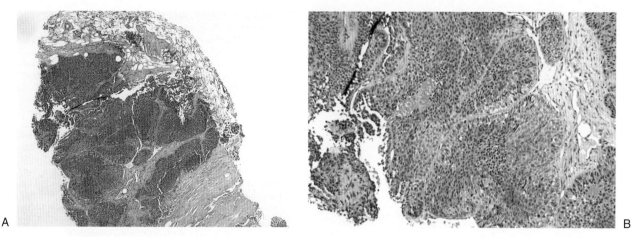

FIGURE 5. Metastatic endometrial carcinoma. A,B: The solid growth pattern subdivided into large alveolar nests in this needle core biopsy specimen of a metastatic lesion resembles the structure of solid papillary mammary carcinoma.

giopericytoma and malignant fibrous histiocytomas may be difficult to distinguish from primary mammary sarcomas and some metaplastic mammary carcinomas (Fig. 6).

The limited sample obtained by needle core biopsy may not contain all the information that would help to distinguish between a primary and a metastatic tumor. A search should be made for *in situ* carcinoma to confirm origin in the breast,

but because this cannot be found in all primary mammary lesions, the absence of *in situ* carcinoma is not conclusive evidence that one is dealing with a metastasis. Metastatic tumor often surrounds and displaces normal-appearing breast parenchyma that typically shows little or no hyperplasia. Lymphatic tumor emboli may result from metastases in the breast as well as from primary breast carcinomas.

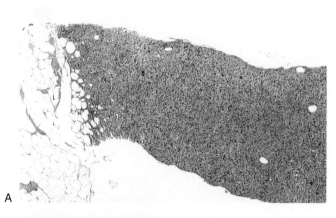

FIGURE 6. Metastatic leiomyosarcoma. A,B: This needle core biopsy specimen shows a dense tumor composed of interlacing spindle cells with eosinophilic cytoplasm. The tumor cells were immunoreactive for smooth-muscle actin. **C:** The source of the metastasis shown here was a primary leiomyosarcoma of the groin resected 1 year earlier.

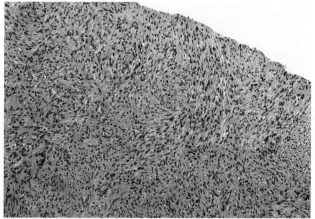

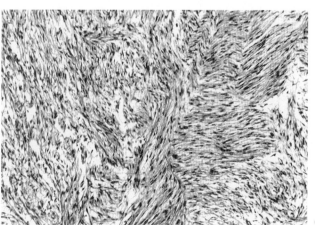

The distinction between a primary breast tumor and a metastasis in the breast is critical for treatment. When an occult extramammary neoplasm presents with a breast metastasis, workup of the patient will be influenced by morphologic features of the tumor that may suggest one or more particular primary sites. Mastectomy is not appropriate for metastatic tumor in the breast in most cases, but it may be performed to obtain local control of bulky or otherwise symptomatic lesions.

REFERENCES

1. Hajdu SI, Urban JA. Cancers metastatic to the breast. *Cancer* 1972;29: 1691–1696.
2. Kelly C, Henderson D, Corris P. Breast lumps: rare presentation of oat cell carcinoma of lung. *J Clin Pathol* 1988;41:171–172.
3. McCrea ES, Johnston C, Haney PJ. Metastases to the breast. *Am J Roentgenol* 1983;141:685–690.
4. Toombs BD, Kalisher L. Metastatic disease in the breast: clinical, pathologic and radiographic features. *Am J Roentgenol* 1977;129: 673–676.
5. Elit LM, Cunnane MF. Breast metastasis from ovarian carcinoma: report of two cases and literature review. *J Surg Pathol* 1995;1:69–74.
6. Ron I-G, Inbar M, Halpern M, Chaitchik S. Endometrioid carcinoma of the ovary presenting as primary carcinoma of the breast. A case report and review of the literature. *Acta Obstet Gynecol Scand* 1992;71: 81–83.
7. Harrist TJ, Kalisher L. Breast metastasis; an unusual manifestation of a malignant carcinoid tumor. *Cancer* 1977;40:3102–3106.
8. Kashlan RB, Powell RW, Nolting SF. Carcinoid and other tumors metastatic to the breast. *J Surg Oncol* 1982;20:25–30.
9. Sneige N, Zachariah S, Fanning TV, Dekmezian RH, Ordonez NG. Fine needle aspiration cytology of metastatic neoplasms in the breast. *Am J Clin Pathol* 1989;92:27–35.
10. Domanski HA. Metastases to the breast from extramammary neoplasms. A report of six cases with diagnosis by fine needle aspiration cytology. *Acta Cytol* 1996;40:1293–1300.
11. Belton AL, Stull MA, Grant T, Shepard MH. Mammographic and sonographic findings in metastatic transitional cell carcinoma of the breast. *AJR Am J Roentgenol* 1997;168:511–512.
12. Alexander HR, Turnbull AD, Rosen PP. Isolated breast metastases from gastrointestinal carcinomas. *J Surg Oncol* 1989;42:264–266.
13. Landon G, Sneige N, Ordonez NG, Mackay B. Carcinoid metastatic to breast diagnosed by fine-needle aspiration biopsy. *Diagn Cytopathol* 1987;3:230–233.
14. Kapila K, Sarkar C, Verma K. Detection of metastatic medulloblastoma in a fine needle breast aspirate. *Acta Cytol* 1996;40:384–385.
15. Hogge JP, Magnant CM, Lage JM, Zuurbier RA. Rhabdomyosarcoma metastatic to the breast. *Br J Ca* 1996;2:270–274.
16. Kwan WH, Choi PHK, Li CK, et al. Breast metastasis in adolescents with alveolar rhabdomyosarcoma of the extremities: report of two cases. *Pediatr Hemat Oncol* 1996;13:277–285.
17. Choudhury M, DeRosas J, Papsidero L, Wajsman Z, Beckley S, Pontes JE. Metastatic prostatic carcinoma to the breast or primary breast carcinoma. *J Urol* 1982;19:297–299.
18. Green LK, Klima M. The use of immunohistochemistry in metastatic prostatic adenocarcinoma to the breast. *Hum Pathol* 1991;22:242–246.
19. Duda RB, August CZ, Schink JC. Ovarian carcinoma metastatic to the breast and axillary node. *Surgery* 1991;110:552–556.

CHAPTER 26

Pathologic Effects of Radiation and Chemotherapy

RADIATION

The breasts may be exposed to radiation during diagnostic procedures, such as mammography and fluoroscopy (1,2), or in the course of radiotherapy administered to another organ, such as mediastinal radiotherapy for Hodgkin's disease (3–6). The low-dose exposure in these situations has been associated with an increased risk for the subsequent development of breast carcinoma (1–3), but no structural changes attributable to this level of radiation are evident when the mammary glandular tissue is examined histopathologically. Patients treated for Hodgkin's disease have carcinomas that tend to be poorly differentiated but otherwise are not significantly different pathologically from tumors that arise in women without prior irradiation (5).

Radiation of the breast for mammary carcinoma in the course of breast-conserving treatment involves levels of exposure that produce alterations in non-neoplastic as well as neoplastic tissues. Radiation-induced histologic changes must be distinguished from recurrent carcinoma in the interpretation of a post-treatment biopsy. When normal breast is compared with a preradiation specimen, the major changes in normal breast are apparent in terminal duct-lobular units (7) (Figs. 1–3). These are (a) collagenization of intralobular stroma, (b) thickening of periacinar and periductular basement membranes, (c) atrophy of acinar and ductular epithelium, (d) cytologic atypia of residual epithelial cells, and (e) relatively prominent acinar myoepithelial cells that tend to be preserved to a greater extent than the epithelial cells. Generally, the effects on the larger ducts are less pronounced than those in lobules following primary radiotherapy. In a minority of specimens, one may also find atypical fibroblasts in the interlobular stroma.

Substantial variation can be observed from one patient to another in the severity of changes in the lobules, and on occasion they may be virtually indistinguishable from physiologic atrophy. In a given patient, most of the glandular tissue responds in a uniform fashion if the entire breast has been radiated.

Fat necrosis and atypia of stromal fibroblasts are more common close to "boosted" or implanted areas (8). Radiation-induced vascular changes are not ordinarily seen after external beam radiotherapy, but they may occur where a boost dose has been delivered. Cytologic and architectural markers of radiation effect in larger blood vessels include fragmentation of elastica, endothelial atypia, and myointimal proliferation that leads to vascular sclerosis. Prominent, cytologically atypical endothelial cells are also apparent in capillaries. Epithelial atypia may occur in the larger ducts of the breast, where it is usually superimposed on preexisting hyperplasia or apocrine metaplasia (Figs. 4,5).

Cytologic atypia in non-neoplastic epithelium can create diagnostic problems if one is unaware of the typical appearance of radiation-induced atrophy of the breast (7,9,10). *In situ* lobular and intraductal carcinoma persisting after radiation therapy remain largely intact, so that the affected lobules and ducts are filled and often expanded with a neoplastic cell population that has an appearance differing little or not at all from the pretreatment appearance of the carcinoma (Figs. 6–8). From time to time, the radiated tumor contains cells with multiple hyperchromatic nuclei, or there is focal necrosis not seen in the pretreatment biopsy specimen, and it may be surmised that these effects are related to irradiation.

CHEMOTHERAPY

Treatment-related histologic changes may be detected in mammary carcinoma and in non-neoplastic breast tissue examined after patients have received chemotherapy. Chemotherapy effect is most often encountered when patients with locally advanced or inflammatory carcinoma have been given high-dose systemic therapy preoperatively (11). The morphologic changes in this situation are often the result of the combined effect of multiple agents administered as neoadjuvant therapy.

In general, the histopathologic effects of systemic chemotherapy can be correlated with the extent of clinical response. The greatest histopathologic alterations are usually found in patients who appear clinically to have complete resolution of their neoplasm (12,13). However, it is not unusual to observe substantial dissociation between the clinical picture and the histologic findings after therapy, as when a patient seems to have a complete response but histologic ex-

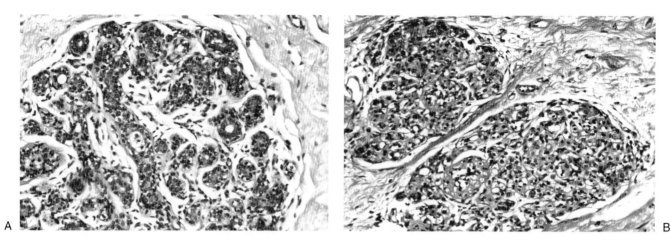

FIGURE 1. Radiation atrophy of lobules. A: A normal lobule in the breast of a 35-year-old woman after lumpectomy for infiltrating duct carcinoma and before the start of radiotherapy. **B:** Lobules in the same breast 3 years after radiotherapy. This needle core biopsy was performed for mammographically detected calcifications in recurrent carcinoma. The posttreatment lobules exhibit changes of radiation atrophy, including sclerosis of intralobular stroma, thickening of basement membranes around lobular glands, atrophy of epithelial cells, and cytoplasmic clearing in myoepithelial cells.

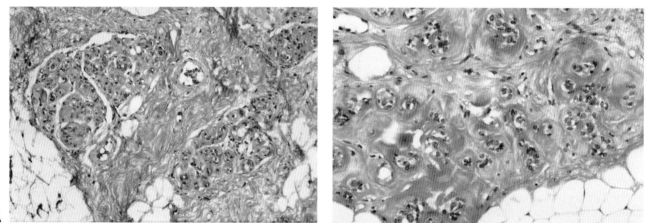

FIGURE 2. Radiation atrophy of lobules. A,B: Two examples of extreme radiation atrophy with marked thickening of basement membranes.

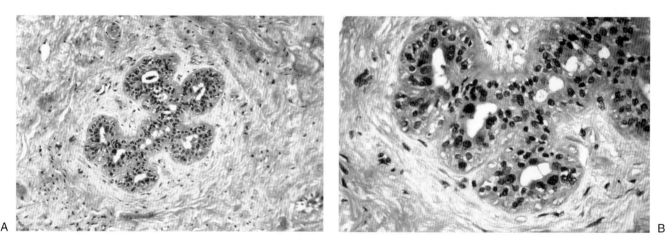

FIGURE 3. Radiation atypia in a small duct. A,B: Isolated epithelial cells bordering on the duct lumen have enlarged, hyperchromatic nuclei. Thickening of the basement membranes is evident.

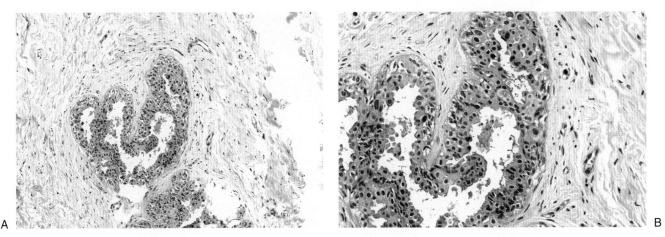

FIGURE 4. Radiation atypia in duct hyperplasia. A,B: Scattered cells in the hyperplastic apocrine epithelium have pleomorphic, hyperchromatic nuclei. Note the even hyperchromatic nuclear chromatin and absence of nucleoli in these atypical nuclei. Disorderly proliferation of myoepithelial cells is also appar-

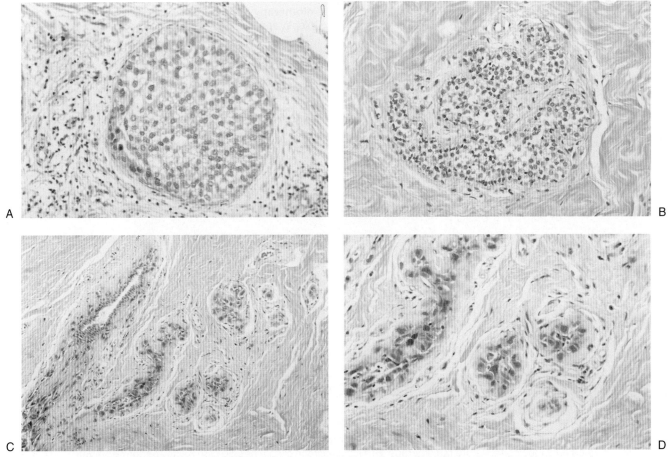

FIGURE 5. Radiation atypia in terminal ducts with atypical lobular hyperplasia. A,B: After an initial excisional biopsy, the patient received radiotherapy. Intraductal carcinoma is shown in (A) and atypical lobular hyperplasia in (B). **C,D:** A needle core biopsy performed 2 years later revealed marked cytologic atypia in these terminal ducts, probably in foci of persisting atypical lobular hyperplasia.

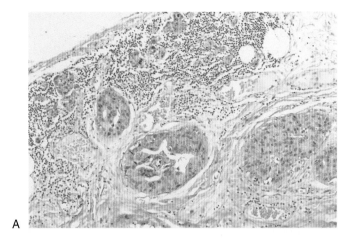

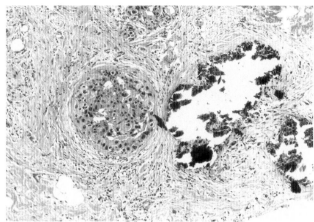

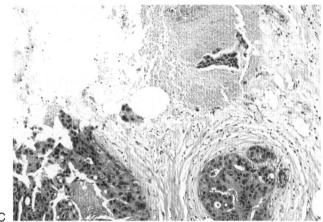

FIGURE 6. Recurrent intraductal carcinoma after radiotherapy. A: Intraductal carcinoma in a needle core biopsy specimen. The patient had a wide excision of the lesional area followed by radiotherapy. **B:** A follow-up mammogram 4 years later revealed calcifications, leading to another needle core biopsy. The specimen illustrated here showed intraductal carcinoma similar to that in (A). **C:** This section is from the excision performed after the diagnosis of recurrent intraductal carcinoma. A tissue defect caused by the needle core biopsy is in the upper left corner. The current carcinoma, shown in (B) and (C), is histologically very similar to the pretreatment lesion.

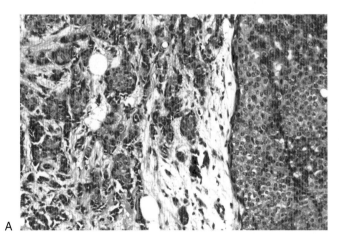

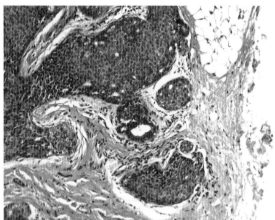

FIGURE 7. Recurrent carcinoma after radiotherapy. A: Intraductal and infiltrating poorly differentiated duct carcinoma before radiotherapy. **B:** This specimen from a needle core biopsy performed 1 year after radiotherapy shows intraductal carcinoma identical to that on the right in (A).

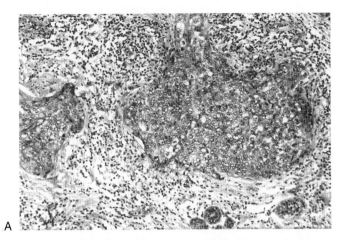
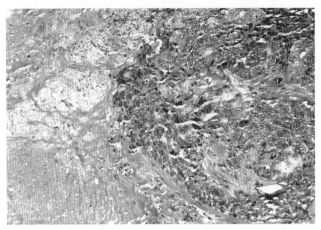

FIGURE 8. Recurrent infiltrating carcinoma. A: Infiltrating poorly differentiated duct carcinoma with a prominent lymphocytic reaction before treatment. **B:** One year after lumpectomy and radiotherapy, carcinoma recurred that was devoid of lymphocytic reaction but otherwise similar to the pretreatment tumor.

amination of the breast reveals residual tumor. Mammography may suggest a response in patients treated with neoadjuvant chemotherapy, but this procedure is not reliable for predicting the pathologic status of the breast. There is no consistent correlation between the pretreatment histologic grade of the tumor and pathologic evidence of response to therapy. When no residual tumor is detectable grossly in the breast, about 60% of patients are found to have persistent carcinoma histologically. Usually, similar chemotherapy effects are found in the primary tumor and in axillary nodal metastases.

The fundamental manifestation of chemotherapy effect is a decrease in tumor cellularity (Fig. 9). In the most extreme situation, no residual carcinoma may be detectable, an oc-

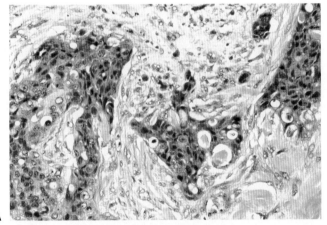
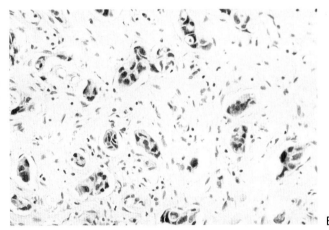
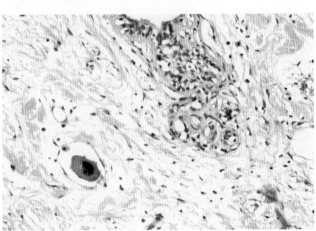

FIGURE 9. Chemotherapy effect. A: Poorly differentiated infiltrating duct carcinoma in a biopsy specimen from a patient who subsequently received doxorubicin (Adriamycin) and radiotherapy. **B:** This needle core biopsy sample was obtained from the breast after the patient had a partial clinical response. Small nests of carcinoma cells with pleomorphic, hyperchromatic nuclei are present in the collagenous stroma. **C:** A markedly enlarged hyperchromatic cell in a lymphatic space is shown near an atrophic lobule. The cytologic changes in the carcinoma are attributable largely to the chemotherapy.

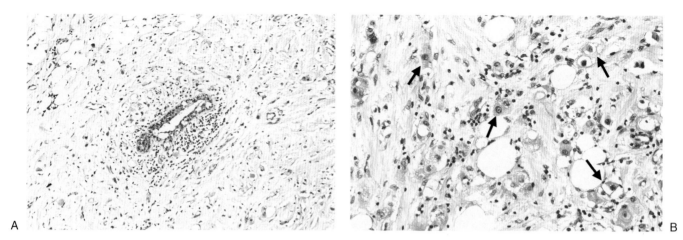

FIGURE 10. Chemotherapy effect in the breast. A,B: This needle core biopsy sample was obtained after a partial clinical response to chemotherapy. Isolated residual carcinoma cells are dispersed in the fibrotic mammary stroma, accompanied by a scattering of lymphocytes.

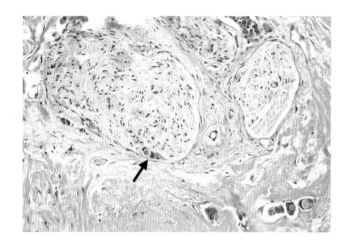

FIGURE 11. Chemotherapy effect in lymphatic tumor emboli. The clusters of carcinoma cells in a nerve (*arrow*) and in lymphatic channels show cytologic changes related to chemotherapy. The patient had a complete clinical response to chemotherapy, and this was the extent of histologically detectable residual carcinoma.

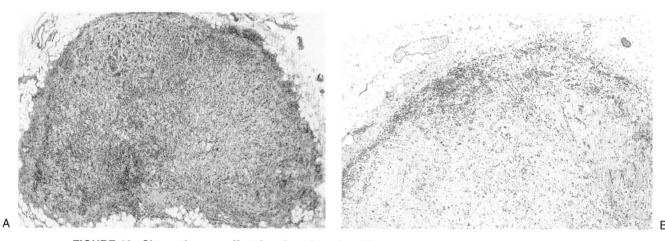

FIGURE 12. Chemotherapy effect in a lymph node with metastatic carcinoma. A: Carcinoma diffusely involves a lymph node before therapy. **B:** After chemotherapy, there are isolated carcinoma cells in a background of fibrosis and lymphoid atrophy.

currence reported in 6.7% to 10.0% of cases (13,14). If the breast of a patient who has a complete clinical response is examined histologically soon after treatment, residual degenerated and infarcted necrotic invasive carcinoma may be recognized by the loss of normal staining properties and decreased architectural detail. With the passage of time, the degenerated invasive carcinoma is absorbed. Healed sites of previous infiltrating carcinoma may be appreciated through residual architectural distortion characterized by fibrosis, stromal edema, increased vascularity composed largely of thin-walled vessels, and a chronic inflammatory cell infiltrate (15) (Fig. 10). There is some evidence that intraductal carcinoma and lymphatic tumor emboli may be relatively more resistant to treatment than invasive carcinoma, so that these sites serve as sanctuaries for persistent carcinoma. In a minority of instances, the residual carcinoma found after complete clinical response in the breast consists only of lymphatic tumor emboli, intraductal carcinoma, or both (Fig. 11). Fibrosis and atrophy of lymphoid tissue are characteristic features of chemotherapy effect at sites of metastatic carcinoma in lymph nodes (16) (Fig. 12).

Residual carcinoma cells may appear morphologically unaltered, but in most cases they exhibit histologic and cytologic changes that reflect chemotherapy treatment effect (12,14,17). The cells are enlarged because of increased cytoplasmic volume. The cytoplasm often contains vacuoles and eosinophilic granules (16). Cell borders are typically well defined, and the cells tend to shrink away from the stroma (see Fig. 10). Some carcinoma cells have enlarged, pleomorphic, and hyperchromatic nuclei (11). The tumor cells retain immunohistochemical reactivity for cytokeratin and epithelial membrane antigen.

Non-neoplastic breast parenchyma is also altered following high-dose cytotoxic chemotherapy, but the changes are more subtle than those induced in the tumor. The glandular elements undergo diffuse atrophy, causing a reduction in the number of lobules and the size of existing lobules (15,16,18). Cytologic atypia may be seen in duct and lobular epithelial cells, but in many cases these changes are not attributable specifically to treatment effect. Comparison with a pretreatment specimen is particularly helpful in this situation. Regressive changes may also be found in the lymphoid tissue of axillary lymph nodes (15).

REFERENCES

1. Boice JD, Manson RR, Rosenstein M. Breast cancer in women after repeated fluoroscopic examinations of the chest. *J Natl Cancer Inst* 1977; 159:823–832.
2. Hildreth NG, Shore RE, Dvoretsky PM. The risk of breast cancer after irradiation of the thymus in infancy. *N Engl J Med* 1989;321: 1281–1284.
3. Anderson N, Lokich J. Bilateral breast cancer after cured Hodgkin's disease. *Cancer* 1990;65:221–223.
4. O'Brien PC, Barton MB, Fisher R, for Australian Radiation Oncology Lymphoma Group (AROLG). Breast cancer following treatment for Hodgkin's disease: the need for screening in a young population. *Australas Radiol* 1995;39:271–276.
5. Yahalom J, Petrek JA, Biddinger PW, et al. Breast cancer in patients irradiated for Hodgkin's disease: a clinical and pathological study of 45 events in 37 patients. *J Clin Oncol* 1992;10:1674–1681.
6. Bhatia S, Robison LL, Oberlin O, et al. Breast cancer and other second neoplasms after childhood Hodgkin's disease. *N Engl J Med* 1996;334: 745–751.
7. Schnitt SJ, Connolly JL, Harris JR, Cohen RB. Radiation-induced changes in the breast. *Hum Pathol* 1984;15:545–550.
8. Girling AC, Hanby AM, Millis RR. Radiation and other pathological changes in breast tissue after conservation treatment for carcinoma. *J Clin Pathol* 1990;43:152–156.
9. Pedio G, Landolt V, Zobeli L. Irradiated benign cells of the breast: a potential diagnostic pitfall in fine needle aspiration cytology. *Acta Cytol* 1989;32:127–128.
10. Peterse JL, Thunnissen FBJM, van Heerde P. Fine needle aspiration cytology or radiation-induced changes in non-neoplastic breast lesions. Possible pitfalls in cytodiagnosis. *Acta Cytol* 1989;33:176–180.
11. Rasbridge SA, Gillett CE, Seymour A-M, et al. The effects of chemotherapy on morphology, cellular proliferation, apoptosis and oncoprotein expression in primary breast carcinoma. *Br J Cancer* 1994; 70:335–341.
12. Brifford M, Spyratos F, Tubiana-Huhn M, et al. Sequential cytopunctures during pre-operative chemotherapy for primary breast cancer. *Cancer* 1989;63:631–637.
13. Feldman LD, Hortobagyi GN, Buzdar AU, Ames FC, Blumenscheinn GR. Pathological assessment of response to induction chemotherapy in breast cancer. *Cancer Res* 1986;46:2578–2581.
14. Frierson HF Jr, Fechner RE. Histologic grade of locally advanced infiltrating ductal carcinoma after treatment with induction chemotherapy. *Am J Clin Pathol* 1994;102:154–157.
15. Sharkey FE, Addington SL, Fowler LJ, Page CP, Cruz AB. Effects of preoperative chemotherapy on the morphology of resectable breast carcinoma. *Mod Pathol* 1996;9:893–900.
16. Aktepe F, Kapucuoglu N, Pak I. The effects of chemotherapy on breast cancer tissue in locally advanced breast cancer. *Histopathology* 1996; 29:63–67.
17. McCready DR, Hortobagyi GN, Kau SW, Smith TL, Buzdar AV, Balch CM. The prognostic significance of lymph node metastases after preoperative chemotherapy for locally advanced breast cancer. *Arch Surg* 1989;124:21–25.
18. Kennedy S, Merino MJ, Swain SM, Lippman ME. The effects of hormonal and chemotherapy on tumoral and non-neoplastic breast tissue. *Hum Pathol* 1990;21:192–198.

CHAPTER 27

Breast Lesions in Men and Children

BENIGN PROLIFERATIVE LESIONS OF THE MALE BREAST

Gynecomastia is the most common clinical and pathologic abnormality of the male breast. Mammary enlargement may be caused by a discrete, nodular increase in subareolar tissue or a diffuse accumulation of tissue. Both breasts are affected in the majority of patients at all ages. Gynecomastia is a frequent adverse side effect of medication used to treat prostatic hyperplasia (1). The initial clinical signs are breast enlargement and a palpable mass that may be accompanied by pain or tenderness. The palpable mass is located in the central subareolar region in most patients. Carcinoma arising in gynecomastia can usually be detected as a localized, asymmetric area of firmness.

Mammography is helpful for distinguishing between gynecomastia and carcinoma and may identify carcinoma developing in gynecomastia (2). Two mammographic patterns associated with gynecomastia are a dendritic retroareolar density with prominent radial extensions into the breast and a triangular subareolar density lacking radiating extensions. Ultrasound has also proved useful in the diagnosis of gynecomastia.

The microscopic features of gynecomastia are similar regardless of etiologic factors (3,4). Three phases of proliferative change have been described. Florid gynecomastia, ordinarily seen soon after onset, is characterized by prominent epithelial proliferation in ducts (Fig. 1). There is usually concomitant myoepithelial cell hyperplasia. The increased amount and cellularity of periductal stroma are accompanied by prominent vascularity, edema, and a round-cell infiltrate. Intermediate gynecomastia has florid and fibrous components. It constitutes a transitional phase in maturation of the lesion (Fig. 2). Fibrous or inactive gynecomastia typically occurs after the lesion has been present for 6 months or longer. The epithelial proliferation tends to be less conspicuous than in the florid phase, but prominent hyperplasia can persist (Fig. 3). The stroma is more collagenous with less edema, and there is reduced vascularity. Pseudoangiomatous hyperplasia of the stroma may be found in any phase of gynecomastia (Fig. 4).

The cytologic features and growth pattern of the epithelial proliferation in ducts may be very atypical. This occurs most often in the florid phase. Atypical features are the development of fenestrated and solid growth patterns and papillary proliferation, in which cytologically atypical cells appear to overgrow the dimorphic population that characterizes florid gynecomastia (Fig. 5). Mitotic activity is variable but may be pronounced in ducts exhibiting atypical hyperplasia. Nuclear estrogen receptor immunoreactivity is present in the epithelial cells in most examples of gynecomastia. Other proliferative epithelial changes found in gynecomastia include lobule formation, pseudolactational hyperplasia, apocrine metaplasia, and squamous metaplasia (Fig. 6).

Intraductal papillomas can arise in the male breast (5). The usual presenting symptom is nipple discharge that is bloody or blood-tinged. Microscopic examination reveals an orderly papillary structure composed of cuboidal or columnar cells. Because of the relatively high proportion of papillary carcinomas of the male breast, all male papillary tumors should be carefully evaluated pathologically. Approximately 5% of the reported examples of *florid papillomatosis* of the nipple have been in men (6). Nearly half of these lesions have contained carcinoma.

Fibroepithelial tumors of the male breast usually arise in a background of gynecomastia. Some lesions classified as *fibroadenoma* or *cystosarcoma* are probably nodular foci of gynecomastia (7,8). Most cystosarcomas in men have been histologically and clinically benign. Some of the male patients with fibroepithelial lesions had been treated with estrogens, resulting in gynecomastia with lobular differentiation (8).

Other benign conditions in the male breast include *duct ectasia* (9) and *fibrocystic changes* (10), both often coexistent with gynecomastia.

CARCINOMA OF THE MALE BREAST

Breast carcinoma in men accounts for not more than 1% of all breast carcinomas (11). There is a straight-line relationship between incidence and age among men (12). This differs from female breast carcinoma, in which the slope is less steep after age 50.

The majority of male breast carcinomas are located centrally in a retroareolar position. The cumulative risk for bilaterality is 3% or less. Carcinoma is found in about 75% of male patients with a mass and bloody discharge. Serous discharge

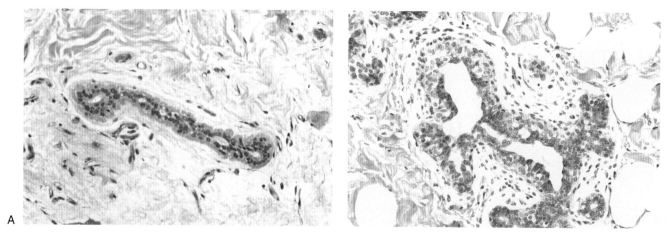

FIGURE 1. Gynecomastia. A: A normal duct in the breast of a 75-year-old man. **B:** Gynecomastia with marked hyperplasia of myoepithelial cells and the periductal stroma.

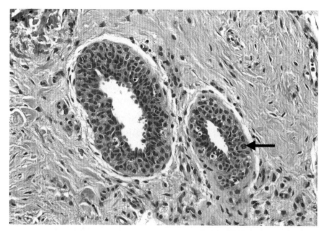

FIGURE 2. Gynecomastia. A lesion with compact epithelial and myoepithelial hyperplasia. An intraepithelial mitotic figure is present (*arrow*). Note the periductal edema and hypervascularity.

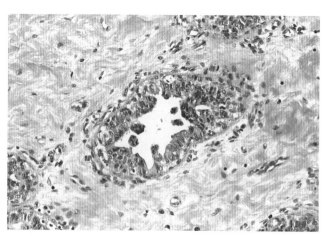

FIGURE 3. Gynecomastia. This focus features atypical micropapillary epithelial hyperplasia and a mild increase in periductal vascularity. The periductal stroma is collagenized.

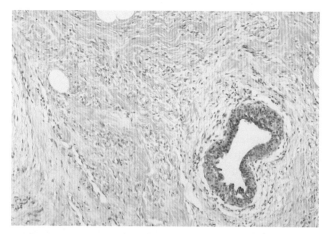

FIGURE 4. Gynecomastia. Pseudoangiomatous hyperplasia of the stroma surrounds a duct with myoepithelial hyperplasia.

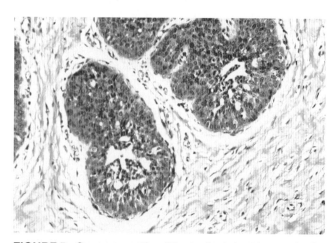

FIGURE 5. Gynecomastia with atypical duct hyperplasia. The proliferation is almost entirely epithelial with a minimal myoepithelial component.

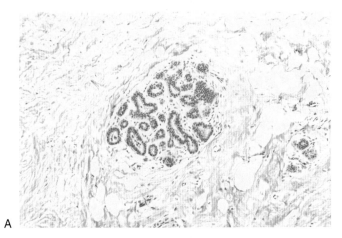
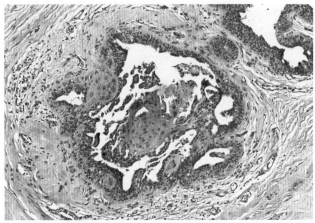

FIGURE 6. Gynecomastia. A: Lobule formation in a male breast. **B:** Florid gynecomastia with squamous metaplasia in the hyperplastic duct epithelium.

alone may indicate intraductal carcinoma (13). Age at diagnosis averages about 60 years, but breast carcinoma has been diagnosed in male adults at virtually all ages. Almost 90% of male breast carcinomas express estrogen receptor (14).

Mammograms of men with breast carcinoma typically reveal distinct lesions with invasive margins that contrast sharply with the surrounding fatty tissue (15,16). Cystic papillary carcinoma produces a discrete round mass that may contain calcifications (17). Microcalcifications are found in 9% to 30% of male breast carcinomas studied mammographically (18,19).

Approximately 85% of male mammary carcinomas are of the ordinary infiltrating duct variety (20,21) (Fig. 7). An intraductal component is found in 35% to 50% of male and 75% of female infiltrating duct carcinomas (20). Extensive intraductal carcinoma of the male breast constituting more than 25% of the tumor and involving surrounding breast is uncommon. The majority of the invasive tumors are moderately or poorly differentiated (21) (Fig. 8), but low-grade and tubular carcinomas have been described (20) (Fig. 9). The structure of male infiltrating duct carcinoma duplicates that of carcinomas in the female breast and includes cribriform, comedo, papillary, solid, and gland-forming patterns. Papillary carcinomas, often with a prominent cystic component, are relatively more common among men than women, constituting 3% to 5% of male carcinomas (20,21) but only 1% to 2% of carcinomas in women (Fig. 10). On occasion, the distinction between a primary carcinoma of the breast and metastatic prostatic carcinoma may be difficult. The immunohistochemical demonstration of prostatic acid phosphatase or prostate-specific antigen is diagnostic of metastatic prostatic carcinoma, whereas the finding of intracellular mucin supports a diagnosis of mammary carcinoma.

The histologic appearances of intraductal carcinoma in men include comedo, cribriform, solid, micropapillary, and papillary patterns (Fig. 11). When intraductal carcinoma arises in gynecomastia, it is sometimes possible to find transitions in the gynecomastia from atypical hyperplasia of

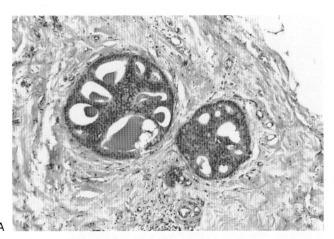
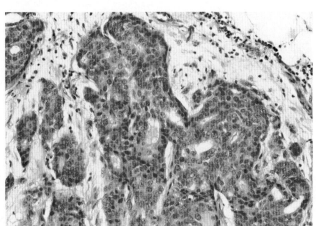

FIGURE 7. Male breast carcinoma. The patient was a 75-year-old man with a palpable tumor. **A,B:** The needle core biopsy sample reveals cribriform intraductal carcinoma and moderately differentiated infiltrating duct carcinoma that has cribriform features.

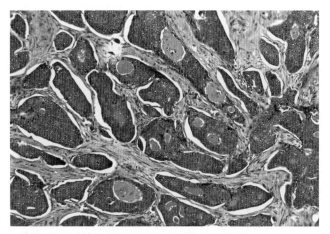

FIGURE 8. Male breast carcinoma. Infiltrating duct carcinoma with focal necrosis and poorly differentiated nuclear grade.

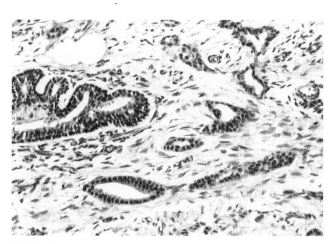

FIGURE 9. Male breast carcinoma. Tubular carcinoma in the male breast is composed of angular glands infiltrating around a duct.

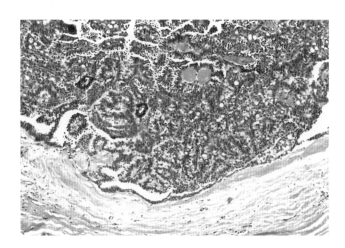

FIGURE 10. Male breast carcinoma. Cystic papillary carcinoma protrudes into the lumen of a greatly dilated duct.

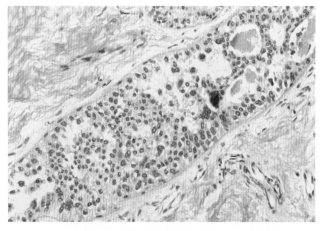

A

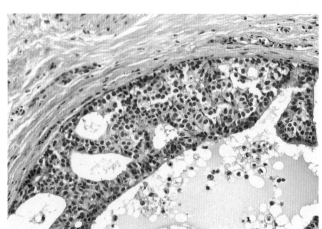

B

FIGURE 11. Male breast carcinoma, intraductal. Two views of cribriform intraductal carcinoma. **A:** The duct is cut longitudinally. One microcalcification is present. The tumor cells have low- to intermediate-grade nuclei. The patient was a 44-year-old man who presented with serous nipple discharge and a mass. **B:** Part of a duct with cribriform intraductal carcinoma cut transversely in a 70-year-old man. The carcinoma cells have a low nuclear grade.

ducts to carcinoma (22). Comedo necrosis and epithelial clear-cell change are features more strongly associated with intraductal carcinoma than with hyperplasia in gynecomastia.

Prognosis is significantly related to stage at diagnosis as determined by tumor size and nodal status (20,23–25). The presence of lymphatic tumor emboli negatively influences prognosis (26). Numerous investigators have concluded that male and female patients with the same stage of disease have a similar prognosis (20,27).

BREAST TUMORS IN CHILDREN

Juvenile papillomatosis (JP) is a localized benign proliferative lesion that usually occurs in women less than 30 years of age; two thirds of the patients are younger than 25. JP is uncommon before puberty and after the age of 40 years (28,29). The typical clinical finding is a solitary, firm, discrete unilateral tumor that is palpably indistinguishable from a fibroadenoma. Bilateral JP, which may be synchronous or metachronous, is occasionally encountered. Very rare instances of multifocal tumors have been reported. Separate, coexistent fibroadenomas are common.

Few descriptions of the mammographic findings in JP are available because mammography is usually not performed preoperatively in these young women. The films reveal a localized area of increased density with a border that is gener-

ally not as well defined as that of a fibroadenoma (29,30). The sonographic appearance of JP is that of an inhomogeneous, ill-defined mass with hypoechoic areas, largely at the periphery (30).

At the time of diagnosis, patients with JP report a frequency of positive family history for breast carcinoma that is similar to that of patients who have mammary carcinoma (31), and with further follow-up, the frequency of positive family history exceeds 50% (32). The female relatives most likely to be affected by breast carcinoma are mothers and maternal aunts of JP patients. Breast carcinoma has only rarely been seen in the sisters of JP patients.

Histologic examination reveals a spectrum of benign proliferative changes that are present in varying proportions in individual cases. Cysts and duct hyperplasia are constant features (Fig. 12). The epithelium of cysts and proliferative foci frequently exhibit apocrine metaplasia. Stasis of secretion in cysts and ducts is manifested by collections of lipid-laden histiocytes. Sclerosing adenosis, lobular hyperplasia, and fibroadenomatoid hyperplasia are variably present. In most cases, the ductal proliferative changes consist of ordinary hyperplasia. Sometimes, ductal hyperplasia has a radial scar pattern. Atypical changes in the ductal hyperplasia include cribriform or micropapillary growth patterns and intraductal necrosis. In one series, significant atypia was detected in 40% of lesions and intraductal necrosis in 15% (32).

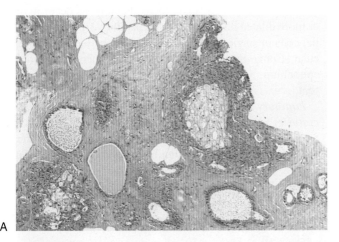

A

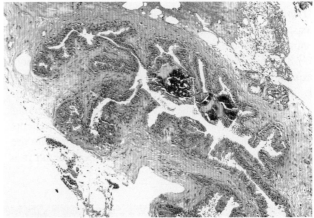

B

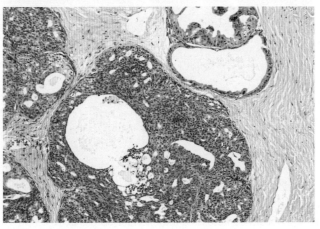

C

FIGURE 12. Juvenile papillomatosis. A–C: This needle core biopsy specimen is from a 2-cm breast tumor in an 18-year-old woman. The diagnostic features are cysts, cystic and papillary apocrine metaplasia, duct hyperplasia, and stasis. Calcifications are present in the papillary apocrine epithelium in (B).

Ten percent to 15% of patients with JP also have breast carcinoma (29,32,33). Virtually all these women have had a positive family history for breast carcinoma, usually affecting their mother or a maternal aunt (32,33). The types of breast carcinoma that have been encountered include intraductal carcinoma, lobular carcinoma *in situ*, infiltrating duct carcinoma, and secretory (juvenile) carcinoma. Most of these patients have had carcinoma and JP diagnosed concurrently. With few exceptions, the carcinoma was within and appeared to arise from the JP. A review of 41 patients with at least 10 years of follow-up after the diagnosis of JP (median age, 14 years) found that breast carcinoma subsequently developed in 4 patients (10%) after an interval of 5 to 15 years (32). These patients were 25 to 42 years old when JP was diagnosed, and thus all were past the mean age for JP. Three of the patients had multifocal or bilateral JP.

Excisional biopsy is often performed for JP with little margin. Incomplete excision probably predisposes to local recurrence, but recurrence may develop even when the margins appear to be adequate histologically. Re-excision of the biopsy site is recommended if the lesion has not been grossly excised or if there is severe atypia. Unless carcinoma is found in the tumor, no treatment is necessary after excisional biopsy. Mammography should be employed judiciously, especially for patients under 35 years of age, during follow-up. Ultrasonography is a useful adjunct to mammography. Female relatives of JP patients, especially on the maternal side, are advised to have regular breast surveillance.

Papillary duct hyperplasia and ***papillomas*** are infrequent breast lesions in patients less than 30 years old (34). The predominantly female patients have a median age of 17 years (35). The majority (70%) are 15 to 25 years of age. The most frequent presenting symptom is a mass. Fewer than 20% of patients have nipple discharge, which may be bloody or clear. Any part of the breast may be affected, but periareolar or subareolar lesions are most common. Very few patients have been subjected to mammography, and the results are nonspecific (35). Microcalcifications have been found in a few cases.

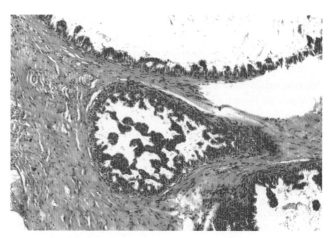

FIGURE 14. Papillomatosis. The patient was a 17-year-old girl with a breast mass. Multiple dilated ducts were present with micropapillary hyperplasia.

Three microscopic growth patterns have been described. ***Sclerosing papilloma*** has been found in nearly 50% of cases. This radial scarlike lesion is fundamentally a papilloma distorted and disrupted by a desmoplastic proliferation of myoepithelial and stromal cells (Fig. 13). Small clusters of epithelial cells incorporated into the stromal proliferation can be mistaken for invasive carcinoma. Lobules may be included in the sclerosing proliferation.

About one third of the lesions are ***papillomas*** without sclerosis, limited to a single focus. Papillomas occur in one or more dilated ducts that contain papillary fronds of epithelial cells in single or multiple layers, supported by fibrovascular stroma. Infrequent mitoses may be encountered in the epithelium. Myoepithelial cell hyperplasia is variably present.

Papillary hyperplasia involving multiple ducts (papillomatosis) is encountered in about 25% of cases. Papillary fronds supported by fibrovascular stroma are seen in some foci, but the hyperplasia often has a solid or micropapillary pattern. In micropapillary areas, the nuclei of hyperplastic epithelial cells tend to become smaller and more hyperchro-

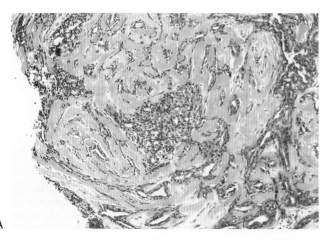

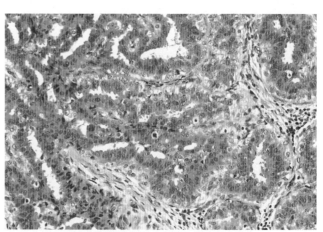

A B

FIGURE 13. Sclerosing papilloma. A: This needle core biopsy specimen from a breast tumor in a 19-year-old woman shows areas of dense sclerosis with epithelium compressed into slender cords. **B:** A portion of the lesion with florid duct hyperplasia.

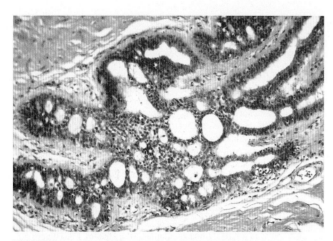

FIGURE 15. Juvenile atypical duct hyperplasia. Laciform hyperplasia is present in this biopsy specimen from an area of breast thickening in a 21-year-old woman.

matic at the tips of individual papillae (Fig. 14). Myoepithelial cell hyperplasia may be present. Some lesions exhibit cytologic atypia.

Most patients with one of the types of papillary duct hyperplasia can be managed by excisional biopsy. In one series, recurrences in the breast were detected in 16% of patients after a median interval of 3 years (35). Information presently available supports the view that papillary duct hyperplasia does not predispose children and young women to the development of breast carcinoma at an early age.

Juvenile atypical duct hyperplasia is a microscopic ductal proliferative lesion that has been described in female patients 18 to 26 years old, with a mean age of 21 years at diagnosis (36). The ductal hyperplasia has been found in biopsy samples of breast "thickening" (four cases) or in specimens from patients who underwent reduction mammoplasty for "mammary hypertrophy" (five cases). Histologic examination reveals widely separated, individual ducts with micropapillary or cribriform epithelial hyperplasia (Fig. 15). In the typical specimen, the area between the hyperplastic

ducts is occupied by dense, collagenous stroma in which there are also widely spaced ducts without hyperplasia and lobules, an important diagnostic feature that is difficult to appreciate in the limited sample obtained by a needle core biopsy (Fig. 16). The hyperplastic changes tend to develop focally in the epithelium of an affected duct. In some ducts, the hyperplastic epithelium forms a lacelike network in the lumen. Myoepithelial cells are present in a continuous or discontinuous fashion.

Fibroadenomas account for at least 75% of breast tumors in children (37). Most are similar histologically to comparable tumors in young adult women (38). Between 5% and 10% of fibroadenomas in adolescent girls attain a substantial size and qualify for the term giant fibroadenoma. Despite their rapid growth and variably cellular stroma, giant fibroadenomas have a benign clinical course. Juvenile fibroadenoma is discussed in Chapter 7.

Cystosarcomas that occur in this age group have the same histologic characteristics as comparable tumors in adults (39). Important features that distinguish cystosarcomas from giant or juvenile fibroadenomas include areas of cellular stromal overgrowth relative to the epithelium, a tendency for cellularity to be greatest in the subepithelial stroma, the presence of stromal mitoses and an invasive border. Although most cystosarcomas in children follow a benign clinical course after excision, instances of local recurrence and systemic metastases have been reported (39).

Breast carcinoma is extremely unusual in children. A literature review published in 1977 listed 74 cases reported between 1888 and 1972 (40). Most of the patients have been girls, with an average age of about 13 years. With few exceptions, the presenting sign has been a mass. Histologically, a substantial number of the tumors have been of the secretory (juvenile) type (see Chapter 18), but other forms of carcinoma commonly found in adults have also been described in children. Small-cell carcinoma of the breast in children is a highly malignant neoplasm that is difficult to distinguish from lymphoma and embryonal rhabdomyosarcoma in rou-

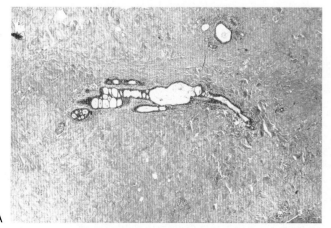
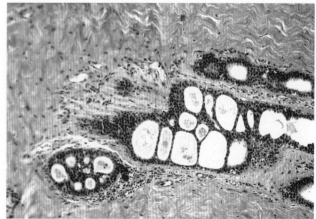

A   B

FIGURE 16. Juvenile atypical duct hyperplasia. A,B: This specimen was obtained from a reduction mammoplasty performed for juvenile hypertrophy in a 23-year-old woman. Laciform hyperplasia is a focal abnormality. Note the broad expanse of collagenous stroma.

tine sections unless *in situ* carcinoma is found. Immunoreactivity for cytokeratin should be detectable, and the cells are not reactive with markers for lymphoma or myosarcoma.

REFERENCES

Benign Proliferative Lesions of the Male Breast

1. Green L, Wysowski DK, Fourcroy JL. Gynecomastia and breast cancer during finasteride therapy. *N Engl J Med* 1996;335:823.
2. Michels LG, Gold RH, Arndt RD. Radiography of gynecomastia and other disorders of the male breast. *Radiology* 1977;122:117–122.
3. Bannayan GA, Hajdu SI. Gynecomastia: clinicopathologic study of 351 cases. *Am J Clin Pathol* 1972;57:431–437.
4. Andersen JA, Gram JB. Gynecomasty. Histological aspects in a surgical material. *Acta Pathol Microbiol Immunol Scand* 1982;90:185–190.
5. Navas MDM, Povedano JLR, Mendivil EA, et al. Intracystic papilloma in male breast: ultrasonography and pneumocystography diagnosis. *J Clin Ultrasound* 1993;21:38–40.
6. Waldo ED, Sidhu GS, Hu AW. Florid papillomatosis of male nipple after diethylstilbesterol therapy. *Arch Pathol* 1975;99:364–366.
7. Ansah-Boateng Y, Tavassoli FA. Fibroadenoma and cystosarcoma phyllodes of the male breast. *Mod Pathol* 1992;5:114–116.
8. Bartoli C, Zurrida SM, Clemente C. Phyllodes tumor in a male patient with bilateral gynecomastia induced by oestrogen therapy for prostatic carcinoma. *Eur J Surg Oncol* 1991;17:215–217.
9. Tedeschi LG, McCarthy PE. Involutional mammary duct ectasia and periductal mastitis in a male. *Hum Pathol* 1974;5:232–236.
10. Banik S, Hale R. Fibrocystic disease in the male breast. *Histopathology* 1988;12:214–216.

Carcinoma of the Male Breast

11. Ewertz M, Holmberg L, Karjalainen S, Tretli S, Adami H-O. Incidence of male breast cancer in Scandinavia 1943–1982. *Int J Cancer* 1989;43:27–31.
12. Hultborn R, Friberg S, Hultborn KA. Male breast carcinoma. I. A study of the total material reported to the Swedish Cancer Registry 1958–1967 with respect to clinical and histopathologic parameters. *Acta Oncol* 1987;26:241–256.
13. Wang Y, Abreau M, Hoda S. Mammary duct carcinoma *in situ* in males: pathological findings and clinical considerations. *Mod Pathol* 1997;10:27A.
14. Rosen PP, Menendez-Botet CJ, Nisselbaum JS, Schwartz MK, Urban JA. Estrogen receptor in lesions of the male breast. *Cancer* 1976;37:1866–1868.
15. Dershaw DD. Male mammography. *AJR Am J Roentgenol* 1986;146:127–131.
16. Chantra PK, So GJ, Wollman JS, Bassett LW. Mammography of the male breast. *AJR Am J Roentgenol* 1995;164:853–858.
17. Sonksen CJ, Michell M, Sundaresan M. Case report: intracystic papillary carcinoma of the breast in a male patient. *Clin Radiol* 1996;51:438–439.
18. Ouimet-Oliva D, Hebert G, Ladouceur J. Radiographic characteristics of male breast cancer. *Radiology* 1978;129:37–40.
19. Dershaw DD, Borgen PI, Deutch BM, Liberman L. Mammographic findings in men with breast cancer. *AJR Am J Roentgenol* 1993;160:267–270.
20. Heller KS, Rosen PP, Schottenfeld D, Ashikari R, Kinne DW. Male breast cancer. A clinicopathologic study of 97 cases. *Ann Surg* 1978;188:60–65.
21. Visfeldt J, Sheike O. Male breast cancer. I. Histologic typing and grading of 187 Danish cases. *Cancer* 1973;32:985–990.
22. Scheike O, Visfeldt J. Male breast cancer. 4. Gynecomastia in patients with breast cancer. *Acta Pathol Microbiol Scand A* 1973;81:359–365.
23. Adami H-O, Hakulinen T, Ewertz M, Tretli S, Holmberg L, Karjalainen S. The survival pattern in male breast cancer. An analysis of 1429 patients from the Nordic countries. *Cancer* 1989;64:1177–1182.
24. Ciatto S, Iossa A, Bonardi R, Pacini P. Male breast carcinoma: review of a multicenter series of 150 cases. *Tumori* 1990;76:555–558.
25. Hultborn R, Friberg S, Hultborn KA, Peterson L-E, Ragnhult I. Male breast carcinoma. II. A study of the total material reported to the Swedish Cancer Registry 1958–1967 with respect to treatment, prognostic factors and survival. *Acta Oncol* 1987;26:327–341.
26. Joshi MG, Lee AKC, Loda M, Camus MG, Heatley GJ, Hughes KS. Male breast carcinoma: an evaluation of prognostic factors contributing to a poorer outcome. *Cancer* 1996;77:490–498.
27. Borgen P, Senie RT, McKinnon WMP, Kinne DW, Rosen PP. Carcinoma of the male breast. Analysis of prognosis compared with matched female patients. *Ann Surg Oncol* 1997;4:385–388.

Breast Tumors in Children

28. Rosen PP, Cantrell B, Mullen DL, De Palo A. Juvenile papillomatosis (Swiss cheese disease) of the breast. *Am J Surg Pathol* 1980;4:3–12.
29. Rosen PP, Holmes G, Lesser ML, Kinne DW, Beattie EJ. Juvenile papillomatosis and breast carcinoma. *Cancer* 1985;55:1345–1352.
30. Kersschot EAJ, Hermans M-E, Pauwels C, et al. Juvenile papillomatosis of the breast: sonographic appearance. *Radiology* 1988;169:631–633.
31. Rosen PP, Lyngholm B, Kinne DW, Beattie EJ Jr. Juvenile papillomatosis of the breast and family history of breast carcinoma. *Cancer* 1982;49:2591–2595.
32. Rosen PP, Kimmel M. Juvenile papillomatosis of the breast: a follow-up study of 41 patients having biopsies before 1979. *Am J Clin Pathol* 1990;93:599–603.
33. Bazzocchi F, Santini D, Martinelli G, et al. Juvenile papillomatosis (epitheliosis) of the breast. *Am J Clin Pathol* 1986;86:745–748.
34. Rosen PP. Papillary duct hyperplasia of the breast in children and young adults. *Cancer* 1985;56:1611–1617.
35. Wilson M, Cranor ML, Rosen PP. Papillary duct hyperplasia of the breast in children and young women. *Mod Pathol* 1993;6:570–574.
36. Eliasen CA, Cranor ML, Rosen PP. Atypical duct hyperplasia of the breast in young females. *Am J Surg Pathol* 1992;16:246–251.
37. Bower R, Bell ML, Ternbergh JL. Management of breast lesions in children and adolescents. *J Pediatr Surg* 1976;11:337–346.
38. Ashikari R, Farrow JH, O'Hara J. Fibroadenomas in the breast of juveniles. *Surg Gynecol Obstet* 1971;32:259–262.
39. Rajan PB, Cranor ML, Rosen PP. Cystosarcoma phyllodes in adolescent girls and young women: a study of 45 patients. *Am J Surg Pathol* 1998;22:64–69.
40. Ashikari H, Jun MY, Farrow JH, Rosen PP, Johnston SF. Breast carcinoma in children and adolescents. *Clin Bull* 1977;7:55–62.

CHAPTER 28

Pathologic Changes Associated with Needling Procedures

The morphologic changes attributable to needling in breast tissue have not, until recently, attracted much attention. In a series of more than 10,000 breast lesions subjected to fine-needle aspiration (23-gauge needle), Us-Krasovec et al. (1) reported that tissue injury was infrequent, consisting only of small areas of hemorrhage. Other studies of changes in the breast associated with fine-needle aspiration have been limited to case reports. Tabbara et al. (2) described a single breast biopsy specimen with extensive intraductal carcinoma after fine-needle aspiration. Clusters of intact, abnormal epithelial cells were present in an inflammatory background in the needle track, simulating stromal invasion. Harter et al. (3) also reported a single case in which fragments of mucinous carcinoma were identified in the needle track of a wire-localized breast biopsy specimen that had been subjected to stereotactic 14-gauge needle core biopsy 2 weeks previously. Grabau et al. (4) found carcinoma cells along a needle track in the skin of a mastectomy specimen after invasive carcinoma had been diagnosed by core needle biopsy 26 days previously.

Virtually all excisional biopsy specimens obtained after needle biopsy or localization contain foci of hemorrhage in the breast stroma (5). Blood within the lumina of ducts and lobules not involved by the pathologic process as well as in epithelial structures in the lesional area is a frequent manifestation of prior needling (6) (Fig. 1). Disruption of the epithelium in the lesion may result in displacement of epithelial cells into the needle track and into stroma in the lesional area to produce a pattern that simulates invasive carcinoma (2,5–8) (Figs. 2,3). Displacement of benign or carcinomatous epithelium is suggested by the finding of scattered, isolated fragments of epithelium in artificial spaces within the breast stroma. At the needle biopsy site, the displaced epithelium is accompanied by hemorrhage, inflammation, hemosiderin-laden macrophages, or granulation tissue. Displaced epithelium that is not in the biopsy site may have no stromal reaction. This effect can lead to the mistaken diagnosis of invasive carcinoma in a benign lesion (Fig. 4). It is not unusual to find fragments of sloughed epithelium in the lumina of ducts and cysts that resemble displaced epithe-

lium in the stroma. Displaced epithelium in vascular spaces is indistinguishable from intrinsic lymphatic or vascular invasions (6,7) (Figs. 5–7). The extent to which current breast needling procedures contribute to the hematogenous or lymphatic dispersal of tumor cells has not been specifically determined.

Stromal epithelial displacement was found in three of five surgical biopsy specimens from patients with intraductal carcinoma and in three of seven papillary carcinomas studied by Boppana et al. (7). Lee et al. (8) drew attention to epithelial displacement in granulation tissue adjacent to a benign papillary tumor, simulating invasive carcinoma. A granulation tissue reaction may also be found around epithelium displaced from carcinoma if sufficient time elapses between the needling procedure and the excisional biopsy. This phenomenon can be difficult to distinguish from invasion when intraductal carcinoma is present (Figs. 5,8,9).

Youngson et al. (5) reported finding displaced epithelium in biopsy specimens of papillary duct hyperplasia and papilloma, as well as in association with various types of intraductal carcinoma, invasive carcinoma, and cystosarcoma phyllodes. The average interval between the needling procedure and excisional biopsy was 10 days, with as long as 28 days elapsing in one case. Intravascular or intralymphatic fragments of benign or malignant epithelium were present in seven cases, six of which also had stromal displacement. One of these women, who had extensive intraductal carcinoma associated with stromal displacement and lymphatic tumor emboli in the breast, also had clusters of carcinoma cells in the subcapsular sinuses of two axillary lymph nodes (Fig. 10).

Epithelial displacement in surgical breast specimens obtained after needling procedures may be encountered with increasing frequency in general surgical pathology practice as the trend toward needle-based diagnosis increases. The clinical significance of this phenomenon is unknown. These alterations present the pathologist with a challenging diagnostic problem. Eliciting a history of a previous needling procedure may help prevent histopathologic confusion and an erroneous tissue diagnosis. A diagnosis of malignancy

Text continues on page 277

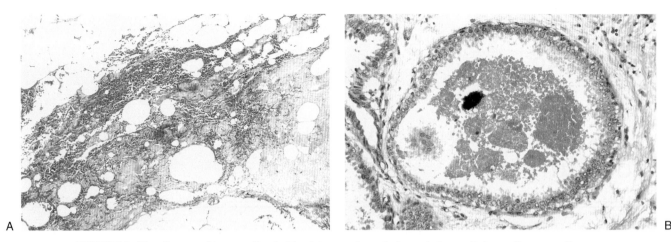

FIGURE 1. Needle core biopsy site. A: Fresh hemorrhage in breast stroma 5 days after a needle core biopsy. **B:** Intraductal hemorrhage with a calcification in the vicinity of a needle core biopsy performed for nonpalpable microcalcifications. The lesion proved to be tubular carcinoma. This duct exhibits columnar cell hyperplasia.

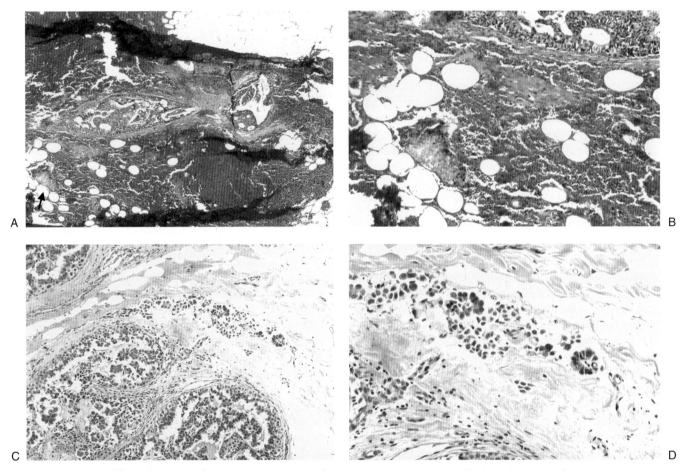

FIGURE 2. Epithelial displacement in postbiopsy excision specimen. A: Intraductal carcinoma is surrounded by hemorrhage at a needle core biopsy site, with a displaced fragment of carcinoma in the lower left corner (*arrow*). **B:** Magnified view of the displaced carcinoma. **C,D:** Displaced fragments of intraductal carcinoma are in the stroma near the site of a needle core biopsy performed 7 days previously. Note the absence of reactive changes in the stroma and the well-preserved cytologic appearance of the displaced tumor cells. The appearance of the displaced epithelium in part resembles lymphatic invasion, but no endothelial cell nuclei are evident around the spaces that contain tumor cells.

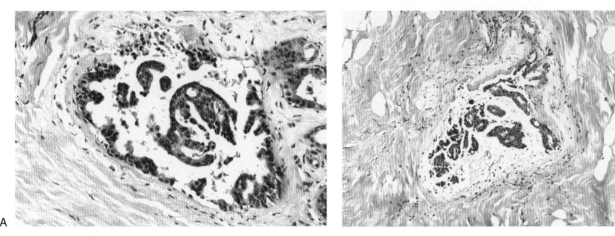

FIGURE 3. Disruption of intraductal carcinoma in a postbiopsy excision specimen. A: Portions of the intraductal carcinoma have been dislodged from the basement membrane and are displaced into the duct lumen after a needle core biopsy. **B:** Another area of the specimen in (A) shows severe disruption of intraductal carcinoma. The detached epithelial fragments have remained within the confines of the basement membrane.

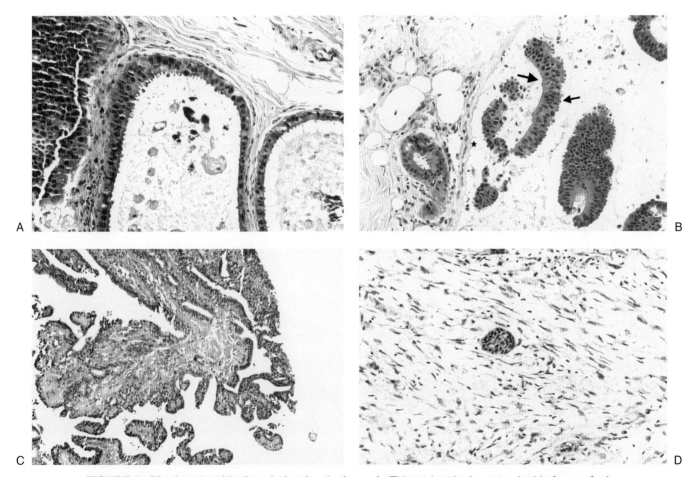

FIGURE 4. Displaced epithelium in benign lesions. A: This patient had a nonpalpable focus of microcalcifications detected by mammography. A needle core biopsy revealed cystic apocrine metaplasia with calcifications and secretion. **B:** The needle core biopsy site in the subsequent excisional biopsy specimen contained these detached fragments of epithelium surrounded by secretion, which led to an erroneous diagnosis of mucinous carcinoma. Note the apocrine "snouts" on the luminal surface (*thin arrow*) and smooth basal edge (*thick arrow*). The basement membrane (*asterisk*) is visible at the junction of the tissue on the left and the cyst lumen on the right. One small, intact gland with calcification is shown on the left. **C:** This needle core biopsy specimen of a papilloma was obtained from a mammographically detected, nonpalpable, 8-mm tumor **(D)**. The excisional biopsy performed 2 weeks later contained residual papilloma and granulation tissue with clusters of displaced benign epithelial cells, one of which is shown here.

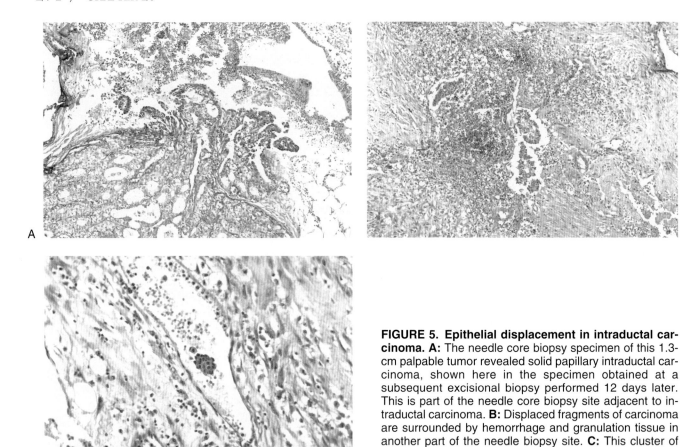

FIGURE 5. Epithelial displacement in intraductal carcinoma. A: The needle core biopsy specimen of this 1.3-cm palpable tumor revealed solid papillary intraductal carcinoma, shown here in the specimen obtained at a subsequent excisional biopsy performed 12 days later. This is part of the needle core biopsy site adjacent to intraductal carcinoma. **B:** Displaced fragments of carcinoma are surrounded by hemorrhage and granulation tissue in another part of the needle biopsy site. **C:** This cluster of carcinoma cells was found in a dilated vascular channel near the needle core biopsy site.

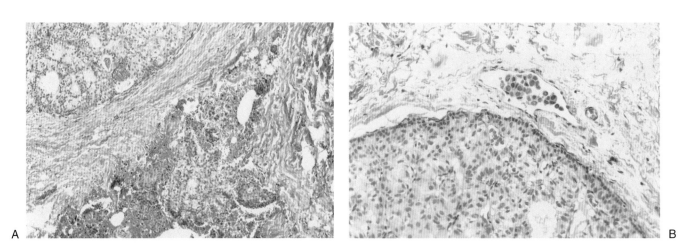

FIGURE 6. Epithelial displacement in intraductal carcinoma. A: This excisional biopsy specimen was obtained after a needle core biopsy performed on a mammographically detected nonpalpable lesion revealed intraductal carcinoma. Shown here is the needle core biopsy site with displaced carcinoma next to cribriform intraductal carcinoma. **B:** A cluster of carcinoma cells is shown in a lymphatic space next to the intraductal carcinoma. Note the absence of changes attributable to the needle core biopsy in this region.

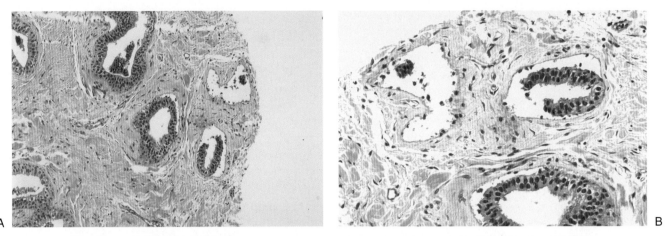

FIGURE 7. Epithelial disruption in a needle core biopsy specimen. A,B: Epithelium in these hyperplastic ducts has been partially dislodged from the basement membranes. The loose fragment in the duct lumen near the edge of the tissue in a needle core biopsy specimen simulates carcinoma in a lymphatic space.

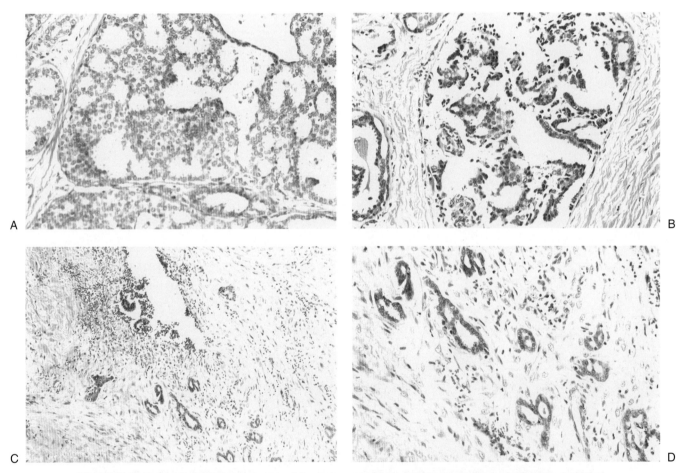

FIGURE 8. Epithelial displacement and invasive carcinoma after a needle core biopsy. A: Cribriform intraductal carcinoma as it appeared in an excisional biopsy specimen obtained 8 days after needle core biopsy of a mammographically detected lesion. **B:** Disrupted intraductal carcinoma in the same speciman as (A). **C,D:** Hemorrhage and displaced epithelial fragments in the needle core biopsy site. Well-differentiated invasive carcinoma is present in the stroma below the needle biopsy site.

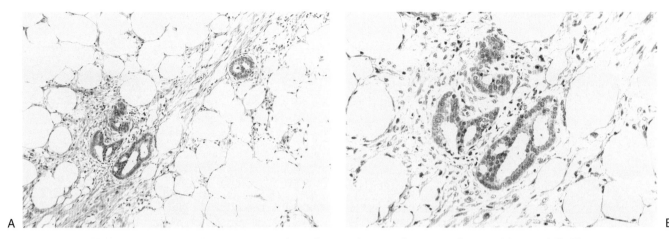

FIGURE 9. Epithelial displacement or invasive carcinoma after a needle core biopsy. A,B: These glands in an excisional biopsy specimen are surrounded by granulation tissue and fat necrosis 13 days after a needle core biopsy showed intraductal carcinoma. Although the possibility of epithelial displacement was considered, this focus was interpreted as representing invasive carcinoma because of the structured appearance of the epithelium and stroma.

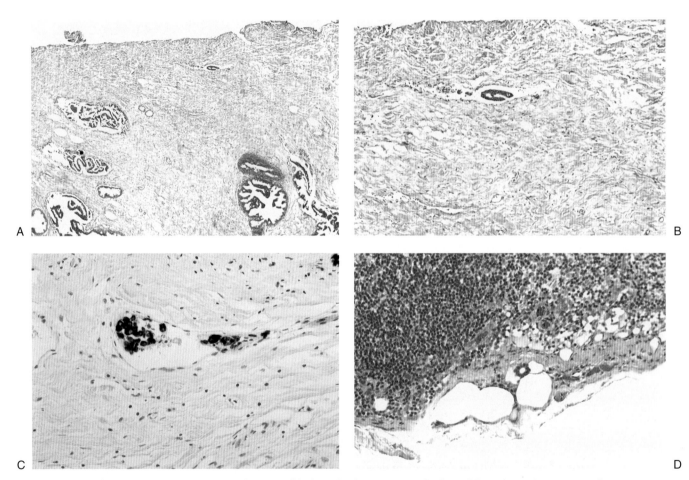

FIGURE 10. Intraductal carcinoma with lymphatic tumor emboli and lymph node metastasis. A,B: This excisional biopsy specimen was obtained 8 days after a needle core biopsy of mammographically detected calcifications revealed intraductal carcinoma. There is a *U*-shaped group of carcinoma cells in the lymphatic space near the upper border of the tissue. **C:** Other cells in lymphatic spaces are shown here to be immunoreactive for cytokeratin (immunoperoxidase: CAM5.2). **D:** Metastatic carcinoma that formed a ring in the subcapsular sinus of a lymph node is shown in this specimen. The axillary lymph node dissection was performed after lymphatic tumor emboli were demonstrated in the excisional biopsy specimen.

should not be based solely on the appearance of epithelium within stroma because epithelial displacement has been observed following needling procedures in benign breast lesions, notably papillary duct hyperplasia and intraductal papilloma.

The significance of carcinomatous lymphovascular emboli remains uncertain in the setting described above. Until further information becomes available, we have interpreted the finding of lymphatic tumor emboli as evidence of invasion in patients with *in situ* carcinoma, even when conventional stromal invasion cannot be identified. We have also interpreted the finding of clusters of carcinoma cells in a lymph node capsule or subcapsular sinus as metastatic carcinoma even when no intrinsic invasion has been found. Such foci may be mistakenly diagnosed as benign ectopic mammary glands. These patients usually also have lymphatic tumor emboli in the breast parenchyma in the vicinity of the needling procedure.

REFERENCES

1. Us-Krasovec M, Golouh R, Auersperg M, Pogacnik A. Tissue damage after fine needle aspiration biopsy. *Acta Cytol* 1992;36:456–457.
2. Tabbara SO, Frierson HF, Fechner RE. Diagnostic problems in tissues previously sampled by fine-needle aspiration. *Am J Clin Pathol* 1991;96: 76–80.
3. Harter LP, Curtis JS, Ponto G, Craig PH. Malignant seeding of the needle track during stereotaxic core needle breast biopsy. *Radiology* 1992; 185:713–714.
4. Grabau DA, Andersen JA, Graversen HP, Dyreborg A. Needle biopsy of breast cancer. Appearance of tumour cells along the needle track. *Eur J Surg Oncol* 1993;19:192–194.
5. Youngson BJ, Cranor M, Rosen PP. Epithelial displacement in surgical breast specimens following needling procedures. *Am J Surg Pathol* 1994;18:896–903.
6. Youngson BJ, Liberman L, Rosen PP. Displacement of carcinomatous epithelium in surgical breast specimens following stereotaxic core biopsy. *Am J Clin Pathol* 1995;103:598–602.
7. Boppana S, May M, Hoda S. Does prior fine-needle aspiration cause diagnostic difficulties in histologic evaluation of breast carcinomas? *Lab Invest* 1994;70:13A.
8. Lee KC, Chan JKC, Ho LC. Histologic changes in the breast after fine-needle aspiration. *Am J Surg Pathol* 1994;18:1039–1047.

CHAPTER 29

Pathologic Examination of Needle Core Biopsy Specimens

Paperwork submitted with the specimen container should specify the following: patient identification data; laterality; clinical indication(s) for the procedure, including relevant history; prior biopsies; clinical diagnosis; sites in the breast sampled; and specifics of the samples, such as the presence or absence of calcifications.

The needle biopsy cores should be placed in fixative by the radiologist promptly after the tissue has been obtained to preserve cytologic detail and minimize degradation of biologic markers, such as hormone receptors. For routine processing in a 24-hour period, 10% neutral buffered formaldehyde can be used. Longer periods of immersion in an aqueous fixative may result in radiographic disappearance of calcifications in needle core biopsy specimens but the impact of apparent radiographic dissolution on the histologic appearance of calcifications was not reported by these authors (1). Preservation of microcalcifications for up to 2 weeks has been described for specimens stored in 74.1% ethanol with 1.0% 2-propanol (1). The dissolution of calcifications may be influenced by specimen size. The author has been able to detect microcalcifications in surgical biopsy specimens after immersion in buffered 10% formaldehyde for periods of 2 or more weeks.

Needle biopsy cores from a lesion with calcifications demonstrated by mammography should be documented by the radiologist with a specimen radiograph. This procedure makes it possible to identify and segregate the core biopsy samples containing calcifications from those without demonstrable calcifications. The cores with and without calcifications from each biopsy site can be placed in separate, properly labeled containers and immersed in fixative. Alternatively, the two sets of cores can be placed into separate tissue cassettes differentiated by color and labeling and submitted in a single container. The method chosen to separate specimens should be standardized within a given institution.

Breast needle core biopsy specimens can be processed in the pathology laboratory together with other specimens by routine methods of paraffin embedding, sectioning, and staining with hematoxylin and eosin. Each set of cores should be embedded in one or more paraffin blocks labeled to correspond to specific specimen identity as described in the accompanying pathology requisition. A gross description should be recorded for each specimen documenting the number of cores, the range of length, and any other notable features. The entire specimen, including blood clot, must be embedded for histologic study. If the material corresponding to a specific sample is too abundant to examine in a single paraffin block, the cores should be separated into groups of approximately equal number and size. Cores are placed in the cassette in a manner that positions all samples at approximately the same plane within the paraffin block. Calcifications can be visualized during roentgenography of paraffin blocks and remain detectable in this condition for an indefinite period of time.

Serial histologic sections are cut at a 5- to 6-μm thickness from two or more levels in each tissue block, depending on the size of the sample. The sections are stained with hematoxylin and eosin for routine diagnostic purposes. It is preferable not to exhaust the tissue specimen in preparing initial histologic sections and to reserve material for additional studies, such as immunohistochemistry for hormone receptors or oncogene expression and other procedures that may assist in reaching a diagnosis (2,3). Estrogen receptors detected by immunohistochemistry in needle core biopsy samples correlated with the receptor status of specimens obtained by subsequent surgical excision in 93% of cases in one study (3). Agreement between the two biopsy specimens for progesterone receptors was observed in 69% of cases, a substantial discrepancy that the authors attributed to greater heterogeneity of receptor expression (3).

The presence or absence of calcifications in the sections should be reported for each specimen. If calcifications were described in the needle core radiograph and none are initially evident histologically, the slides should be examined for birefringent calcium oxalate crystals under polarized light (4). Radiographic study of the paraffin blocks may also be helpful to determine the location of calcifications (5). A detailed comparison of histologic sections of needle core biopsy specimens and corresponding specimen radiographic studies revealed that calcifications smaller than 100 μm detected microscopically were not visible radiographically (6). Consequently, histologically detected calcifications of this small dimension cannot be assumed to constitute the calcifications seen in a clinical mammogram. In the same study, calcifications described as linear and interpreted radiographically as having a "ductal" distribution had a ductal distribution histologically in 67% of the core biopsy specimens, whereas 24% were in the stroma and 9% were in other sites. Radiographically clustered calcifications also had a predominantly ductal distribution histologically.

The pathology report should describe the diagnostic features in a manner that presents the findings in a concise and clinically relevant form. It is not necessary to give a detailed microscopic description of the histologic findings as long as the specific components are clearly identified. For example, it is sufficient to report a diagnosis of "fibroadenoma" without offering a microscopic description of the individual microscopic characteristics that define such a lesion. Microscopic details may be added to the diagnosis to convey additional information, as, for example, in the diagnosis "fibroadenoma with cellular stroma; recommend excision to rule out cystosarcoma." The most frequent benign lesions are fibroadenoma, papilloma, sclerosing adenosis, duct hyperplasia, apocrine metaplasia, and radial scar. Fat necrosis, scar, lymph nodes, and pseudoangiomatous stromal hyperplasia are also encountered. The findings in specimens from 1,061 consecutive needle core biopsies performed at Memorial Hospital and reviewed by the author are given in Tables 1 through 3.

Standardized forms listing the majority of potential diagnoses are a useful method for reporting breast pathology findings in many routine cases. Having such a checklist is an efficient method for recording the diagnosis in a comprehensive manner. A major drawback, however, to the use of most formatted diagnoses is rigidity of the report, which usually gives equal weight to all components by presenting the findings in a predetermined sequence. In a particular case, certain diagnoses may require emphasis and should be given priority in the sequence of the report as well as additional commentary. If the preformatted report does not have sufficient flexibility to permit rearranging the diagnostic components when necessary, the pathologist may choose to issue a nonstructured diagnosis. This is especially important if critical information cannot be conveyed by amplifying the formatted text with comments. When atypical hyperplasia is diagnosed by needle core biopsy, the pathologic report

TABLE 2. *Pathology of 1,061 consecutive needle core biopsy specimens of the breast: 319 benign neoplasms (30%)*

Fibroadenoma	265
Papilloma	21
Pseudoangiomatous stromal hyperplasia	13
Cystosarcoma	13
Hemangioma	3
Fibromatosis	2
Granular-cell tumor	1
Lipoma	1

should recommend consideration of prompt surgical biopsy of the lesional area because approximately 50% of these patients are found to have carcinoma in the subsequent excisional specimen (7–9).

When carcinoma is diagnosed, the presence or absence of invasion must be noted (see Table 3). For *in situ* carcinoma, the diagnosis should state the type (ductal or lobular), nuclear grade, the architecture if the carcinoma is ductal (e.g., cribriform, solid), and the presence or absence of calcification. A high degree of concordance in the classification of intraductal carcinoma has been found between needle core and excisional biopsy specimens in the same patient. Jackman et al. (8) found intraductal comedocarcinoma in 91% of excisional specimens after a needle core diagnosis of comedocarcinoma and in 15% of excisional specimens following a needle core diagnosis of intraductal non-comedocarcinoma. Major benign findings should also be cited.

When invasive carcinoma is diagnosed, the subtype of tumor (ductal, lobular, or special type, such as tubular or mucinous), associated *in situ* carcinoma, nuclear and histologic grade, and vascular invasion should be described, in addition to any significant benign proliferative lesions and the distribution of calcifications. Comparison of the grading of invasive ductal carcinomas in needle core and excisional biopsy specimens of the same tumor reveals a tendency to assign a lower grade on the basis of the needle core biopsy (7). Difficulty in distinguishing invasive ductal and lobular carcinomas may be encountered when tubule formation is not apparent in the core biopsy specimen (7).

Needle core biopsy is highly accurate for the diagnosis of most breast lesions. However, it cannot be relied on to pro-

TABLE 1. *Pathology of 1,061 consecutive needle core biopsy specimens of the breast: 346 proliferative lesions (32%)*

Adenosis/sclerosing	63	Fibrosis/scar	38
Apocrine metaplasia	46	Negative breast	47
Atypical duct hyperplasia	32	Fat necrosis	19
Duct hyperplasia	38	Fat	9
Cysts	14	Lymph node	8
Fibroadenomatoid hyperplasia	9	Calcification	8
Atypical lobular hyperplasia	7		
Mucocele	5		
Secretory hyperplasia	3		

TABLE 3. *Pathology of 1,061 consecutive needle core biopsy specimens of the breast: 396 malignant neoplasms (38%)*

Carcinoma—387 (36%)				
Invasive ductal	229	Lymphoma	2
Intraductal	92	Sarcoma	2
Invasive lobular	31	Cystosarcoma	1
Tubular	13	Metastatic	4
Papillary	7		
Lobular *in situ*	7		
Mucinous	4		
Apocrine	2		
Adenoid cystic	1		
Medullary	1		

vide comprehensive data equal to what can be obtained from a surgically excised specimen. The pathologic report for a breast needle core biopsy specimen must be integrated with other patient data, including the clinical history, laboratory results, and physical and mammographic findings, to develop a treatment plan for the individual patient (10). As these judgments are made, consideration must be given to the potential advantages and limitations of needle core biopsy diagnosis that have been stressed throughout this volume.

REFERENCES

1. Moritz JD, Luftner-Nagel S, Westerhof JP, Oestmann J-W, Grabbe E. Microcalcifications in breast core biopsy specimens: disappearance at radiography after storage in formaldehyde. *Radiology* 1996;200: 361–363.
2. Dahlstrom JE, Jain S, Sutton T, Sutton S. Diagnostic accuracy of stereotactic core biopsy in a mammographic breast cancer screening programme. *Histopathology* 1996;28:421–427.
3. Zidan A, Christie Brown JS, Peston D, Shousha S. Oestrogen and progesterone receptor assessment in core biopsy specimens of breast carcinoma. *J Clin Pathol* 1997;50:27–29.
4. Stein MA, Karlan MS. Calcifications in breast biopsy specimens: discrepancies in radiologic-pathologic identification. *Radiology* 1991; 179:111–114.
5. Rebner M, Helvie MA, Pennes DR, Oberman HA, Ikeda DM, Adler DD. Paraffin tissue block radiography: adjunct to breast specimen radiography. *Radiology* 1989;173:695–696.
6. Dahlstrom JE, Sutton S, Jain S. Histologic-radiologic correlation of mammographically detected microcalcification in stereotactic core biopsies. *Am J Surg Pathol* 1998;22:256–259.
7. Dahlstrom JE, Sutton S, Jain S. Histological precision of stereotactic core biopsy in diagnosis of malignant and premalignant breast lesions. *Histopathology* 1996;28:537–541.
8. Jackman RJ, Nowels KW, Shepard MJ, Finkelstein SI, Marzoni MA Jr. Stereotaxic large-core needle biopsy of 450 nonpalpable breast lesions with surgical correlation in lesions with cancer or atypical hyperplasia. *Radiology* 1994;193:91–95.
9. Tocino I, Garcia BM, Carter D. Surgical biopsy findings in patients with atypical hyperplasia diagnosed by stereotaxic core needle biopsy. *Ann Surg Oncol* 1996;3:483–488.
10. Morrow M. When can stereotactic core biopsy replace excisional biopsy? A clinical perspective. *Breast Cancer Res Treat* 1995;36:1–9.

CHAPTER 30

Techniques for Imaging-Guided Needle Core Biopsy

D. David Dershaw

A variety of techniques are available, and others are in development, that make it possible to remove varying amounts of breast tissue percutaneously under imaging guidance. The menu of procedures from which the biopsy technique is chosen in any individual case is best understood by separating the imaging modality used to guide the biopsy probe into the lesion from the actual biopsy instrument used to retrieve tissue from the breast. For the pathologist, only the latter half of this process, the biopsy probe technology, may be evident. However, constraints dictated by the patient or by lesion configuration and conspicuity under varying imaging technologies can influence the physician's selection of the biopsy probe and thereby the character of the specimen obtained.

Before a decision to perform a biopsy is made, a complete imaging workup of nonpalpable lesions should be undertaken (1). It should not be the role of the biopsy procedure to replace such a workup. If a lesion presents as a palpable mass, the algorithm of the workup is modified by findings on physical examination. Because the development of a new, palpable breast mass is indicative of lesion growth, biopsy is often indicated for these lesions, unless it can be demonstrated that the mass is a cyst.

IMAGING TECHNOLOGIES FOR BREAST BIOPSY

Stereotactic Imaging

Stereotactic imaging employs radiographic (mammographic) imaging to triangulate the location of a lesion within the breast. Equipment is designed to obtain equally angled radiographic views of the suspected lesion (Fig. 1). When the lesion is located on these images, its depth from the skin surface can be calculated based on the following formula:

$$\Delta z = \frac{\Delta z}{2 \tan (15°)} = 1.866 \, \Delta x$$

As the x-ray beam is angled along the x-axis, or horizontal axis, there will be increasing change in the position of the lesion as it is located more deeply in the breast. Fifteen degrees is the standard angulation of the x-ray beam, although some manufacturers have altered this, and for equipment in which the x-ray tube is angled more steeply, the denominator of the formula is altered appropriately. Based on this formula, the z-axis, or depth of the lesion within the breast, is calculated (2). The vertical location of lesion, or y-axis, as well as the location of the lesion on the horizontal axis, or x-axis, is evident on the nonoblique (0° angulation) scout view of the breast. This view is also needed to determine if the lesion is in the field of view of the stereotactic unit. Calculation of the position of lesion in the x-, y- and z-axes is accomplished by feeding the location of the site at which the biopsy probe is to be positioned on the equally angled oblique or stereotactic views into a computer incorporated into the biopsy unit (Fig. 2).

Because the images for stereotactically guided biopsy are obtained with x-rays, as are mammograms, any lesion seen mammographically can potentially be sampled with stereotactic technique. Calcifications, which are not reliably seen with sonography or other imaging modalities, are readily imaged with stereotaxis. Abnormalities that are characterized by calcifications on the mammogram should therefore be sampled using this technology (3). Lesions that are seen only with sonography or magnetic resonance (MR) imaging cannot be sampled stereotactically with current technology.

Although mammographic abnormalities can be imaged with stereotaxis, in some situations, these may not be easily appreciated during the biopsy procedure. The field of view during the procedure can be as small as 4 × 5 cm; in most units with digital imaging, the field of view is 5 × 5 cm. This sometimes limits the ability of the physician to correlate the lesion seen during the biopsy easily with that found when the full breast is imaged with x-rays for a mammogram. On occasion, biopsy of the wrong lesion can result from this limited field of view. Areas of asymmetric tissue are particularly

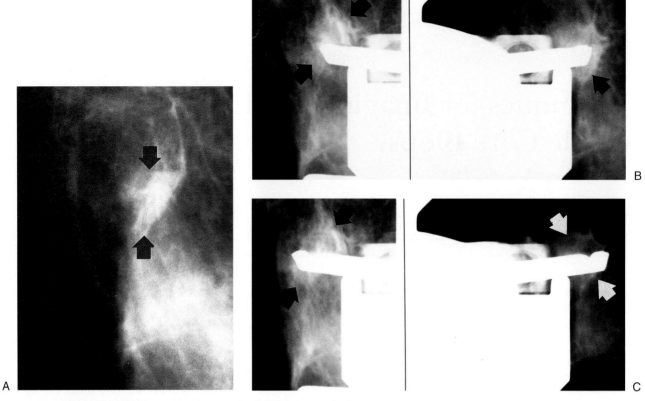

FIGURE 1. Stereotactic biopsy of a breast mass. A: Zero-degree angled scout film shows an irregular, uncalcified breast mass. The location of the mass in the horizontal and vertical axes is apparent on this image, but its depth in the breast cannot be determined. **B:** Fifteen-degree angled views of the same lesion (*arrows*) with a 14-gauge biopsy needle in the prefire position. Note how the configuration of the lesion changes with different angulation of the x-ray tube and alteration of the window and level (brightness and contrast) of the digital images. **C:** The postfire 15° angled views document that the biopsy needle has coursed through the lesion. Based on the prefire and postfire images, it can be determined that the tissue retrieved during the biopsy was derived from the lesion in question. Histologic assessment of the specimen showed fibrosis.

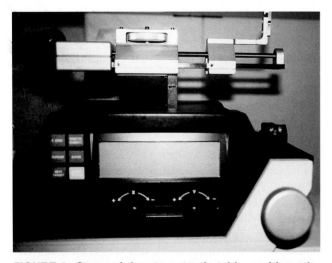

FIGURE 2. Stage of the stereotactic table positions the needle accurately within the breast. The gun is attached to the upper portion of this device, and the biopsy probe can be positioned manually or automatically at the desired x-, y-, and z-axes, as shown in Fig. 4. This stage is positioned between the x-ray tube and the breast, which is compressed against the imaging receptor.

difficult to localize in this setting. Architectural distortion can also be very difficult to localize. In some situations, it may be desirable to sample these lesions with preoperative needle localization rather than stereotactically guided core technique.

Digital Imaging

The use of digital imaging can influence the ability to localize areas during stereotactic biopsy. With digital imaging, information in the image can be collected and stored electronically, so that it is not necessary to rely on film development. The x-ray image of the breast is therefore more rapidly available and can be viewed in as little as 3 seconds rather than the 3 to 5 minutes required with film (4). One obvious advantage of this is that the patient is less likely to move during the procedure, so that the initial calculation of the lesion location in the field of view remains accurate. Patient tolerance is increased with shorter duration of the procedure. However, because this technology is expensive, it is not universally available.

Digital imaging also enables the image to be windowed

and leveled, with adjustment of brightness and darkness, as well as the amount of contrast in the picture. Although some lesions become more conspicuous with such manipulation, others can become more difficult to differentiate from background breast tissue. Although this situation should be unusual, it can result in biopsy of the wrong breast lesion. Digital imaging technology also sacrifices some image resolution. For this reason, some fine detail readily appreciated with film mammography can be difficult or impossible to appreciate digitally. This issue becomes important when faint microcalcifications are the biopsy target and the ability to localize these lesions accurately is limited.

Calcifications

When calcifications are sampled under stereotactic imaging, confirmation that they have been sampled should be obtained with specimen radiography. This is comparable to documenting removal of a lesion during a needle-localized breast biopsy procedure. If calcifications are not present in the initial cores removed from the breast, it is routine to continue sampling the breast until calcification is obtained (Fig. 3). However, prolongation of the biopsy procedure can be limited by patient tolerance. Also, if calcifications are not present in the initial 5 to 10 specimens, it is unlikely that continued attempts to obtain calcifications will be successful, particularly with gun-needle biopsy probes, because progressive destruction of breast architecture and hemorrhage into the area resulting from repeated passage of the core needle through a small volume of tissue decreases the ability to retrieve a cohesive piece of tissue from a site within the breast. The failure to obtain calcifications in lesions in which they have been characterized mammographically can considerably diminish the likelihood of making a diagnosis. In the assessment of any single core, this has been shown to decrease the ability to make a diagnosis based on that core from 82% to 40% (5). The significance of retrieval of calcification in core biopsy specimens appears to be as an indicator that the correct site within the breast has been sampled, even though the abnormality containing the lesion can be uncalcified. Failure to retrieve calcifications strongly suggests that the correct site in the breast has not been sampled.

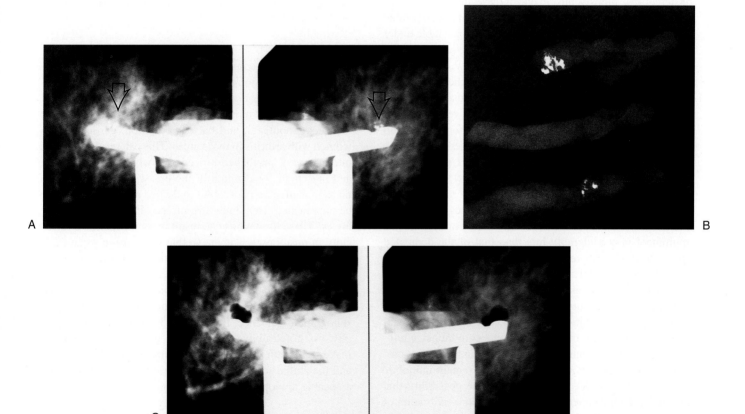

FIGURE 3. Stereotactic biopsy of breast calcifications. A: A small cluster of heterogeneous microcalcifications (*arrows*) is positioned adjacent to a vacuum-suction biopsy probe collection chamber on 15° angled stereotactic images. These views document accuracy of positioning before tissue removal begins. **B:** Specimen radiography of three of the cores removed during this biopsy demonstrates that targeted calcifications are present in two of the cores. **C:** A stereotactic pair taken at the end of the procedure shows that all calcifications have been removed, and a small cavity is now present at the biopsy site. This postbiopsy change can resolve within a few days. The calcifications were in a fibroadenoma.

It is reasonable for the pathologist to expect that the physician performing the biopsy will communicate whether the lesion in question contained calcification and whether calcification was obtained at the time of biopsy. If desired, it should be possible for cores containing calcification to be submitted separately from those without calcium. As with specimens obtained at surgical biopsy, it is possible to obtain x-ray images of the paraffin block if calcifications are not appreciated on routine sectioning. This can be done to guide the pathologist in obtaining further sections for microscopic examination. It is not routine for specimen radiography of uncalcified lesions to be performed, as it is in surgical biopsy. Successful biopsy of these lesions is documented by imaging the location of the needle and its relationship to the breast mass after tissue has been obtained. X-ray imaging of the paraffin block to localize the area of interest within the fixed cores has also not been reported. Of course, the final determination of the success of the biopsy for any type of lesion awaits histopathologic interpretation.

Upright versus Prone Dedicated Stereotactic Units

Current equipment design offers two major configurations of stereotactic biopsy units. In one of these, the add-on or upright unit, a stereotactic device attaches to a mammographic unit. In the other type, the patient lies prone on a table under which a mammographic unit is located; this type is designed exclusively to perform breast biopsies.

Upright equipment is designed to be attached to a mammographic unit, modifying it so that it can be used to perform stereotactic biopsies (6). This equipment is removable, so that the unit can be used for regular mammography. With this equipment design, a room need not be dedicated to the performance of stereotactic breast biopsies. Upright equipment design makes it possible to obtain biopsy specimens of certain lesions located in the posterior breast near the chest wall or in the axilla, areas that are sometimes inaccessible when tables and the prone position are used. The price of this equipment is considerably less than that of the dedicated table, about $35,000 versus $140,000, so that facilities with a limited budget or space can more readily perform stereotactic biopsies with this equipment than with tables (7).

The major disadvantage of upright stereotactic units is the limited space available for performance of the biopsy procedure. Because of the bulkiness of some core biopsy equipment, this can be technically limiting during the biopsy procedure. The patient is required to sit and remain immobile during the procedure, which increases the possibility that movement by the patient will cause the initial calibration of lesion location to be incorrect. Also, because patients are sitting and can view the biopsy procedure as it is being performed, vasovagal reactions sometimes occur, and these have been reported in 1% to 5% of procedures (8).

Dedicated tables provide the physician with greater working space during the procedure (Fig. 4). Because the patient is prone during the biopsy, the incidence of vasovagal reac-

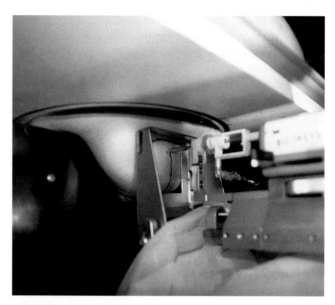

FIGURE 4. Stereotactic biopsy. A close-up view of a stereotactic biopsy shows the patient on the top of the photograph, lying prone, with her breast hanging through a hole in the table. The breast is compressed against the digital imaging receptor. The biopsy probe is attached to a stage (Fig. 2) that accurately positions it in three dimensions. The biopsy needle is in place within the breast to remove tissue from the lesion in question.

tions is essentially reduced to none. Patient anxiety is also reduced by inability to see the biopsy being performed. However, because the patient is required to lie prone on a padded metal table for 20 minutes and often longer, discomfort in the neck, shoulders, and back is common, particularly in women with arthritis in these areas. This can result in patient intolerance of prolonged procedures, which causes motion and inaccurate localization of the breast lesion. Of the two major manufacturers of tables, only one allows the lesion to be approached from anywhere on the circumference of the breast. These limitations can result in rare instances of difficulty in positioning women, so that it is hard in some cases to compensate for breast thickness that is insufficient to accommodate the movement of gun-needle core biopsy probes during biopsy. In this situation, the biopsy must be converted to a fine-needle aspiration procedure or performed under sonographic guidance, if the lesion is visible with sonography. As noted above, prone table equipment design can make it difficult to access the posterior aspect of the breast and the axilla, so that lesions in these locations may not be amenable to biopsy with this type of equipment.

Sonographically Guided Breast Biopsy

In most situations in which either stereotactic or sonographic guidance can be used for core biopsy, many radiologists prefer to use sonographic imaging. These procedures are often more direct and do not require computerized calculation of lesion location. They are also free of many of the limitations of approach to a lesion associated with stereotactic biopsies that may result from the location of a lesion or from the configuration of the breast (9).

One of the advantages of sonographically guided biopsy is the availability of biopsy equipment. Any facility performing diagnostic breast imaging with sonographic equipment can perform these biopsies, obviating the need for additional expenditure to acquire special biopsy equipment. Although core biopsies of the breast can be performed with specially designed needle probes that guide the needle into the lesion, these direct the needle toward the chest wall, making it possible to cause a pneumothorax during the procedure. They are therefore not recommended, and no special imaging equipment needs to be acquired to perform these procedures.

Sonographically guided breast biopsy is usually performed with a "free-hand" technique. After the lesion is visualized, the physician is able to guide the needle into position for the biopsy without special equipment. Some physicians use a coaxial system, placing a guiding sheath in position at the time of the initial core biopsy. Successive biopsies are performed by reinserting the needle into the breast through this sheath. At least theoretically, this limits the ability of the physician to direct the biopsy needle into various sites within the lesion to sample it entirely.

During sonographically guided core biopsy, the patient is in a supine position and the breast is flattened against the chest wall. Issues of adequate breast thickness to accommodate movement of the needle are eliminated by such positioning. Because the position of the ultrasound transducer is not restricted, an infinite number of approaches to the lesion are possible. Because the patient is supine, vasovagal reactions do not occur. Although the patient's view of the biopsy procedure is not obstructed, she usually turns her head away as the procedure is performed. In some cases, patients view the procedure on the sonography screen. Patient cooperation during the procedure is usually excellent, and the discomfort that women experience from lying on the stereotactic table for long periods is eliminated. Core biopsy is usually performed more quickly under sonographic guidance. Patient positioning is rapid; imaging is performed in real time, with no delay between obtaining and viewing the images, and the relationship between lesion and needle is easily appreciated on the images.

The major limitation of sonographically guided core biopsy is the inability to visualize microcalcifications reliably. Although some newer, high-frequency transducers can image microcalcifications, it is difficult to be certain that microcalcifications seen sonographically correspond to those seen mammographically. At the present time, experience with biopsy of microcalcifications under sonographic guidance is extremely limited, and the appropriateness of sonographic guidance for biopsy of these lesions is unknown. Depending on the resolution capabilities of various equipment, the ability to see some masses sonographically can also be limited. It is to be expected that with almost all equipment,

at least some solid lesions may be sonographically inapparent and therefore cannot be sampled under sonographic guidance.

Breast Biopsy Guided by Magnetic Resonance (MR) Imaging

It should be expected that in the near future percutaneous biopsy procedures will be performed under MR imaging guidance. Guidance systems for MR are in development but have not become commercially available. Non-ferromagnetic biopsy probes are needed to operate in the strong magnetic field. Successful performance of preoperative needle localization procedures and fine-needle aspirations with MR imaging guidance have been reported (10,11). Experience with core biopsy under MR imaging has not been reported, but it is expected that the technology will be developed to enable these procedures to be performed in the near future.

BIOPSY PROBES

A variety of technologies are available to perform large-core breast biopsy. Equipment choice will influence the diameter and length of core specimens submitted to the pathologist (Fig. 5). Depending on the choice of the biopsy probe, the volumetric relationship of successive cores to each other and the amount of hemorrhage as larger numbers of cores are obtained can sometimes be altered. Decisions regarding choice of a biopsy probe in any individual case will be influenced by whether or not the lesion is to undergo biopsy with sonographic or stereotactic guidance, the thickness of the breast under compression, whether the lesion appears as a mass or calcifications, and cost considerations.

Automated Gun-Needle Combinations

The traditional needle for core biopsy has been a cutting needle that fits into an automated spring-loaded gun. A needle gauge no smaller than 14 should be used. In a study in which surgically excised malignant lesions underwent core biopsy with needles of varying caliber, it was found that the

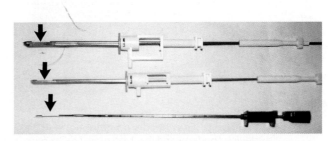

FIGURE 5. Core biopsy needles. Three commonly used breast biopsy needles are (*from the bottom*) a 14-gauge "Tru-Cut" type needle, a 14-gauge vacuum-suction probe, and an 11-gauge vacuum-suction probe. The collection chamber of each needle is indicated (*arrow*).

sensitivity for diagnosis was 100%, 92%, and 65% for 14-, 16-, and 18-gauge needles from the same manufacturer (12). Fibroadenomas were also more readily diagnosed with 14-gauge needles than with smaller ones. Specimens obtained with 14-gauge core biopsy needles will also vary depending on the manufacturer of the biopsy instrument. In biopsies performed on cadaveric breast tissue, the mean specimen volume was found to range from 9.9 to 17.9 mm³ when 14-gauge core biopsy instruments from five different manufacturers were tested (13). For women undergoing stereotactic biopsy of masses with these needles, results are optimized when at least five cores are obtained. This has been demonstrated to result in a 99% diagnostic yield (14). As previously noted, when microcalcifications are sampled, cores should be obtained until calcifications are retrieved, as documented with specimen radiography (5).

The TruCut type of cutting needles used with the spring-loaded gun are made of stainless steel and consist of an inner tissue sampling needle and an outer cutting needle. This gun-needle combination was first used for prostate biopsies. Core needles are generally manufactured in longer (16 cm) and shorter (10 cm) lengths. The tissue-collection slot in the needle is located 4 mm from the needle tip. In the longer needle, the tissue-collection slot is 17 mm long, and in shorter needles the collection chamber measures 11 mm. The movement of the needle through the breast is accomplished by a biopsy gun, and the distance the needle travels is described as its "throw." "Long-throw" needles advance 21 to 25 mm during the biopsy, whereas "short-throw" needles advance 10 to 15 mm. The shorter throw is sometimes inadequate to provide diagnostic sampling of breast tissue, and these needles are therefore not routinely recommended for breast biopsy. However, in a situation in which calcifications are the biopsy target and the breast compresses to less than the throw of the long-throw needle, a short-throw needle may be the only method of performing core biopsy.

The spring-loaded gun acts when fired to advance the inner sampling needle into the breast automatically (Fig. 6). Because the cutting tip of the needle is beveled downward,

as the needle advances forward, it is deflected slightly downward. Downward deflection is increased with increasing needle gauge. The outer cutting needle is then automatically advanced, drawing the needle upward and compressing tissue into the collection slot near the end of the inner needle. As the outer needle advances over the inner component, tissue in the collection slot of the inner needle is cut away from the rest of the breast. At the completion of the biopsy, the needle must be removed from the breast to retrieve the specimen. Each core is obtained by repositioning the biopsy needle within the breast. For masses, the needle should be positioned so that cores are obtained from the center, top, bottom, and right and left sides of the mass.

When calcifications undergo biopsy, sampling of several cubic millimeters of breast tissue at the site of calcifications is attempted. Because of the forward and downward motion of the needle and because of the very small size of calcifications undergoing biopsy, it is often more difficult to obtain calcifications than to sample tissue from a mass. Successful targeting of calcifications can also be compromised when minimal heterogeneity in the individual calcific forms makes it difficult to select the same form on both stereotactic views so that targeting is correct. When calcifications are loosely clustered rather than in close proximity, it can also be more difficult to capture any calcification in the collection chamber of the needle because despite accurate targeting, the course of the needle through breast tissue can be deflected by angulation of the beveled needle tip and resistance to the passage of the needle in some dense tissues.

Because the needle is withdrawn from the breast after each core is obtained, continuous retrieval of adjacent cores from the volume of the lesion does not occur. Also, because of the serial puncturing of tissue, repetitive biopsy causes hemorrhage in the area undergoing sampling. The continued needling of a small volume of the breast can also result in some tissue being displaced. As noted above, multiple cores are obtained to guarantee adequate sampling of the lesion (15). It is not uncommon in lesions containing calcification to obtain more than 10 cores in an attempt to retrieve some

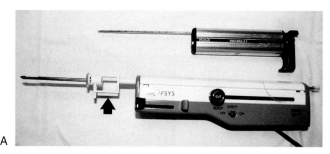
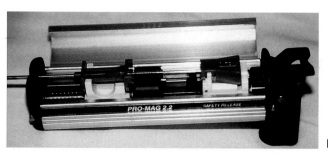

A   B

FIGURE 6. Gun-needle combinations A: Two commonly used sets are the 11-gauge vacuum-suction device (*bottom*) and the 14-gauge TruCut type of device (*top*). With the vacuum-suction device, the needle can be rotated 360° to collect tissue adjacent to the needle circumferentially. This is done by rotating the plastic dial to the left of the tissue collection area (*arrow*) of the probe. Multiple specimens can be retrieved without removal of the needle from the breast. **B:** The spring-powered gun of the TruCut type first advances an outer needle into the breast and then an inner cutting needle. The needle must be removed each time it is fired to retrieve each core.

calcium. Despite the noncontiguous biopsy pattern, it is possible to excise small lesions fully with this technique. Some have argued that lesions smaller than 5 mm should not be sampled with the 14-gauge core biopsy probe because of this possibility (16). If totally excised, it may be difficult or impossible to localize the site within the breast that contained the lesion if a surgical excision is performed (17).

Directional Vacuum-Suction Biopsy Probes

A more recently developed needle biopsy technology has made it possible to remove contiguous core specimens, making removal of entire lesions a more common occurrence. These newer probes (Biopsys, Irvine, CA) are commonly used in 14- and 11-gauge needle sizes (Fig. 7). With these probes, the needle is positioned within the breast, and a vacuum pulls tissue into the cutting chamber of the probe. A hollow cutting needle is advanced into this chamber; rotating at high speed, it cuts the core specimen from the breast and then withdraws it through the outer needle. This makes it possible to remove the specimen while the biopsy probe remains in place within the breast. The probe can be rotated 360°, making it possible to obtain circumferential biopsy specimens. Serial specimens can be obtained at 45° intervals so that eight adjacent cores can be retrieved at each rotation (18). Depending on the strength of the vacuum and the resistance of the tissue, serial circumferential tissue removal is possible. Usually, two rotations of the biopsy probe will result in tissue retrieval, yielding 16 cores. With the larger, 11-gauge probe, at least one more rotation of the probe will usually continue to result in tissue removal (19).

Differences in Cores Removed with Varying Biopsy Probes

The volume of the core specimen removed with directional, vacuum-suction biopsy probes is more than twice as large as that retrieved with automated gun-needle probes. In one study, core weight was increased from 17.2 mg when a

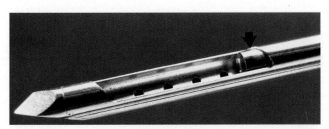

FIGURE 7. The vacuum-suction needle draws tissue into the collection chamber by a vacuum that acts through small holes in the collection chamber. A hollow cutting needle (*arrow*) is then advanced while it rapidly rotates, cutting tissue from the breast and withdrawing it to a collection area (Fig. 6) outside the breast. Multiple adjacent cores can be collected without removing this probe from the breast. (Photograph courtesy of Biopsys Medical/Ethicon Endo-Surgery, Inc., Johnson and Johnson, Cincinnati, OH.)

14-gauge Biopsys gun-needle combination was used to 31.9 mg when a Biopsys vacuum-suction probe was used (20). This more than twofold increase in the weight of individual cores has been confirmed by other investigators (21). They also found that when an 11-gauge vacuum-suction probe was used, the weight of the specimen increased to an average of 94.4 mg, a 2.6-fold increase over the weight of the 14-gauge specimen removed with the vacuum-suction probe, and a more than 5-fold increase over the weight of the specimen retrieved with the 14-gauge gun-needle probe. Increases in the length of individual cores tended to parallel increases in their weight, with mean specimen lengths ranging from 6 to 27 mm. Likewise, specimen diameters showed progressive increase with larger specimen size, ranging from 1.5 mm for the gun-needle 14-gauge probes to 2.6 mm for the 11-gauge vacuum-suction probe. However, fragmentation of specimens was also shown to increase with larger core size. Smaller cores have been documented to be removed as a single piece of tissue, whereas large cores are often removed in two or more fragments.

OTHER TECHNICAL FACTORS AFFECTING SPECIMEN QUALITY

A variety of other factors during patient preparation, positioning, and biopsy can affect the specimen submitted for histologic analysis. These factors can alter the nature of the specimen submitted or the ability to sample the lesion in question.

Depending on the technique used to perform a biopsy, the volume of anesthetic injected into the volume of the breast undergoing sampling can be dramatically altered. With gun-needle probes, usually only a few cubic centimeters of local anesthetic is injected into the breast. However, with vacuum-suction devices, 10 to 20 ml of local anesthetic and epinephrine are commonly used during the procedure, and the anesthetic may be directly injected into the biopsy site before tissue is removed.

When lesions do not contain calcification, fluid around the lesion can obscure it during the biopsy procedure, making it difficult to determine the relationship of the biopsy probe to the target lesion. This can be caused by hemorrhage at the biopsy site or the injection of anesthetic around the lesion. Often, uncalcified lesions become progressively obscured during tissue sampling. This occurs during both sonographic and stereotactically guided procedures and can compromise accurate positioning of the biopsy probe. In this circumstance, it can be difficult for the physician performing the biopsy to determine whether or not the lesion in question has been successfully sampled (22).

Several technical factors can result in failure to obtain an adequate tissue sample. Accurate needle positioning during stereotactic biopsy requires that the biopsy probe be appropriately positioned on the biopsy stage of the stereotactic unit. Otherwise, the needle tip is not in the position in which the computer assumes it is located, and the needle tip does not advance to the expected site within the breast. Inapparent patient movement during the biopsy causes the target lesion to move, also resulting in inaccurate targeting. It is also possible for the lesion to move within the breast as the needle approaches, so that a sample is not obtained.

IMPACT OF TECHNICAL FACTORS ON SPECIMENS SUBMITTED

In the specimen that is submitted to the pathologist, only the choice of the biopsy probe will be evident. This affects specimen size, fragmentation, volumetric relationship of the cores to each other, and perhaps the number of cores submitted. Other factors are important only in regard to the ability to perform the biopsy and the accuracy of needle positioning. A final assessment of the accuracy of needle positioning and adequacy of tissue sampling depends on correlation of the histopathologic findings with the imaging (and, if appropriate, clinical) findings. This assessment may require the pathologist and the physician performing the biopsy to discuss their findings with each other to decide whether or not an accurate, final diagnosis can be made based on the core specimens.

REFERENCES

1. Bassett L, Winchester DP, et al. Stereotactic core-needle biopsy of the breast: a report of the joint task force of the American College of Radiology, American College of Surgeons, and College of American Pathologists. *CA Cancer J Clin* 1997;47:171–190.
2. Hendrick RE, Parker SH. Stereotaxic imaging. In: Haus AG, Yaffe MJ, eds. *Syllabus: a categorical course in physics. Technical aspects of breast imaging.* Oak Brook, IL: Radiological Society of North America, 1994:263–274.
3. Parker SH, Dennis MA, Stavros AT. Critical pathways in percutaneous breast intervention. *Radiographics* 1995;15:946–950.
4. Dershaw DD, Fleischman RC, Liberman L, Deutch B, Abramson AF, Hann L. Use of digital mammography in needle localization procedures. *AJR Am J Roentgenol* 1993;161:559–562.
5. Liberman L, Evans WP III, Dershaw DD, et al. Radiography of micro-calcifications in stereotaxic mammary core biopsy specimens. *Radiology* 1994;190:223–225.
6. Walker TM. Impalpable breast lesions: stereotactic core biopsy with an "add-on" unit. *Breast* 1997;6:126–131.
7. Dershaw DD. Stereotaxic breast biopsy. *Semin Ultrasound CT MR* 1996;17:444–459.
8. Fajardo L. Equipment considerations: stereotaxic and digital systems. In: Dershaw DD, ed. *Interventional breast procedures.* New York: Churchill Livingstone, 1996:45–53.
9. Parker SH, Stavros AT, Dennis MA. Needle biopsy techniques. *Radiol Clin North Am* 1995;33:1171–1186.
10. Orel SG, Schnall MD, Newman RW, Powell CM, Torosian MH, Rosato EF. MR imaging-guided localization and biopsy of breast lesions: initial experience. *Radiology* 1994;193:97–102.
11. Fischer U, Vosshenrich R, Doler W, Hamadeh A, Oestmann JW, Grabbe E. MR imaging-guided breast intervention: experience with two systems. *Radiology* 1995;195:533–538.
12. Nath ME, Robinson TM, Tobon H, Chough DM, Sumkin JH. Automated large-core needle biopsy of surgically removed breast lesions: comparison of samples obtained with 14-, 16- and 18-gauge needles. *Radiology* 1995;197:739–742.
13. Krebs TL, Berg WA, Severson MJ, et al. Large-core biopsy guns: comparison for yield of breast tissue. *Radiology* 1996;200:365–368.
14. Liberman L, Dershaw DD, Rosen PP, Abramson AF, Deutch BM, Hann LE. Stereotaxic 14-gauge breast biopsy: how many core specimens are needed? *Radiology* 1994;192:793–795.
15. Brenner RJ, Fajardo L, Fisher PR, et al. Percutaneous core biopsy of the breast: effect of operator experience and number of samples on diagnostic accuracy. *AJR Am J Roentgenol* 1996;166:341–346.
16. Dershaw DD, Caravella BA, Liberman L. Limitations and complications in the utilization of stereotaxic core breast biopsy. *Breast J* 1996;2:13–17.
17. Hann LE, Liberman L, Dershaw DD, Cohen MA, Abramson AF. Mammography immediately after stereotaxic breast biopsy: is it necessary? *AJR Am J Roentgenol* 1995;165:59–62.
18. Parker SH, Klaus AJ. Performing a breast biopsy with a directional, vacuum-assisted biopsy instrument. *Radiographics* 1997;17:1233–1252.
19. Liberman L, Dershaw DD, Rosen PP, Morris EA, Abramson AF, Borgen PI. Percutaneous removal of malignant mammographic lesions at stereotactic vacuum-assisted biopsy. *Radiology* 1998;206:711–715.
20. Burbank F, Parker S, Fogarty T. Stereotactic breast biopsy: improved tissue harvesting with the Mammotome. *Am Surg* 1996;62:738–744.
21. Berg WA, Krebs TL, Campassi C, Magder LS, Sun CJ. Evaluation of 14- and 11-gauge directional, vacuum-assisted biopsy probes and 14-gauge biopsy guns in a breast parenchymal model. *Radiology* 1997;205:203–208.
22. Berg WA, Hruban RH, Kumar D, Singh HR, Brem RF, Gatewood OMB. Lessons from mammographic-histopathologic correlation of large-core needle breast biopsy. *Radiographics* 1996;16:1111–1130.

CHAPTER 31

Impact of Percutaneous Imaging-Guided Core Biopsy on the Clinical Management of Breast Disease

Laura Liberman

Percutaneous imaging-guided needle core biopsy is being used increasingly in the diagnosis of breast lesions (1–15). Tissue-acquisition devices for percutaneous core biopsy include spring-loaded guns and automated needles (usually 14-gauge) and directional vacuum-assisted biopsy devices (14- or 11-gauge); equipment that obtains larger volumes of tissue is also available. Guidance methods for percutaneous core biopsy include stereotaxis (1–12), ultrasonography (10–15), and magnetic resonance (MR) imaging (16–23).

Stereotactic core biopsy may be employed for all types of mammographic lesions (masses and calcifications) but requires the use of dedicated equipment. Ultrasound-guided core biopsy, used primarily for masses, has several advantages, including lack of ionizing radiation, real-time visualization of the needle, accessibility to all parts of the breast and axilla, and multipurpose use of equipment. MR-guided biopsy is in the developmental stage and currently is performed mostly in a research setting for the evaluation of lesions detected primarily with MR imaging. The choice of guidance modality depends on several factors, including lesion visibility and accessibility, equipment availability, and patient and radiologist preference.

Early studies of stereotactic automated needle core biopsy showed an 87% to 96% concordance between the results of stereotactic core biopsy and surgery (Table 1). The best results were observed by investigators who obtained multiple specimens with a 14-gauge needle and a long excursion gun. In a 1993 study of ultrasound-guided 14-gauge automated needle large-core biopsy, Parker et al. (13) reported 100% concordance between results of core biopsy and surgery in 49 lesions that went to surgery, and no carcinomas were identified at 12- to 36-month follow-up in 132 lesions after a benign finding on needle core biopsy.

The patient care advantages of percutaneous needle core breast biopsy are numerous. The procedure is less invasive and less expensive than surgical biopsy, and it can be performed rapidly. Less tissue is removed, resulting in no deformity of the breast and less scarring evident on subsequent mammograms. Percutaneous needle core biopsy can obviate the need for surgery in women with benign lesions, and it can reduce the number of surgical procedures performed in women with breast cancer. Complications of percutaneous core biopsy are unusual, with the frequency of hematoma and infection each less than 1 in 1,000 (11).

CLINICAL ADVANTAGES OF PERCUTANEOUS CORE BIOPSY

Indications for Needle Core Biopsy

Percutaneous needle core biopsy is most frequently employed to evaluate nonpalpable lesions identified by screening mammography. The Breast Imaging Reporting and Data System (BI-RADS) lexicon of the American College of Radiology defines final assessment categories, a group of terms used to describe the level of suspicion regarding a mammographic lesion (24) (Table 2). Routine (annual) follow-up is warranted for lesions classified as BI-RADS category 1 or 2. Short-interval follow-up (at 6 months for the ipsilateral breast, followed by examination of both breasts at 1, 2, and 3 years after the initial mammogram) is suggested for lesions in BI-RADS category 3. Biopsy is suggested for lesions classified as category 4 or category 5.

Percutaneous needle core biopsy is most often used in the assessment of category 4 lesions, many of which are benign (25,26) (Table 3). If the needle core biopsy of a category 4 lesion yields a benign diagnosis concordant with the imaging characteristics, the patient is spared the need for diagnostic surgery in most instances. The utility of needle core biopsy for the evaluation of category 5 lesions depends on the clinical setting. They account for a minority of lesions warrant-

TABLE 1. *Studies correlating results of stereotactic automated needle core biopsy and surgery*

Investigator/year (ref.)	No. lesions	No. cancers	Needle gauge	Gun	No. passes	Stereo equipment	No. concordant (%)	No. insufficient (%)	No. cancers missed (%)[c]
Parker/1990 (1)	103 [102][a]	16	18-G (n = 65) 16-G (n = 9) 14-G (n = 29)	Short (n = 2) Long (n = 101)	3 or 4	Upright (n = 30) Prone (n = 73)	89 (87)	1 (1)	1 (6)
Parker/1991 (2)	102	23	14-G	Long	3 or 4	Prone	98 (96)	0 (0)	1 (4)
Dowlatshahi/1991 (6)	250	76	20-G[d]	Short (n = 120) Long (n = 130)	2 or 3	Prone	167 (67)	43 (17)	19 (25)
Dronkers/1992 (3)	70 [53][a]	45	18-G	Short	2	Upright	48 (91)	3 (6)	2 (4)
Elvecrog/1993 (4)	100	35[b]	14-G	Long	≥5	Prone	95 (95)	0 (0)	1 (3)

[a] No. cases with surgical correlation.
[b] Excludes 1 case of lobular carcinoma *in situ*.
[c] No. cancers yielding benign (not atypical, suspected, or insufficient) results at core biopsy, expressed as percentage of surgically confirmed cancers.
[d] Patients underwent fine-needle aspiration, 2 to 3 passes with a 20-G needle, prior to 20-G core biopsy.

ing biopsy, but most are malignant (25,26) (see Table 3). Because it was customary in the absence of needle core biopsy to perform a diagnostic surgical biopsy, followed by a second (therapeutic) surgical procedure if carcinoma was found, performing a needle core biopsy before the therapeutic excision can spare patients with category 4 or 5 lesions a surgical procedure.

The role of needle core biopsy in the evaluation of category 3 lesions has been a matter of debate (27–30). The traditional management of category 3 lesions has been short-term mammographic follow-up. The frequency of carcinoma in these lesions is 0.5% to 2% (31,32). Sickles (32) reported results in 3,189 lesions classified as "probably benign" (equivalent to BI-RADS category 3) that underwent short-term follow-up mammography. Carcinoma was detected in 17 (0.5%) lesions, on the basis of interval change in a follow-up mammogram in 15 and by palpation in 2. Most tumors were small invasive carcinomas (median size, 1.3 cm); 15 (88%) had negative axillary lymph nodes and none had distant metastases. These data indicate that BI-RADS category 3 lesions have an extremely high likelihood of being benign, and that the few category 3 malignant lesions can be diagnosed at an early stage if short-term follow-up mammography is performed.

Percutaneous image-guided needle core biopsy is also helpful in the evaluation of palpable lesions, particularly if the lesion is deep, mobile, or vaguely palpable (10). Performing the biopsy under image guidance can help ensure that the lesion has been sampled.

Fewer Operations

It can be estimated that 1 million breast biopsies will be performed in the United States in 1998. At least 30% (300,000) will be for nonpalpable lesions identified by screening mammography (33,34). Approximately 70% (210,000) of the 300,000 nonpalpable lesions will be benign (35). If percutaneous needle core biopsy yields a benign diagnosis concordant with imaging characteristics, a woman is spared the need for a surgical biopsy.

When percutaneous needle core biopsy successfully removes a patient with benign disease from the pool of women who undergo operative biopsy, the positive predictive value of needle localization/surgical biopsy (i.e., the percentage of needle-localized lesions that prove to be malignant) should increase. This effect of percutaneous needle core biopsy was

TABLE 2. *Breast imaging reporting and data system (BI-RADS) lexicon: final assessment categories*

Category	Interpretation	Recommendation
1	Normal mammogram	Routine annual mammography
2	Benign finding	Routine annual mammography
3	Probably benign	Short-interval mammographic follow-up
4	Suspected abnormality	Biopsy ("Biopsy should be considered."[a])
5	Highly suggestive of malignancy	Biopsy ("Appropriate action should be taken."[a])

[a] From ref. 24, with permission.

TABLE 3. *BI-RADS categorization as a predictor of malignancy*

Investigator/ year (ref.)	No. lesions referred for biopsy (% of lesions that had biopsy)	Lesions with cancer (%)
Orel/1997 (26)		
Category 2	13 (2)	0
Category 3	75 (13)	3
Category 4	427 (71)	29
Category 5	83 (14)	94
Total	598 (100)	34
Liberman/1998 (25)		
Category 3	8 (2)	0
Category 4	355 (72)	34
Category 5	129 (26)	81
Total	492 (100)	46

BI-RADS, Breast Imaging Reporting and Data System.

demonstrated in a study of 200 patients by Rubin et al. (12), in which 200 patients had an imaging-guided percutaneous needle core breast biopsy under ultrasound (n = 167) or stereotactic (n = 33) guidance. The positive predictive value of needle localization/surgical biopsy increased from 35% just before needle core biopsy was introduced to 55% after needle core biopsy was employed. For masses, the positive predictive value increased from 43% to 72%.

Percutaneous needle core biopsy can also decrease the number of surgical procedures necessary in women with breast cancer. Liberman et al. (36) found that a single surgical procedure was performed in 84% of women for whom the diagnosis of cancer was made by percutaneous needle core biopsy, compared with 29% of those for whom the diagnosis was made by surgical biopsy. The likelihood of undergoing a single surgical procedure was significantly higher for women whose cancer was diagnosed by percutaneous needle core biopsy than by surgical biopsy, regardless of whether the mammographic lesion was a mass or calcifications, or whether the needle core biopsy diagnosis was ductal carcinoma *in situ* (DCIS) or invasive cancer. Jackman et al. (37) reported that a single surgical procedure was performed in 90% of patients whose cancers were diagnosed by core biopsy and in only 24% of patients with cancers diagnosed by surgical biopsy. Smith et al. (38) noted that the average number of surgical procedures was 1.25 in women whose cancers were diagnosed by core biopsy and 2.01 in women with cancers diagnosed by needle localization and surgical biopsy ($p < .001$).

For women with multiple lesions demonstrated mammographically or clinically, needle core biopsy of two or more areas can help determine if carcinoma is present at a single site or multiple sites. This information may influence the decision regarding the optimal surgical therapy because the presence of carcinoma in two different quadrants is often an indication for a mastectomy (39,40). When needle core biopsy is performed for multiple lesions, each biopsy sample is obtained separately with separate equipment, including the needle and anesthetic syringe. The material must be sent in separate containers that are individually labeled, and each specimen should be described by a separate diagnosis.

Percutaneous needle core biopsy can decrease the number of surgical procedures in women with new mammographically detected lesions after breast-conserving therapy (41). If the needle core biopsy yields a benign diagnosis concordant with the imaging characteristics, a surgical biopsy may be avoided, and if the procedure reveals recurrent carcinoma, the patient may proceed with definitive surgery, often a salvage mastectomy.

Lower Cost

Substantial savings can result from the use of needle core biopsy instead of surgical biopsy for the evaluation of BI-RADS category 4 or 5 lesions. Lindfors and Rosenquist (42), in a theoretical model, found that the marginal cost per year of life saved by screening was reduced a maximum of 23% (from $20,770 to $15,934) with the use of needle core biopsy instead of surgery. In clinical practice, Liberman et al. (43) found that stereotactic core biopsy spared a surgical procedure in 77% of women with BI-RADS 4 or 5 lesions. Stereotactic biopsy spared a surgical procedure in 93% of women whose needle core biopsy finding was benign without atypia, 81% of women with carcinoma documented by needle core biopsy, 84% of women who had a mass at mammography, and 66% of women with lesions evidenced by calcifications. Needle core biopsy resulted in a greater than 50% decrease in the cost of diagnosis. On the basis of these data, the estimated annual national savings from use of stereotactic biopsy for the diagnosis of nonpalpable lesions approached $200 million (43).

The cost savings of stereotactic biopsy as a function of mammographic findings were assessed by Lee et al. (44). These authors found that 81% of patients were spared a surgical procedure, resulting in a mean savings of $741 per patient. A surgical procedure was avoided by using needle core biopsy in 87% of patients with a mass and 72% of those with calcifications. It was possible to avoid a surgical procedure in 88%, 75%, and 69% of women with indeterminate, suspected, or highly suspected lesions, respectively, and in 74%, 81%, and 84% of women with lesions measuring less than 5 mm, 5 to 10 mm, and more than 10 mm, respectively. Cost savings (based on Medicare estimates) were observed in all groups, with the magnitude depending on the mammographic features. Savings were least for calcifications ($630 per case) and highly suspected (BI-RADS category 5) lesions ($637 per case), and greatest for masses ($807 per case) and indeterminate (BI-RADS category 4) lesions ($825 per case).

Cost savings for ultrasound-guided needle core biopsy may exceed those of stereotactic biopsy. In a study of 151 women who underwent ultrasound-guided core biopsy of nonpalpable masses, 128 (85%) were spared a surgical procedure (15). To calculate cost savings, Medicare figures of $385 for ultrasound-guided core biopsy, $610 for stereotactic core biopsy, and $1,332 for needle localization and surgical biopsy were used. Ultrasound-guided needle core biopsy resulted in cost savings when compared with surgical biopsy of $744 per case, a 56% decrease in the cost of diagnosis. If stereotactic rather than ultrasound-guided core biopsy had been used, the cost savings would have been $519 per case, a 39% decrease in the cost of diagnosis in comparison with surgical biopsy. This study suggests that both stereotactic core biopsy and ultrasound-guided core biopsy are less expensive than surgery, but that the savings are greater if the biopsy is performed under ultrasound guidance.

Needle core percutaneous biopsy is more expensive than short-term mammographic follow-up for category 3 lesions. In an analysis of 3,184 patients with "probably benign" (BI-RADS category 3) lesions, Brenner and Sickles (30) found that the ratio of the cost of needle core biopsy to the cost of surveillance mammography was 8:1.

Less Scarring

Mammographic changes after surgical biopsy are common and include calcifications, skin thickening or retraction, hematoma, and architectural distortion. These changes may decrease the sensitivity and specificity of mammography. Needle core biopsy causes minor and transient mammographic alterations. Hann et al. (45) reported minimal biopsy-related changes on 76% of mammograms performed immediately after stereotactic 14-gauge needle core biopsy, including decreased lesion size in 10%, air at the biopsy site in 42%, and hematoma in 51%. In follow-up mammograms performed 6 months after a benign finding on stereotactic automated 14-gauge needle core biopsy in 25 women, Kaye et al. (46) reported that three (12%) lesions had changes related to sampling (fewer calcifications in two lesions and a defect in one mass). There was no evidence of fat necrosis, architectural distortion, or scarring. In a study of 132 lesions with follow-up mammograms obtained an average of 6.6 months after a benign finding on 14-gauge directional vacuum-assisted needle core biopsy, Burbank (47) reported no residual deformity at the biopsy site.

Complete Removal of the Mammographic Lesion

The directional vacuum-assisted stereotactic biopsy instrument acquires larger volumes of tissue than the automated needle (48–50) (Table 4). In some instances, a percutaneous breast biopsy removes the entire lesion observed on the mammogram, a situation more likely after directional vacuum-assisted biopsy than after automated core biopsy (47,48,51–53) (Table 5). In a study of mammographic findings immediately after 14-gauge stereotactic biopsy, Liberman et al. (51) reported complete removal of the mammographic lesion in 13% of cases after a vacuum biopsy and in 4% following an automated needle core biopsy ($p = .02$). In a study of mammographic findings at first imaging follow-up, Burbank (47) described complete removal of the mammographic lesion in 48% patients who underwent a stereotactic 14-gauge vacuum biopsy and in 15% after an automated core biopsy ($p < .0001$). The average follow-up interval was 6.6 months for vacuum biopsy and 8.6 months for automated core biopsy. It has not yet been determined whether total excision of the mammographic findings associated with the original lesion is advantageous in terms of diagnostic yield or patient management.

Complete removal of the mammographic lesion does not ensure complete excision of the pathologic abnormality. Liberman et al. (54) described 15 carcinomas in which the mammographic lesion had been entirely removed at stereotactic 11-gauge directional vacuum-assisted breast biopsy. Surgery revealed residual carcinoma in 11 (73%) of 15 cases. In four noncomedo DCIS lesions, the biopsy site was identified in the surgical specimen and no residual carcinoma was found. Currently, percutaneous biopsy is suitable for breast diagnosis. Prospective clinical studies with surgical correlation and follow-up will be required before percutaneous needle techniques can be used for therapy.

Placement of a Localizing Clip

A 2×2-mm radiopaque, stainless steel localizing clip can be placed through the 11-gauge probe after a percutaneous vacuum-assisted biopsy. This clip, easily visible on mammograms and specimen radiographs, marks the biopsy site for subsequent surgical excision if the mammographic findings associated with the original lesion have been removed (Fig. 1). The surgeon and radiologist should inform the pathologist about the presence of the clip because it should be identified in the surgical specimen obtained after a percutaneous directional vacuum-assisted biopsy and clip placement.

Clip placement is more accurate through the 11-gauge probe than after 14-gauge biopsy. Liberman et al. (55) analyzed stereotactic images obtained immediately after clip placement and found that the distance from clip to lesion site was less than 1 cm in 40 of 42 lesions (95%) following clip placement through an 11-gauge probe and in 11 of 15 lesions (73%) when the clip was placed after a 14-gauge vacuum biopsy ($p < .04$). The biopsy site was identified in the surgical specimen in 19 of 19 (100%) and 5 of 6 (83%) lesions following clip placement after 11-gauge and 14-gauge vacuum biopsy, respectively.

Burbank and Forcier (56) also reported that a localizing clip can be placed in close proximity to the biopsy site after directional vacuum-assisted breast biopsy. They used a masking method to calibrate a system for measuring the clip-to-lesion distance on mammographic images. The baseline variability in location over time for 22 benign lesions was 8 mm. Among 149 clips placed after directional vacuum-as-

TABLE 4. *Mean specimen weights with different percutaneous breast biopsy instruments[a]*

Investigator/year (ref.)	Subject	14-G ALCBB	14-G DVABB	11-G DVABB
Burbank/1996 (48)	Human	17	34	NA
Berg/1997 (49)	Turkey breast	18	37	94
Burbank/1997 (50)	Human	NA	40	96

G, gauge; ALCBB, automated large-core breast biopsy; DVABB, directional vacuum-assisted breast biopsy; NA, not applicable.

[a] Numbers reflect weight per biopsy specimen in milligrams.

TABLE 5. *Complete removal of the mammographic lesion by stereotactic directional vacuum-assisted breast biopsy*

Investigator/ year (ref.)	Probe	Mean no. specimens	When assessed	No. lesions removed/ total no. lesions (%) (all lesions)	No. lesions removed/ total no. lesions (%) (lesions ≤5 mm)
Burbank/1996 (48)	14-G	15	Immediate	166/345 (48)	92/117 (79)
Liberman/1997 (51)	14-G	14	Immediate	14/108 (13)	11/19 (58)
Burbank/1997 (52)	14-G	27	Immediate	23/40 (58)	14/15 (93)
Burbank/1997 (47)	14-G	25	Delayed[a]	63/132 (48)	NS (73)
Liberman/1998 (53)	11-G	14	Immediate	51/112 (46)	31/43 (72)

NS, not stated; G, gauge.
[a] Mean, 8.6 months.

sisted biopsy, initial clip deployment averaged 5 mm above baseline from the center of the target lesion. The biopsy site was found in each of the 36 lesions that underwent subsequent surgery. Thirty-one clips examined by mammography at a mean of 8.6 months after a benign finding on biopsy remained in place. The long-term stability of clip placement is yet to be determined.

LIMITATIONS OF PERCUTANEOUS NEEDLE CORE BIOPSY

Retrieval of Calcification

When stereotactic needle core biopsy is performed for lesions manifested as calcifications, it is necessary to document that calcifications were retrieved in specimen radio-

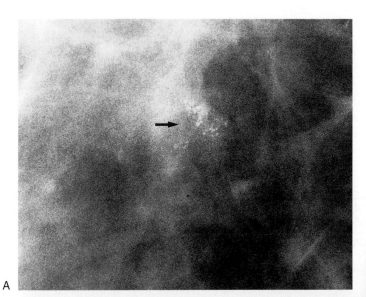

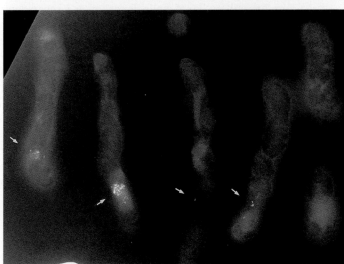

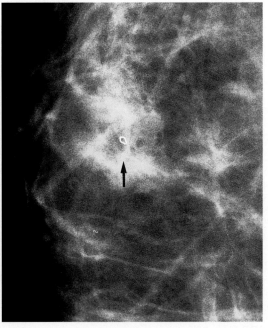

FIGURE 1. A: Collimated, magnified (×1.5), mediolateral oblique view left mammogram in a 45-year-old woman demonstrates a cluster of pleomorphic microcalcifications (*arrow*) measuring 0.5 cm in the longest dimension. **B:** Radiographs of specimens obtained during stereotactic 11-gauge directional vacuum-assisted breast biopsy demonstrate calcifications (*arrows*). Histopathologic analysis yielded ductal carcinoma *in situ*, solid type. **C:** Collimated, mediolateral oblique view left mammogram obtained after stereotactic biopsy demonstrates the radiopaque clip placed to mark the biopsy site (*arrow*). Although all the calcifications were removed, subsequent needle localization and surgical excision demonstrated residual solid ductal carcinoma *in situ*.

A

B

C

graphs and by histopathologic analysis. It is important for the pathologist to note the histopathologic distribution of calcifications in tumor, non-neoplastic breast tissue, or both. Liberman et al. (57) found that diagnostic material was obtained in 81% of needle core biopsy specimens that demonstrated calcifications on specimen radiographs and in only 38% of specimens that did not show calcifications when calcifications were the indication for the procedure.

In previous studies of stereotactic 14-gauge automated large-core biopsy, calcifications were not retrieved in 6% to 12% of cases (44,57–59). If calcifications are not retrieved and the diagnosis is benign, rebiopsy is warranted. Calcification retrieval with the automated needle is challenging because calcifications present a tiny and discontinuous target. The automated needle acquires tissue only along the line of fire; if the calcifications are not precisely in line with the needle, they may be missed. The directional vacuum-assisted needle core biopsy instrument acquires larger volumes of tissue than the automated needle and can obtain tissue from outside the line of fire. Several investigators have found that the directional vacuum-assisted biopsy instrument is superior to the automated needle in the retrieval of calcifications (58,59) (Table 6).

Underestimation of Diagnosis

Stereotactic core biopsy may underestimate the degree of pathology in lesions containing atypical ductal hyperplasia (ADH) and DCIS. When the core biopsy specimen obtained

TABLE 6. *Calcification retrieval by stereotactic breast biopsy*

Investigator/ year (ref.)	14-G ALCBB[a]	14-G DVABB[a]	11-G DVABB[a]
Liberman/1994 (57)	65/72 (90)	NA	NA
Lee/1997 (44)	133/151 (88)	NA	NA
Liberman/1997 (51)	NA	50/55 (91)[b]	NA
Meyer/1997 (58)	118/130 (91)	106/106 (100)[c]	NA
Jackman/1997 (59)	1122/1196 (94)	1195/1209 (99)	720/723 (>99)[d]
Liberman/1998 (53)	NA	NA	106/112 (95)

NA, not applicable; ALCBB, automated large-core breast biopsy; DVABB, directional vacuum-assisted breast biopsy; G, gauge.
[a] Numbers in parentheses are percentages.
[b] Frequency of calcification retrieval was 19/24 (79%) in the first half of the 8-month study period and 31/31 (100%) in the second half.
[c] $p < .001$.
[d] Frequency of retrieving calcifications was significantly higher for 14-G DVABB than for 14-G ALCBB ($p < .0001$) and significantly higher for 11-G DVABB than for 14-G ALCBB ($p < .0001$) but did not differ significantly for 11-G vs. 14-G DVABB ($p = .15$).

TABLE 7. *Atypical duct hyperplasia (ADH) underestimates by percutaneous breast biopsy*

Investigator/ year (ref.)	14-G ALCBB[a]	14-G DVABB[a]	11-G DVABB[a]
Jackman/1994 (7)	9/16 (56)	NA	NA
Liberman/1995 (60)	11/21 (51)	NA	NA
Burbank/1997 (52)	8/18 (44)	0/8 (0)[b]	NA
Jackman/1997 (63)	26/54 (48)	13/74 (18)	4/31 (13)[c]
Liberman/1998 (53)	NA	NA	1/10 (10)

ALCBB, automated large-core breast biopsy; DVABB, directional vacuum-assisted breast biopsy; NA, not applicable; G, gauge.
[a] Numbers in parentheses are the percentages of lesions yielding ADH at core biopsy in which surgery revealed carcinoma.
[b] $p = .03$.
[c] $p < .0001$.

with a 14-gauge automated needle indicates ADH, approximately 50% of subsequent surgical biopsies reveal carcinoma (7,60). Among 144 surgically confirmed cancers that had previously undergone stereotactic 14-gauge automated needle core biopsy in a study by Liberman et al. (61), the core biopsy diagnosis was atypical hyperplasia in 21 (15%). The diagnosis of atypical hyperplasia was more frequently observed in needle core biopsy specimens of malignant calcifications than in biopsy specimens of masses (30% vs. 5%; $p < .0001$), more often in DCIS than in invasive carcinoma (33% vs. 7%; $p = .0002$), and more often in noncomedo than in comedo DCIS (60% vs. 9%; $p = .0008$) (61). The needle core biopsy diagnosis of ADH in a lesion that contains carcinoma has been termed an ADH underestimate. The high frequency of obtaining a core biopsy diagnosis of ADH when a carcinoma is sampled reflects the difficulties inherent in distinguishing ADH from DCIS in a small volume of lesional tissue (61).

Among lesions diagnosed as DCIS by stereotactic 14-gauge automated needle large-core biopsy, approximately 20% are found to have invasive carcinoma in the subsequent surgical excision (7,62). This may require that the patient return for axillary lymph node dissection as a separate procedure. The finding of invasive carcinoma at surgery in a lesion that yielded DCIS in a percutaneous needle core biopsy has been termed a DCIS underestimate.

The directional vacuum-assisted biopsy instrument, which acquires larger volumes of tissue, provides more accurate characterization of ADH and DCIS lesions. Among lesions diagnosed as ADH by directional vacuum-assisted biopsy, 0% to 18% have been found to contain carcinoma at surgery (52,63) (Table 7), and among lesions reported to be DCIS with a directional vacuum-assisted biopsy instrument, 0% to 5% have been demonstrated to contain invasive carcinoma at surgery (52,53) (Table 8).

Rebiopsy

In several studies of percutaneous needle core biopsy, a repeated biopsy (rebiopsy) was recommended in 11% to

TABLE 8. *Ductal carcinoma in situ (DCIS) underestimates by percutaneous breast biopsy*

Investigator/ year (ref.)	14-G ALCBB[a]	14-G DVABB[a]	11-G DVABB[a]
Jackman/1994 (7)	8/43 (19)	NA	NA
Liberman/1995 (62)	3/15 (20)	NA	NA
Burbank/1997 (52)	9/55 (16)	0/32 (0)[b]	NA
Liberman/1998 (53)	NA	NA	1/21 (5)

ALCBB, automated large-core breast biopsy; DVABB, directional vacuum-assisted breast biopsy; NA, not applicable; G, gauge.

[a] Numbers in parentheses are percentages of lesions yielding DCIS at core biopsy in which surgery revealed invasive carcinoma.

[b] $p = .02$.

18% of cases because the material did not provide a definitive diagnosis (15,44,64,65). Reasons for rebiopsy include discordance between pathologic findings and imaging characteristics, presence of ADH, inadequate tissue, and the pathologist's recommendation for wider sampling (Table 9). Benign lesions for which surgical excision is suggested include radial scars (66,67) and fibroepithelial tumors, in which it is difficult to distinguish fibroadenoma from phyllodes tumor (Table 10). Some have suggested that surgical excision be performed for benign papillary lesions diagnosed by percutaneous biopsy because the sampling might not detect coexistent carcinoma. However a follow-up study of seven lesions diagnosed as benign papillomas by 14-gauge biopsy revealed only papilloma at surgery (12).

TABLE 10. *Benign lesions for which excision may be warranted after percutaneous needle core biopsy*

Lesion	No. excised	Surgical pathology
Fibroepithelial tumor: fibroadenoma vs. phyllodes tumor		
Dershaw/1996 (64)[a]	7	3 (43%) benign phyllodes tumors,[b]
Meyer/1998 (65)	9	2 (22%) malignant phyllodes tumors[b]
Liberman/1998 (15)	3	1 (33%) malignant phyllodes tumor,[b]
Radial scar		
Jackman/1995 (67)	6	2 (33%) carcinoma
Lee/1997 (44)	4	1 (25%) carcinoma
Meyer/1998 (65)	4	0 (0%) carcinoma
Dershaw/1996 (64)	1	0 (0%) carcinoma
Liberman/1998 (15)	1	0 (0%) carcinoma

[a] Investigator/year (ref.).

[b] The other fibroepithelial tumors were fibroadenomas at surgery.

Equipment that obtains larger volumes of tissue, such as the directional vacuum-assisted biopsy instrument, may improve lesion characterization by percutaneous biopsy and decrease the number of lesions referred for rebiopsy (68,69).

Follow-Up

Follow-up is essential after percutaneous needle core breast biopsy. Kopans (70) has criticized a multiinstitutional

TABLE 9. *Repeated biopsy after percutaneous breast biopsy: frequency, reasons, and results*

Investigator/ year (ref.)	Method	No. cases	No. rebiopsies suggested (%)	Reasons for rebiopsy	No. rebiopsies done	No. malignant (% of rebiopsies)
Dershaw/1996 (64)	Stereotactic 14-G ALCBB	314	56 (18)	ADH (n = 30)	28	15 (54)
				Discordance (n = 15)	11	4 (36)
				Wider sampling (n = 10)	10	0 (0)
				Radial scar (n = 1)	1	0 (0)
				All	50	19 (38)
Lee/1997 (44)	Stereotactic 14-G ALCBB	405	71 (18)	Insufficient (n = 24)	14	3 (21)
				Atypical hyperplasia (n = 22)	20	6 (30)
				Discordance (n = 18)	9	0 (0)
				Radial scar (n = 4)	4	1 (25)
				Wider sampling (n = 3)	3	0 (0)
				All	50	10 (20)
Meyer/1998 (65)	Stereotactic (n = 824) Ultrasound (n = 208) 14-G ALCBB (n = 718) 14-G DVABB (n = 106)	1,032	112 (11)	Possibly missed (n = 41)	41	2 (5)
				Wider sampling (n = 40)[a]	40	16 (40)
				Discordance (n = 24)	24	0 (0)
				Other (7)	7	0 (0)
				All	112	18 (16)
Liberman/1998 (15)	Ultrasound 14-G ALCBB	151	16 (11)	Wider sampling (n = 7)	7	1 (14)
				Discordance (n = 5)	4	1 (25)
				Inadequate (n = 2)	2	0 (0)
				ADH (n = 1)	1	0 (0)
				Growth on follow-up (n = 1)	1	0 (0)
				All	15	2 (13)

ADH, atypical ductal hyperplasia; ALCBB, automated large-core breast biopsy; DVABB, directional vacuum-assisted breast biopsy.

[a] Includes 31 cases yielding ADH or atypical features at core biopsy, of which 14 (45%) yielded carcinoma at surgical excision, and 9 fibroepithelial tumors, 2 (22%) of which were malignant phyllodes tumors at surgery.

study of 6,152 lesions by Parker et al. (11) because follow-up data were available in only 3,765 lesions (clinical follow-up in 2,402; surgical follow-up in 1,223). Goodman et al. (71) noted that noncompliance with follow-up recommendations was an important problem in a study of 160 breast lesions that underwent percutaneous core biopsy. In that study, only 52 (74%) of 70 lesions referred for surgical excision had documented surgical outcomes. Among 90 lesions referred for mammographic surveillance, 10 (11%) were resolved at the time of the study, 49 (54%) were on track toward 3-year lesion stability, 21 (23%) were being followed up elsewhere, 4 (4%) were lost to physicians, and 6 (7%) were lost to follow-up for other reasons.

Jackman et al. (67) reported the results of follow-up after stereotactic 14-gauge automated needle large-core biopsy of 483 consecutive nonpalpable lesions, including 143 with carcinoma, 21 with atypical hyperplasia, and 319 with benign findings. The 319 benign lesions underwent rebiopsy (n = 31) or mammographic follow-up at 4 to 45 months (n = 283). Follow-up revealed carcinoma in 6 (2%) of 319 benign lesions, including 2 (33%) of 6 radial scars and 4 (1%) of 313 other benign lesions. Follow-up failed in 15 (5%) of 319 benign lesions, including 11 (20%) of 54 outside referrals and 4 (2%) of 265 internal referrals.

A substantial commitment of time and resources is necessary to acquire follow-up data, but this endeavor is necessary for patient care and to improve our understanding of the false-negative rate of percutaneous core biopsy of the breast (72).

NEW TECHNOLOGY IN PERCUTANEOUS BREAST BIOPSY

The advanced breast biopsy instrumentation (ABBI) system (US Surgical, Norwalk, CT) is a tissue-acquisition device that offers a variety of cannula sizes up to 2 cm. With these, it is possible to obtain specimens extending from the subcutaneous tissue to beyond the lesion (73–80). The ABBI system has the advantage of potentially removing the entirety of a small lesion in a single specimen rather than multiple fragments. The disadvantage of the ABBI system is that the large volumes of tissue obtained can cause more cosmetic deformity and higher complication rates, without benefiting the majority of women who undergo needle core biopsy, as they have benign lesions.

Chesbrough et al. (76) state that for an ABBI procedure to be performed, the patient should be able to lie prone for at least 1 hour, the compressed breast thickness must exceed 30 mm, and the lesion must be at least 20 mm from the chest wall. These stringent requirements may limit the number of women who can undergo ABBI biopsy. This was illustrated in a study by Baum et al. (77), who found that among women with nonpalpable lesions warranting biopsy, 15% to 20% were potential ABBI candidates and 10 of 64 patients scheduled for ABBI biopsy had the procedure canceled for technical reasons.

Ferzli et al. (74) also have demonstrated some practical limitations of the ABBI system. Nine (16%) of 58 patients with nonpalpable breast lesions referred for ABBI biopsy were excluded because of problems with positioning or lesion visualization, and two procedures (3%) could not be completed. As for the remaining 47 lesions, which had a mean specimen volume of 12.7 cm^3, in 14 cases (30%) the procedure was converted to an open manual excision with surgical instruments on the stereotactic table because of mechanical problems with the ABBI system. Five (63%) of eight patients who underwent an open surgical biopsy previously said that the ABBI procedure was more traumatic and painful than surgery. Chesbrough et al. (76) reported complications in 5 (16%) of 32 women who underwent ABBI biopsy, including two postprocedure hematomas, two arterial lacerations requiring surgical ligation, and one pneumothorax.

More encouraging results with the ABBI system have been described by D'Angelo et al. (75), who reported that 2 (9%) of 23 women who underwent ABBI biopsy had the procedure converted to an excision with scissors. Mean specimen weight was 7 ± 3 g for ABBI biopsies and 12 ± 7 g for needle localization and surgical biopsy. Blood loss averaged 14 ± 10 ml for ABBI biopsy and 20 ± 10 ml for needle localization and surgical biopsy. Subjective comfort of ABBI biopsy was reported as excellent by 21 (91%) patients and good by two (9%). No complications were encountered.

Although a theoretical advantage of the ABBI system is the potential ability to remove an entire lesion in a single specimen, it is unusual to obtain clear histopathologic margins of resection with the ABBI procedure. Carcinoma was present at the margins of the ABBI biopsy specimen in each of five carcinomas reported by D'Angelo et al. (75) and in five (71%) of seven carcinomas reported by Chesbrough et al. (76). Margins were close or positive in five (83%) of six carcinomas in a study by Leibman and Frager (78).

The ABBI device, like all percutaneous breast biopsy equipment, is currently approved for the diagnosis but not the treatment of breast lesions. If carcinoma is found, surgery is necessary to ensure clear histologic margins of resection. For most lesions, large-core biopsy with an automated needle or directional vacuum-assisted device provides material adequate for diagnosis more quickly, less invasively, and at lower cost than does the ABBI device. The role of the ABBI technology in breast diagnosis is still under investigation.

CONCLUSION

Percutaneous imaging-guided needle core biopsy is a less invasive and less expensive alternative to surgical biopsy for the evaluation of breast lesions. Needle core biopsy can obviate the need for surgical biopsy in many women. It can be performed quickly and causes less scarring than surgical biopsy. Percutaneous biopsy can remove an entire mammographic lesion, but this does not ensure complete excision of the pathologic process. The limitations of needle core biopsy include occasional difficulties in retrieving calcifications and underestimation of lesions containing ADH and DCIS, both of which are lessened with the use of the directional vacuum-assisted biopsy instrument. Further work is necessary to define the role of newer technologies for tissue acquisition in the management of women with benign and malignant breast disease.

REFERENCES

1. Parker SH, Lovin JD, Jobe WE, et al. Stereotactic breast biopsy with a biopsy gun. *Radiology* 1990;176:741–747.
2. Parker SH, Lovin JD, Jobe WE, Burke BJ, Hopper KD, Yakes WF. Nonpalpable breast lesions: stereotactic automated large-core biopsies. *Radiology* 1991;180:403–407.
3. Dronkers DJ. Stereotaxic core biopsy of breast lesions. *Radiology* 1992;183:631–634.
4. Elvecrog EL, Lechner MC, Nelson MT. Nonpalpable breast lesions: correlation of stereotaxic large-core needle biopsy and surgical biopsy results. *Radiology* 1993;188:453–455.
5. Gisvold JJ, Goellner JR, Grant CS, et al. Breast biopsy: a comparative study of stereotaxically guided core and excisional techniques. *AJR Am J Roentgenol* 1994;162:815–820.
6. Dowlatshahi K, Yaremko ML, Kluskens LF, Jokich PM. Nonpalpable breast lesions: findings of stereotaxic needle-core biopsy and fine-needle aspiration cytology. *Radiology* 1991;181:745–750.
7. Jackman RJ, Nowels KW, Shepard MJ, Finkelstein SI, Marzoni FA. Stereotaxic large-core needle biopsy of 450 nonpalpable breast lesions with surgical correlation in lesions with cancer or atypical hyperplasia. *Radiology* 1994;193:91–95.
8. Caines JS, McPhee MD, Konock GP, Wright BA. Stereotaxic needle core biopsy of breast lesions using a regular mammographic table with an adaptable stereotaxic device. *AJR Am J Roentgenol* 1994;163:317–321.
9. Brenner RJ, Fajardo L, Fisher PR, et al. Percutaneous core biopsy of the breast: effect of operator experience and number of samples on diagnostic accuracy. *AJR Am J Roentgenol* 1996;166:341–346.
10. Parker SH, Burbank F. A practical approach to minimally invasive breast biopsy. *Radiology* 1996;200:11–20.
11. Parker SH, Burbank F, Jackman RJ, et al. Percutaneous large-core breast biopsy: a multi-institutional study. *Radiology* 1994;193:359–364.
12. Rubin E, Dempsey PJ, Pile NS, et al. Needle localization biopsy of the breast: impact of a selective core needle biopsy program on yield. *Radiology* 1995;195:627–631.
13. Parker SH, Jobe WE, Dennis MA, et al. US-guided automated large-core breast biopsy. *Radiology* 1993;187:507–511.
14. Liberman L, Feng TL, Morris EA, Zakowski MF, Abramson AF, Dershaw DD. Ultrasound-guided core biopsy of the breast: rebiopsy rates, reasons, and results. *AJR Am J Roentgenol* 1998;170(Suppl):83–84(abst).
15. Liberman L, Feng TL, Dershaw DD, Morris EA, Abramson AF. Ultrasound-guided core breast biopsy: use and cost-effectiveness. *Radiology* 1998;208:717–723.
16. Fisher U, Vosshenrich R, Keating D, et al. MR-guided biopsy of suspect breast lesions with a simple stereotaxic add-on device for surface coils. *Radiology* 1994;192:272–273.
17. Orel SG, Schnall MD, Newman RW, Powell CM, Torosian MH, Rosato EF. MR imaging-guided localization and biopsy of breast lesions: initial experience. *Radiology* 1994;193:97–102.
18. Schnall MD, Orel SG, Connick TJ. MR-guided biopsy of the breast. *Magn Reson Imaging Clin N Am* 1994;2:585–589.
19. Fischer U, Vosshenrich R, Doler W, Hamadeh A, Oestmann JW, Grabbe E. MR imaging-guided breast intervention: experience with two systems. *Radiology* 1995;195:533–538.
20. Orel SG, Schnall MD, Powell CM, et al. Staging of suspected breast cancer: effect of MR imaging and MR-guided biopsy. *Radiology* 1995;196:115–122.
21. Wald DS, Weinreb JC, Newstead G, Flyer M, Bose S. MR-guided fine needle aspiration of breast lesions: initial experience. *J Comput Assist Tomogr* 1996;20:1–8.
22. Doler W, Fischer U, Metzger I, Harder D, Grabbe E. Stereotaxic add-on device for MR-guided biopsy of breast lesions. *Radiology* 1996;200:863–864.
23. Kuhl CK, Elevelt A, Leutner CC, Gieseke J, Pakos E, Schild HH. Interventional breast MR imaging: clinical use of a stereotactic localization and biopsy device. *Radiology* 1997;204:667–675.
24. American College of Radiology (ACR). *Breast imaging reporting and data system (BI-RADSTM)*, 2nd ed. Reston, VA: American College of Radiology, 1995.
25. Liberman L, Abramson AF, Squires FB, Glassman RJ, Morris EA, Dershaw DD. The breast imaging reporting and data system: positive predictive value of mammographic features and final assessment categories. *AJR Am J Roentgenol* 1998;171:35–40.
26. Orel SG, Sullivan DC, Dambro TJ. BI-RADS categorization as a predictor of malignancy. *Radiology* 1997;205(P):447(abst).
27. Sickles EA, Parker SH. Appropriate role of core breast biopsy in the management of probably benign lesions. *Radiology* 1993;188:315.
28. Logan-Young WW, Janus JA, Destounis SV, Hoffman NY. Appropriate role of core breast biopsy in the management of probably benign lesions. *Radiology* 1994;190:313.
29. Sickles EA, Parker SH. Reply. *Radiology* 1994;190:313–314.
30. Brenner RJ, Sickles EA. Surveillance mammography and stereotactic core breast biopsy for probably benign lesions: a cost comparison analysis. *Acad Radiol* 1997;4:419–425.
31. Varas X, Leborgne F, Leborgne JH. Nonpalpable, probably benign lesions: role of follow-up mammography. *Radiology* 1992;184:409–414.
32. Sickles EA. Periodic mammographic follow-up of probably benign lesions: results of 3,184 consecutive cases. *Radiology* 1991;179:463–468.
33. Landis SH, Murray T, Bolden S, Wingo PA. Cancer statistics, 1998. *CA Cancer J Clin* 1998;48:6–29.
34. Osteen RT, Cady B, Chmiel JS, et al. 1991 national survey of carcinoma of the breast by the Commission on Cancer. *J Am Coll Surg* 1994;178:213–219.
35. Kopans DB, Moore RH, McCarthy KA, et al. Positive predictive value of breast biopsy performed as a result of mammography: there is no abrupt change at age 50 years. *Radiology* 1996;200:357–360.
36. Liberman L, LaTrenta LR, Dershaw DD, et al. Impact of core biopsy on the surgical management of impalpable breast cancer. *AJR Am J Roentgenol* 1997;168:495–499.
37. Jackman RJ, Marzoni FA, Finkelstein SI, Shepard MJ. Benefits of diagnosing nonpalpable breast cancer with stereotactic large-core needle biopsy: lower costs and fewer operations. *Radiology* 1996;201(P):311.
38. Smith DN, Christian R, Meyer JE. Large-core needle biopsy of nonpalpable breast cancers: the impact on subsequent surgical excision. *Arch Surg* 1997;132:256–259.
39. Liberman L, Dershaw DD, Rosen PP, Morris EA, Cohen MA, Abramson AF. Core needle biopsy of synchronous ipsilateral breast lesions: impact on treatment. *AJR Am J Roentgenol* 1996;166:1429–1432.
40. Rosenblatt R, Fineberg SA, Sparano JA, Kaleya RN. Stereotactic core needle biopsy of multiple sites in the breast: efficacy and effect on patient care. *Radiology* 1996;201:67–70.
41. Liberman L, Dershaw DD, Durfee S, et al. Recurrent carcinoma after breast conservation: diagnosis with stereotaxic core breast biopsy. *Radiology* 1995;197:735–738.
42. Lindfors KK, Rosenquist CJ. Needle core biopsy guided with mammography: a study of cost effectiveness. *Radiology* 1994;190:217–222.
43. Liberman L, Fahs MC, Dershaw DD, et al. Impact of stereotaxic core biopsy on cost of diagnosis. *Radiology* 1995;195:633–637.
44. Lee CH, Egglin TIK, Philpotts LE, Mainiero MB, Tocino I. Cost-effectiveness of stereotactic core needle biopsy: analysis by means of mammographic findings. *Radiology* 1997;202:849–854.
45. Hann LE, Liberman L, Dershaw DD, Cohen MA, Abramson AF. Mammography immediately after stereotaxic breast biopsy: is it necessary? *AJR Am J Roentgenol* 1995;165:59–62.
46. Kaye MD, Vicinanza-Adami CA, Sullivan ML. Mammographic findings after stereotaxic biopsy of the breast performed with large-core needles. *Radiology* 1994;192:149–151.
47. Burbank F. Mammographic findings after 14-gauge automated needle and 14-gauge directional, vacuum-assisted stereotactic breast biopsies. *Radiology* 1997;204:153–156.
48. Burbank F, Parker SH, Fogarty TJ. Stereotactic breast biopsy: improved tissue harvesting with the Mammotome. *Am Surg* 1996;62:738–744.
49. Berg WA, Krebs TL, Campassi C, et al. Evaluation of 14- and 11-gauge

directional vacuum-assisted biopsy probes and 14-gauge biopsy guns in a breast parenchymal model. *Radiology* 1997;205:203–208. 1997.

50. Burbank F. Stereotactic breast biopsy: comparison of 14- and 11-gauge Mammotome probe performance and complication rates. *Am Surg* 1997;63:988–995.

51. Liberman L, Hann LE, Dershaw DD, Morris EA, Abramson AF, Rosen PP. Mammographic findings after stereotactic 14-gauge vacuum biopsy. *Radiology* 1997;203:343–347.

52. Burbank F. Stereotactic breast biopsy of atypical ductal hyperplasia and ductal carcinoma *in situ* lesions: improved accuracy with a directional, vacuum-assisted biopsy instrument. *Radiology* 1997;202:843–847.

53. Liberman L, Smolkin JH, Dershaw DD, Morris EA, Abramson AF, Rosen PP. Calcification retrieval at stereotactic 11-gauge vacuum-assisted breast biopsy. *Radiology* 1998;208:251–260.

54. Liberman L, Dershaw DD, Rosen PP, Morris EA, Abramson AF, Borgen PI. Percutaneous removal of malignant mammographic lesions at stereotactic vacuum-assisted biopsy. *Radiology* 1998;206:711–715.

55. Liberman L, Dershaw DD, Morris EA, Abramson AF, Thornton CM, Rosen PP. Clip placement after stereotactic vacuum-assisted breast biopsy. *Radiology* 1997;205:417–422.

56. Burbank F, Forcier N. Tissue marking clip for stereotactic breast biopsy: initial placement accuracy, long-term stability, and usefulness as a guide for wire localization. *Radiology* 1997;205:407–415.

57. Liberman L, Evans WP III, Dershaw DD, et al. Radiography of microcalcifications in stereotaxic mammary core biopsy specimens. *Radiology* 1994;190:223–225.

58. Meyer JE, Smith DN, Dipiro PJ, et al. Stereotactic breast biopsy of clustered microcalcifications with a directional, vacuum-assisted device. *Radiology* 1997;204:575–576.

59. Jackman RJ, Burbank FH, Parker SH, et al. Accuracy of sampling microcalcifications by three stereotactic breast biopsy methods. *Radiology* 1997;205(P):325(abst).

60. Liberman L, Cohen MA, Dershaw DD, Abramson AF, Hann LE, Rosen PP. Atypical ductal hyperplasia diagnosed at stereotaxic core biopsy of breast lesions: an indication for surgical biopsy. *AJR Am J Roentgenol* 1995;164:1111–1113.

61. Liberman L, Dershaw DD, Glassman JR, et al. Analysis of cancers not diagnosed at stereotactic core breast biopsy. *Radiology* 1997;203:151–157.

62. Liberman L, Dershaw DD, Rosen PP, et al. Stereotaxic core biopsy of breast carcinoma: accuracy at predicting invasion. *Radiology* 1995;194:379–381.

63. Jackman RJ, Burbank FH, Parker SH, et al. Atypical ductal hyperplasia diagnosed by 11-gauge, directional, vacuum-assisted breast biopsy: how often is carcinoma found at surgery? *Radiology* 1997;205(P):325(abst).

64. Dershaw DD, Morris EA, Liberman L, Abramson AF. Nondiagnostic stereotaxic core breast biopsy: results of rebiopsy. *Radiology* 1996;198:323–325.

65. Meyer JE, Smith DN, Lester SC, et al. Large-needle core biopsy: nonmalignant breast abnormalities evaluated with surgical excision or repeat core biopsy. *Radiology* 1998;206:717–720.

66. Rosen PP. Radial sclerosing lesions. In: Rosen PP. *Rosen's breast pathology.* Philadelphia: Lippincott–Raven Publishers, 1997:76–81.

67. Jackman RJ, Finkelstein SI, Marzoni FA. Stereotaxic large-core needle biopsy of histologically benign nonpalpable breast lesions: false-negative results and failed follow-up. *Radiology* 1995;197(P):203(abst).

68. Liberman L, LaTrenta LR, Dershaw DD, et al. Stereotactic 14-gauge biopsy of breast calcifications: comparison of vacuum vs. automated core biopsy techniques. *Radiology* 1997;205(P):325(abst).

69. Philpotts LE, Shaheen NA, Carter D, Lee CH. Comparison of rebiopsy rates after stereotaxic breast core biopsy with 11-gauge vacuum suction probe vs. 14-gauge needle and automated gun. *AJR Am J Roentgenol* 1998;170(Suppl):83(abst).

70. Kopans DB. Caution on core. *Radiology* 1994;193:325–328.

71. Goodman KA, Birdwell RL, Ikeda DM. Compliance with recommended follow-up after percutaneous breast core biopsy. *AJR Am J Roentgenol* 1998;170:89–92.

72. Berlin L. Tracking for breast cancer. *AJR Am J Roentgenol* 1998;170:93–95.

73. Bird RE. A prospective and retrospective evaluation of the potential usefulness of the 2-cm core ABBI technology in breast biopsy. Presented at the Third Postgraduate Course of the Society of Breast Imaging, San Diego, CA, April 16–19, 1997.

74. Ferzli GS, Hurwitz JB, Puza T, Vorst-Bilotti SV. Advanced breast biopsy instrumentation: a critique. *J Am Coll Surg* 1997;185:145–151.

75. D'Angelo PC, Galliano DE, Rosemurgy AS. Stereotactic excisional breast biopsies utilizing the advanced breast biopsy instrumentation system. *Am J Surg* 1997;174:297–302.

76. Chesbrough R, Rebner M, Gregory N. Initial surgical experience with the advanced breast biopsy instrument (ABBI). *AJR Am J Roentgenol* 1998;170(Suppl):82(abst).

77. Baum JK, Raza S, Keeler B, Collette C, Houlihan MJ. ABBI breast biopsy: early experience using a combined radiological-surgical approach. *AJR Am J Roentgenol* 1998;170(Suppl):83(abst).

78. Leibman AJ, Frager D. Experience with breast biopsy using the advanced breast biopsy instrumentation (ABBI) system. *AJR Am J Roentgenol* 1998;170(Suppl):85(abst).

79. Kelley WE Jr, Schwartzberg BS, Uddo JF. Advanced breast biopsy instrumentation [Letter; Comment]. *J Am Coll Surg* 1997;185:604–605.

80. Ferzli GS. Advanced breast biopsy instrumentation: in reply. *J Am Coll Surg* 1997;185:605.

Subject Index

Page numbers followed by *f* and *t* refer to figures and tables, respectively.